Rachel Summer

Feed Yourself Right

BOOKS BY LENDON SMITH, M.D.

The Children's Doctor
The Encyclopedia of Baby and Child Care
New Wives' Tales
Improving Your Child's Behavior Chemistry
Feed Your Kids Right
Foods for Healthy Kids
Feed Yourself Right

Feed Yourself Right

LENDON SMITH, M.D.

McGRAW-HILL BOOK COMPANY
New York   St. Louis   San Francisco
Toronto   Mexico   Hamburg

This book is not intended to replace the services of a physician. Any application of the recommendations set forth in the following pages is at the reader's discretion and sole risk.

3 4 5 6 7 8 9 D O C D O C 8 7 6 5 4 3

ISBN 0-07-058499-0

LIBRARY OF CONGRESS CATALOGING IN PUBLICATION DATA

Smith, Lendon H., 1921–
Feed yourself right.
1. Orthomolecular therapy.   2. Nutrition.   I. Title.
RM235.5.S64   1983   616.8'54   83-959
ISBN 0-07-058499-0

Book design by Roberta Rezk

I HAVE DEDICATED each of my books to my dear, supportive wife; I would like to do the same with this one. If you should stumble onto this page, Julie, I love you and I'm sorry I didn't pay much attention to you when I was doing this.

Acknowledgments: In this book I hope I open a few doors for readers, patients, and health professionals in teaching our children and ourselves to eat properly and exercise sufficiently to maintain health. I believe the methods suggested here are well-documented, safe, and simple enough for widespread use. With any luck and the proper nutritional management, we should be able to take care of ourselves until we have served out our time at age 120.

This book was obviously not done in a vacuum. The following people helped with content, form, and readability:

Dr. Wayne Anderson, a naturopathic physician in Portland, has been more than helpful in introducing me to alternative therapeutic modalities. He has helped make this book instructive for people looking to feel better in a safe, natural way.

Mr. Larry A. Grant, Director of Ortho-Eco-Communications in Trail, Oregon, has shown me better ways of being persuasive.

Mrs. Tracy S. La Placa, an editor in New York, knows from personal experience how proper metabolic balance can improve physical and mental performance. Her insights and encouragement and stylistic changes have been invaluable. Anastasia Chehak, R.D., of Edmond, Oklahoma, has further reinforced my belief that nutrition can help almost every living thing.

Kathryn Dopler-Elverum did much for the ambience of the manuscript and helped it to flow—linearly, of course.

Nancy Hoffman forced me to see the error of some of my writing ways; she really helped.

Peggy Moss is still helping me, as she has with every book. Her intelligence is appreciated by me and, I'm sure, by my readers.

Thank you all.

CONTENTS

Abdominal Discomfort *81* • Abortion *90* • Achalasia
90 • Aches *91* • Achlorhydria *93* • Acne *93* • Addiction *97* • Adrenal Gland Failure *99* • Aggressive Behavior *100* • Alcoholism *104* • Allergies, Sensitivities,
and Intolerances *114* • Alopecia *137* • Alzheimer's
Dementia *139* • Anal Fissure *140* • Anemia *140* • Anorexia *143* • Anxiety *146* • Apathy *148* • Arthritis *150*
• Ataxia *158* • Autoimmune Diseases *160* • Bed Con-

CHAPTER 6 ☐ Find Yourself (Or Skip This if You Are in Perfect Health) *Continued*

CONTENTS

PREFACE

WE DON'T REALLY KNOW who we are until we are somewhere between the ages of twenty and thirty (some of us not even then).

As a child I was usually nice enough, but I had mood swings—from elation and noisy ebullience to quiet withdrawal or pouting. My mother didn't care that I was difficult, odd, a bed-wetter, a changeling, inconsistent. She thought all boys were supposed to act that way. "It's a phase" was her favorite response to my irrationalities.

Because Mom didn't pressure me to shape up, I had no idea that my headaches, somnolence, inappropriate responses, and emotional lability meant that something was wrong. I had no chance to live in another person's body and to experience his perceptions.

By mid-adolescence, though, we have usually gotten some input from people who are not as nice as our mothers. As a high-school student, I tried to imitate my heroes. I needed to win.

When the coach of my football team said to me, "Smith, you ain't worth a fart in a whirlwind," I decided to seek another way to feel good about myself.

We all need to hear the truth sometimes (though not necessarily in those terms), and that is my purpose in writing this book. Over the years in my life and in my medical practice, I have learned some hard truths about what makes us the individuals we are—specifically about the roles of diet and nutrition in our personality, behavior, and sense of well-being. I call these truths "hard" because many in the medical profession remain close-minded on the subject (as they were taught to be), and because many people reading this book will see the need for drastic changes in their eating habits and lifestyles. For some it will mean giving up the very thing they love most.

Many people feel rotten much of the time. They go to the doctor, who tells them they are reasonably average. He has the statistics to prove it: "Everyone gets mono," or "It's OK to have five cavities by the age of fifteen and be edentulous by sixty." But is "average" normal? Is "average" even healthy? You and I know people who have all their teeth, who never get a cold, and who have no obvious allergies. Is it possible for all of us to attain this level of health?

We must stop fooling ourselves. The people who live to age ninety-two, who remain active, alert, and useful, are the normal ones. We should all be at that norm. An allergy, a cold, a virus infection, insomnia, a cavity, slow and weepy days, are all deviations from normal. If an accident, a stress, or a disappointment triggers the problem, we have to accept that. But if our state of mental distraction causes us to forget to eat properly or not to take care of our physical selves, the problem will only get worse. Any stress has the potential of exhausting the adrenal glands. Unless we give them extra support during those times, a variety of somatic problems can surface.

I have found that sickness and feeling punk are the results of a multiplicity of factors: morbid genetics, a mother's stressful pregnancy, accidents, inadequate nutrients in the diet, a poorly functioning absorption mechanism, occult food and chemical allergies, stress, lack of exercise, and the absence of a faith, mantra, or obtainable goal. No one has the answers to all the problems of living, but enough is known to help each one of us to achieve his or her potential more fully.

Parents used to beat children for wetting the bed; many of those children grew up to be criminals. Children who stuttered or had tics and twitches were scorned by their peers. Kids who rocked the bed or twisted their hair were told they were bad; many of them lived to fulfill this appellation. Hyperactive kids really got the shaft. They were scolded for not sitting still and were flunked because they were distractible and could not work up to their potential. They quit school. Many of them became depressed or alcoholic. Some went into prison. What was going on with all these patients? What was wrong with me? Did our mothers do all this to us? Did we "deserve" the punishment we got because we were bad, or because we were screwed up biochemically? Surely we can't blame *all* the troubles in the world on bad parenting skills.

Over the years, to placate parents who were concerned about these minor symptoms in their kids, I prescribed medication or ordered diagnostic testing. As I realize now, I rarely put my finger on the physiological or chemical imbalance that was causing the symptom to appear. Today good evidence suggests that nutrition plays a significant role in the production of symptoms and signs of even the most surprising kind.

About ten years ago I began to change my mode of treatment. A thirty-year-old woman came to see me in my office who claimed that she had been an alcoholic for fifteen years. She wanted me to give her a vitamin shot. I had never done such a useless thing in my professional life, and I was a little embarrassed to think that she considered me to be the kind of doctor who would do that sort of thing.

She told me that a doctor a few years previously had given her a shot and that it had helped. I ordered a vial of B complex from my pharmacist, who was nice enough not to giggle. I gave the woman 0.5 cc of the stuff in her arm muscle, and with a "Good luck—let me hear from you," I sent her home.

I became a believer when the next day she returned smiling. Her cheeks had turned from gray to pink. She was ecstatic, but not from booze. "I walked by three bars and I didn't have to go in," she said.

The theory runs that alcoholics drink because they have unresolved oral drives and are dependent upon their parents. It was therefore hard to believe that a few vitamins could improve a "psychiatric" problem so obviously, so safely, so quickly. The recovery was *not* a placebo effect. It suggested to me that there were other coincidences I could take as working hypotheses. *Is* it true that colicky babies are hypertonic and simply built that way? *Are* people allergic because it runs in the family? *Do* people have insomnia because they worry? *Do* heart attacks occur only in type-A people? *Do* kids wet the bed because they hate their mothers?

People have a right to better answers than they have been getting. Physicians and other health professionals have an obligation to study the correlation between diet and symptoms and to consider what can be done to improve health through nutritional supports—through eating the right foods, staying away from the wrong foods, and supplementing to meet individual needs. These approaches work. The results are attested to in our own standard literature. Biochemically sophisticated laboratory tests show these results to be more than a series of anecdotes; improvement is more than a placebo effect.

I hope this book will give fresh insights into old problems. Instead of treating the *symptoms*, we must all strive to remove the *reasons* for the symptoms. Of course we all need the doctor and his diagnostic skills, but his therapy usually is limited to relieving the symptoms and falls short of the mark. Until the medical profession has all the answers, the patient has to take some of the responsibility for his or her own health needs.

Big problems usually begin at one time as little problems. I want to educate readers so that they will be able to look for and evaluate the little signs that can easily be reversed before the big problems overwhelm the body and demand medical attention with all the expense and side effects that come with it.

The doctor, the x-ray, and the laboratory usually cannot detect the slight deviations from the normal. This means that it is up to you to make the necessary adjustments in your diet, habits, exercise, and environment to remove the nagging symptom. If lifestyle changes are not made, the barely detectable symptoms soon form constellations called diseases. Once these diagnostic signs are labeled as one of the biggies (hypertension, obesity, diabetes, gallstones, allergy, infection, anxiety, depression), the problem is difficult to reverse without resorting to surgery or drugs.

An ear infection requires treatment with an antibiotic, but there is a reason behind the infection and that reason has to be discovered before another infection comes along. A food or inhalant allergy plus low levels of vitamin C and possibly vitamin A are to blame. The cause of the pus behind the eardrum is the growth of a common bacterium in that dark, moist, friendly cave. But what allergic or immunological fault allowed the invasion and growth of the bacteria? We know malnourished third-world people get sick frequently and seriously. Are our children similarly deficient in some nutrient that allows these earaches to recur?

An inflamed appendix is a symptom of a low-roughage diet. It is too late at this stage for a nutritional approach, but this must be initiated postsurgically to avoid future difficulties with hemorrhoids, fissures, diverticulitis, and possible bowel cancer, all related to diet.

Frequently the same deficiencies or special needs run in families. If a mother seems to have symptoms of a calcium deficiency, her child is more likely to be similarly affected. (A mother's backache during pregnancy suggests that her baby's colic is due to low calcium.) A family allergy calls for aid to the adrenal glands to help relieve the sneeze, the wheeze, and the itch.

Many symptoms are not dramatic. They are little signs that only you, the owner of your body, can perceive. Yet they are clues to something that is taking place. Perceiving bodily changes means that the body is asking the brain for help. Something you are eating or doing is causing an overload somewhere which the routine homeostatic mechanisms of the body cannot handle. If you get gas when you eat beef, a rash from strawberries, or a runny nose from milk, your body is telling you that these foods are "poison" to you. The therapist (and sometimes your mother) can figure out what antispasmodic, antihistamine, or decongestant will make you comfortable, but you should not be satisfied until you have improved your body's condition to the point that these symptoms no longer appear.

See if you can find yourself in this book. I am sure that you have a few symptoms you would like to get rid of. Why not try? Feeling good is your birthright. Most people know that if they gave up their fatty, salty, sugary foods, their booze, and their sedentary lives, they would feel better and lose a few pounds along with some of their nagging symptoms.

You could compromise with your addictions, cutting down on the offenders instead of getting rid of them entirely. That won't work as well as doing the total program, but in a month you should see and feel a change. Look up your symptom or sign, try the nutritional suggestions—swallow some B-vitamin complex, dump the sugar, use the stairway instead of the escalator—and see what happens. Try eating a handful of nuts at bedtime. If you get out of bed more easily in the morning, then you know your body is salvageable and worth feeding better. You may even improve your self-image and discover that you are a decent, worthwhile person. Feeding yourself right may turn out to be a pleasure. Learning about yourself, correcting deficiencies with diet and exercise, and achieving a positive attitude can be your most rewarding achievement. Whatever else happens in your life, *that* is something you have the power to do for yourself.

PART
1

PART
1

1

No such thing as a little bit sick

WHEN I FIRST began to change the diets of hyperactive children ten years ago, something odd began to happen. Mothers would volunteer the information that "Charlie is eating half as much food and gaining weight."

Aha, I thought, that must mean he had an absorption problem. *Aha* again: that's why the hair tests were low in calcium and magnesium. Another *aha* when I figured out why some of these children were helped with thyroid—not because thyroid is a stimulant, but because it is necessary at the cell-wall level to let nutrients in. Then came reports that stress interferes with absorption, which means that we can swallow nutrients but they won't necessarily get to the bloodstream and the cells. That seemed to explain why many of us do not stay healthy with just the Recommended Daily Allowances (RDAs) of the various vitamins and minerals. You have to be healthy to be healthy.

I began to see adults who were fatigued, crabby, dissatisfied, and mildly depressed; even though they were doing all the proper things—in megadoses—they just could not get their old zip back. I would try a vitamin B complex injection (0.5 cc in the muscle), and the majority would tell me that the next day they'd had a good one or two hours. "So, that's no good, eh, Doc?"

I would try to cheer them: "Even a few minutes of improvement means that your body is restorable. The wherewithal is lying around inside you. We just have to fuel it more consistently." We would arrange with a neighborhood nurse to administer two injections a week for three weeks and then reevaluate. To help rule out the placebo effect, I tried *not* to suggest how the patient would feel. (Many people get well if the doctor just says "How are you doing?")

But many of these patients improved in areas I had not even thought were related. When I treated fatigue or depression with vitamin shots, their allergies improved. Or insomnia disappeared. *Aha,* I thought, I'm making the whole body better. Those little enzymes in the intestinal wall that digest and absorb the food floating by are dependent on B-complex vitamins. But the unhealthy person (because of stress or prolonged poor diet) cannot absorb the vitamins to help the enzymes absorb the vitamins.

I found that the key organs involved are the adrenals, pancreas, and liver. They all need vitamins and minerals to do their work. They are all stressed when the blood sugar bounces around as a result of eating the wrong foods. Stress increases the need for vitamins B and C, calcium, magnesium, and zinc.

When I realized I could help the sleep habits, allergies, gas, and infection rate, as well as the restlessness, of these hyperactive children, I began to "treat" the adults who complained of headaches, allergies, hypertension, infections, depression, and undesirable behavior in somewhat the same way, that is, by changing their eating habits and lifestyles.

The results have been exciting, but I can't make the nutritional approach work on everyone. I discovered in my practice that if the child or adult had hay fever, asthma, or eczema, usually I could help control the symptoms by assuming that the adrenals were not working well enough to produce sufficient cortisol. I gave heroic doses (intravenously) of calcium, B_6, and C because these patients were in such a deep nutritional hole.

I also made the assumption that once a disease becomes established, the stress of the disease itself is enough to perpetuate it. Removing the stress may not be sufficient at this stage of decompensation. *Aha*, I thought, that's why the RDAs are inadequate for most of us who have a few symptoms or stress. The RDAs are only for those who are well, who have no stress (or at least are not perceiving it), and are absorbing all the nutrients they are swallowing. They are not enough for those of us who have special needs.

I know a man who worked with chemicals that contain alcohol. After he was divorced a few years ago, he started searching the bars for female companionship. It would always take a few drinks before he could be convivial and make the pick-up. Then he had to drive the woman to his apartment and perform before the alcohol limited his abilities. A delicate balance. One night the police found him driving the wrong way on a one-way street. The alcohol in his blood was high enough to convict him. The judge ordered him to take Antabuse for five years. Alcohol becomes a sickening chemical to people on Antabuse, and this man was unable to continue with his work. Today, on vitamins and a good diet, he no longer needs the drug, nor does he need to drink. He is looking for women elsewhere.

I thought my headaches were due to stress and my conscientious attitude. When I stopped the half-pound of cookies I was eating daily (because the dentist said my mouth was a mess), the headaches stopped.

Aha happened again just now, as I talked to a woman over the phone. She had a stress a few months ago, developed bronchitis, took several different antibiotics, but didn't get well until she upped the vitamin C and A. But she had felt so drawn and spacey that she stopped the vitamins and then she got worse, really exhausted. She wanted to know if she could be addicted to the vitamins because she feels miserable without them. I thought to ask her about her memory. "Gone." The combination of stress, antibiotics, fatigue, and memory loss told me that the woman's problem is a yeast infestation. (She will probably do well with nystatin.) Had she gone to a psychiatrist, the evaluation might have been "a neurotic withdrawal from life." Had she tried to treat her bronchitis with vitamins C and A and thymus gland in the first place, she might not have developed the complication.

If you have an ache or a pain, taking aspirin is OK, but at the same time see if you can find a physiological reason for the pain. A headache may mean that your blood sugar is falling and the blood vessels in your skull are dilating to get more blood into the brain. You don't have to assume you have unresolved aggression.

What I have come to understand in the ten years since the woman alcoholic walked into my office is that we can't separate any one part of our body from any of the other parts. They all work together. Let one part break down and the effect begins to spread. That's why we say that you have to be healthy to be healthy.

It seems fairly obvious to me that you can't have good health with bad nutrition—and by *health* I mean the capacity to live a long and zestful life free of illnesses and untimely degeneration of body tissue. Good nutrition may not guarantee this, but it is, I believe, an absolute requisite for that goal.

2

YOU ARE A TOSSED SALAD

HEALTH MIGHT BE a simple matter if all we had to worry about was what Dr. Jonathan Miller calls "the body in question." But the fact is, none of us is completely contained inside our skin. Things that are outside of us and things that existed before we did have a lot to do with how healthy we are and how healthy we can be. We are a toss-up of many factors: the genes we began with at conception; the biochemical influences on us at pregnancy; any physical injuries we may have sustained at birth; and the variety of emotional, physical, chemical, and nutritional forces we have been subjected to since birth. Tossed salad!

Just look at our genetic makeup. We can see Grandfather's nose in the six-year-old, Aunt Bess in her laugh, and Cousin Jody's expressive fingers. Genetic quirks show up in structure, color, and in action. Recent twin studies have shown the power of genetics to find expression in thoughts and deeds.

My whole interest in nutrition stemmed from the observation that many hyperactive children were fair-complexioned—blue- or green-eyed blonds or redheads. These characteristics suggested a genetic factor, yet until recently, hyperactivity was believed to be caused by some subtle or not-so-subtle hurt to the nervous system at birth. I had sense enough to ask if there were some diseases lying around in the relatives of these restless, goosey kids. I found that 60 percent of family members had one or all of these sugar-related conditions: diabetes, obesity, and alcoholism.

Then I found out what the hyperactives were eating. It all seemed to fit. Genetically these children are high-insulin makers, and they have to remedy their low blood sugar with more quick-sugar foods. So the blood sugar bounces around, and as they mature either they develop the family disease or else they figure out their biochemistry and eat nutritiously and perhaps beat the family curse. Nutrition can be used in a preventive, protective fashion.

I know a young man who had colic from milk as an infant, then asthma as a toddler from dairy products. His mother solved a bed-wetting problem by stopping milk when he was seven, and now at age twenty-seven he gets "whiteheads" on his face if he drinks a couple of glasses of milk a day. I know what the cause is; he knows what the cause is. If he sees a dermatologist, he is likely to be sent away with an antibiotic and a salve.

The young man's father had a mastoid operation as a child and now gets a bloody nose whenever he drinks milk. A genetic link is clear, because this father and son share the same general facial appearance. The precipitating event for the son may have been a stressful pregnancy. He was born eleven months after his healthy, nonallergic brother, and may have been denied all the nutrients that would have made strong adrenal glands to protect him from allergies.

The point is this: if you know a little of your genetic background and what your mother was doing when you were in her uterus, and if the obstetrician had to spank you at birth (stress), you will have something to work from. You will be able to understand your symptoms, vague and subtle though they may be, and be able to decide what remedial, logical, nutritional action you have to take.

If you have assumed that your mother's surliness, backache, and indifference to you was due to calcium deficiency, you may logically conclude that your insomnia and occasional muscle cramps are due to low calcium also. You take calcium and find in two to three weeks that you sleep better and the cramps are gone. The history allows for a quicker, more accurate diagnosis than if you had gone to the doctor. The doctor is trained to treat the symptoms, so he will give you a prescription for a bedtime sedative and will tell you your cramps are due to jogging and to cut it out. The blood tests are all normal.

The doctor is trained to treat diseases that are obvious, palpable, and confirmed by the laboratory. He doesn't want to fool around with the aches and pains of "hypochondriacs." But these aches and pains are the harbingers of more recognizable disease entities. A little gas and an occasional loose stool today may be colitis in five years. A sneeze and an itchy nose now may become asthma later. They don't *have* to—but why wait? A little care now will save you grief later on. And you have to be the one to do it, because the doctor cannot recognize the early signs of most diseases and he cannot project himself into your body and feel your symptoms. You have to be in charge.

But you have to be armed with the facts about your genetics, and what happened in the pregnancy in your early years. See if you can find out a few things from your mother (and father); it should give some personal insights and help you with your own children. I have found these questions helpful in my practice:

Is there diabetes anywhere in your family? One out of four of us has inherited the genes for diabetes. There is some evidence that hypoglycemia, or at least chronic ingestion of quick sugars, is the preliminary state to diabetes. Mood swings, Jekyll and Hyde behavior, is the give-away clue to blood sugar swings. If you find yourself craving sugar treats, you may be trapped by the family genes, but there are nutritional ways out.

Is there obesity in any relative? It is known that if both parents are obese, 80 percent of the children will have a weight problem. If both parents are thin, only 10 percent of the children will have to fight the bulge. The problem is multifactorial. Most obese people have more than average amounts of insulin floating about in their bloodstream. Insulin puts ingested carbohydrates into storage as fat. The trick is to keep the sugar and empty calories out of the house, nibble on nourishing, wholesome food every two to four hours, and maintain an exercise program. If you have ever had a few extra pounds hanging about your stomach and hips, you know you have the family tendency, especially if you have short tapering fingers and thick lips. Those clues are supposed to mean that you have a long (30- to 40-foot) intestinal tract which is very efficient, soaking up every last calorie.

Is there alcoholism in the family or is there much drinking? There is no "prealcoholic personality" that goes on to alcoholism. Alcoholics were all social drinkers who began to drink a little faster and more frequently than their peers. Are you looking forward to the next drink? If you are, or have ever had a scary blackout, and there is alcoholism in the family, you don't *have* to join A.A. yet, although it would be a good idea. You can help yourself and your biochemistry by eating in such a way that you will never have a dip in your blood sugar. If both parents are alcoholic, 50 percent of their sons and 10 percent of their daughters will follow the pattern.

Are allergies rampant in either side? Allergies do run in families. Inheriting a tendency to allergies is not the same as inheriting odd toenails. Children with allergies frequently come from mothers who had stress in the pregnancy or who loaded their system with one food, such as milk or wheat, thereby stimulating the allergy. Disturbing events may have been minimized later but during the pregnancy many have been *perceived* as stress. When the neocortex of the brain perceives stress, it sends messages to the pituitary gland and then to the adrenals. Adrenalin and cortisol are called out to handle the emergency. If the proper vitamins and minerals are not ingested, the adrenals have difficulty remaking the hormones. Allergies might appear, since cortisol, especially, has the ability to suppress allergy symptoms. A pregnant woman should avoid allergens and eat the foods she likes (milk, soy, corn, wheat, citrus, eggs) in rotation—once every three or four days.

Did your mother eat nourishing food during her pregnancy with you and gain at least 25 pounds? The baby's long-term health is determined in large part by its nourishment in the uterus. The nutrients must be in the mother's bloodstream in order to get to the baby.

Did she have much nausea, vomiting, muscle cramps, respiratory or urinary infection during that pregnancy? Did she drink or take drugs? If your mother's body was deficient in B vitamins, minerals, and vitamin C, you may have started life with a deficiency in those same elements. If drink or drugs were taken, you and your mother may actually have a dependency. Diuretics alter the chemical and nutritional balance and are dangerous to an unborn infant.

Can you identify any stress during those nine months? Was your mother under seventeen or over thirty-seven years of age? Was she happy about being pregnant with you? Was the delivery traumatic? Was she heavily sedated? Were you a Caesarean-section baby? Could she nurse you? For how long? Were her pregnancies close together?

Did you have many formula changes as a baby? If this occurred, it suggests a milk allergy; if you are a heavy milk drinker now, a milk allergy could explain your present symptoms. The allergy may move from one organ or system to another. Intestinal colic in infancy may become nasal phlegm and sinusitis in an adult.

Did you rock the bed or suck your thumb or show some rhythmical activity as a child? Or do you now? That history suggests a low level of calcium or magnesium, which could be still causing restlessness.

Were you sickly as a child? Many ear, throat, respiratory infections? Tonsils and adenoids removed? Allergies often show up through repeated infections. Milk allergy is the common one. Although you think you can drink milk now because these respiratory symptoms have disappeared, your colitis or skin rash may be related to dairy-product ingestion. There are people who sneeze with hay fever when the ragweed is blowing *only* if they are also drinking milk or eating sweets. The body's ability to handle allergies can be overloaded.

Any operations, injuries, accidents, or hospitalizations? These would constitute stress, especially if no attempt was made to build up the adrenals, liver, pancreas, and brain. Sickness (due to a defective immune system), allergies (due to fatigued adrenals), or any one of a number of psychosomatic illnesses might appear. The latter could include arthritis, psoriasis, colitis, depression, hyperactivity, shingles, and gas. The organ that is hit is genetically determined. The reason it happens is that the body cannot sufficiently filter out or disregard the stimuli coming in to the brain; the brain responds by setting up a further stimulation in the body which perpetuates the stress. (The flu that follows the final exams. The migraine that came on the last note of the piano recital. The soldiers who get paralyzed from the waist down when given orders for Alaska.) The mind affects the body and the body affects the mind.

Many people sick enough to be hospitalized are treated with antibiotics, cortisone, sugar in their veins, and a bland diet—pudding, gelatine, and white bread. A yeast begins to grow and an allergy to this develops. At a time when maximum nutrition is mandatory for a pleasant and rapid convalescence, the patient frequently is denied protein, vitamins, and minerals—known healers. Thus the stress of the treatment compounds the stress of the disease that required the hospitalization.

Genetic weaknesses are present in all of us. The stresses of life (injury, poor nutrition, surgery, emotional upsets) will permit the weaknesses to initiate some symptoms or signs. Controlling these minor clues is superior to allowing them to coalesce into an obvious disease.

3

WHAT IS YOUR BODY SAYING?

WE WERE TAUGHT in medical school that the patient's history is the most important diagnostic aid. The laboratory, the physical exam, and the x-rays only confirmed the diagnosis and helped us push our accuracy level to above 90 percent. By itself, the story the patient tells should reveal the disease more than 70 percent of the time. The Canadian physician Sir William Osler said, "If you listen to the patient long enough, he will tell you what he has." The statement is true—if the patient has a "good" disease, that is, one of the well-charted entities.

But what if the patient says he is *tired* and little else? That symptom goes with fifty diseases, including anemia, infection, allergy, stress, and low thyroid function. So the doctor uses the laboratory in the hope that it will turn up something specific or at least rule out the obvious negatives. Most of us trained in the "laboratory era" made our diagnoses by first getting all the lab work we could order and *then* talking to the patient. We put the diagnosis together from what the lab reported, then maybe confirmed it by the patient. This made it more "scientific," because the patient was an unreliable witness to his own disease. If the patient's history was vague—like "burning hair roots" and a "sense of pressure in my liver"—*and* if the lab found nothing and the exam was all normal, off we packed the patient to the psychiatrist, who seems to thrive on vague symptoms.

Today we are asking some—not all—of those patients back, because the vague early-warning signs and symptoms are beginning to form diagnostic constellations that have real meaning for the present (we can help faster if we get to it earlier) as well as significant implications for the future. As a pediatrician with the opportunity to make some long-term observations, I can see that if we doctors had initiated more prophylactic and preventive measures in the patients' early years, we could have averted some of the exhausting and expensive diseases and psychopathology that came to them later on.

At every moment of the day or night, your body is telling you something. If you have no symptoms, if you sleep soundly, if you are feeling great and are used to feeling that way, your body is telling you that you are one of the healthy ones.

Most of us are not so fortunate, however. Usually there is something we are aware of that isn't quite as it should be. Or it may be giving us real trouble—not necessarily catastrophic trouble, but something that complicates our life.

Read your body. If you have symptoms that match descriptions in Chapter 6, it means that someone or something is affecting you. You and your body are not able to screen out the world, and your brain perceives the stresses. This perception puts the pituitary, adrenal, and other glands into action in an attempt to minimize the stress. The body sends a message to the brain that a biochemical fault has appeared.

The body tries to rebalance, but it doesn't have what it needs to do this. If you follow the tilt, eventually it will lead to a mechanical problem or a diagnosable disease. With simple nutritional means or lifestyle changes, you and your doctor might be able to remedy the initial fault and stop the cycle at the beginning. Which possibility do you prefer?

SAY YOU ARE a reasonably healthy, active female of thirty years. You have two children and may have more. You love to cuddle them, feed them, and nest in your house, but you have a part-time job. Occasionally you get exhausted, which is understandable. What drives you wild, though, are the once-a-week insomnia attacks that last all night. Also, it gets to you when the children make noise (walking on their heels). You have a sister who is two years older and in good health. Your relatives, Scandinavians, tend to live forever. Your mother is in good health, as she was before and during her pregnancy with you. If she has a fault it is that she uses too much sugar when she cooks. You had crippling eczema on your arms, face, and legs in your first few years. It is now a little scaly thickness in the front part of your elbows and on your ankles, and you control it with a little cortisone ointment and a special oil in your bath water. You crave salty and sour food; sugar makes you ill. Bronchitis once a year. Joint aches and pains come and go.

What your history and your body are telling you is that you need calcium and magnesium. The infantile eczema is a genetic manifestation indicating that your adrenals were and are fatigued from your mother's pregnancy and her sugary diet. Salt cravers often have fatigued adrenals. Stress allows calcium to leave the body, and calcium and magnesium seem to help the body to notice less, to disregard things. Calcium has a calming effect on the nervous system; magnesium allows people to respond less to noises. Vitamin C helps the adrenals and should cut down on the bronchitis. The B complex should be helpful, especially B_6 and pantothenic acid, since they help the adrenals combat allergy.

Your formula would be: vitamin C, 1000 mg (increase until stools are slightly loose); calcium, 1000 mg (taken an hour before bedtime); magnesium, 500 mg; B complex, 50 mg of each; zinc, 30 mg; and vitamin A, 20,000 units; Folic acid, 0.4 mg.

In two months you report only a rare restless night. You have to cut your nails, whereas before you wore them out with scratching. You had a cold but no bronchitis. You have fewer cravings, your arthritis is minimal, and you have been able to quit smoking because you are calmer. Noises bother you less (children off to school helped). Your only stress now is your husband, who noisily chews nuts.

HERE'S ANOTHER ONE. You are mean and surly, the terrible-tempered Mr. Bang. You work hard as a contractor, your wife is OK, your teenage sons are lippy, and you occasionally feel the need to deck them when they talk back. You get no respect, or you have to fight to get it. You admit to mood swings. You justify your hostility on the basis that you work hard running your own business; it makes you tense. You have a steel beam as the rear bumper on your pickup which you use as a weapon; you stop suddenly and let a tailgating car fold around the beam. You drive off gleefully listening to glass and chrome hit the concrete. You are a touchy, green-eyed redhead. There is diabetes and alcoholism in the family. You had croup as a child and they took your tonsils out. You were a Jekyll-and-Hyde in school and had to see the principal frequently. You learned to hate school. You have a chip on your shoulder.

You see the doctor because of stomachaches, and an x-ray reveals a hiatal hernia (the top part of the stomach pushing up into the diaphragm). He says you are turning your aggression in on yourself. (It doesn't make sense, since so much of your anger is external already.) He wants to operate. You examine your life and family background and decide to change your diet.

You stop the sugar cookies and cola drinks; you try nibbling on seeds, nuts, raw vegetables, and fruit. You stop milk because you suspect it is causing an allergic stomach reaction. You add the B complex, digestive enzymes, calcium, and magnesium. In a month your stomach is better and you stop knocking your sons down. You feel better; the world is not so irritatingly close.

A COMMON ONE: You are a nice, gentle woman of twenty-six with two young children and a routine husband—not perfect but OK. You are depressed off and on for no good reason. You have a home, you're content with your sex life, your parents check on you but are not pests, you have friends. There is really no burning problem to write Ann Landers about. Still, you are feeling awful about 30 percent of the time. There are days when nothing gets done, and then you feel guilty because you didn't do your jobs. You are often tired, and that makes you depressed. It is worse after childbirth and before your periods. A psychiatrist says it's buried hostility and would like you to try Elavil.

You can find no helpful family clues. Some grandparent had pernicious anemia, but your mother said you were wanted and loved. No special allergies. You love coffee and chocolate. Gas is a problem.

Laboratory tests are available, but you may be one of those who need supplements despite "normal" test values. The answer for you may be B_{12} and folic acid, and the best results may be achieved by injections: 1 mg of B_{12} and 1 mg of folic acid intramuscularly every two to three days for a couple of weeks, then once a week, then maybe once a month during the week prior to your period.

ONE MORE: You are an active sixty-year-old woman who has recently retired after teaching school for thirty-five years. You have an alert, inquiring mind—or you did until recently—and would like to pursue your intellectual interests if you weren't so tired and depressed all the time. Your doctor says it is "normal" at your age to be this way. You refuse to believe that and will not take the Valium® he prescribes. Your mother's history is negative for any physical or mental symptoms. Some family members have had hay fever and asthma, but other than some seasonal sneezing, you are free from symptoms.

You have eliminated the sugar and empty calories from your diet. Using no artificial foods and flavors helped, but you are still more tired and depressed than you feel you are entitled to be. You upped your vitamins, had shots of B_{12} and folic acid, took some minerals on the basis of a hair test, added thyroid because your morning temperature was low. All these things helped, but you still are not right.

You try one more thing: the four-day fast. It is tough getting by with only water. You have headaches and anxiety on the third day, which suggests you are on to something, and, sure enough, on the fourth day you feel good inside *and* out—the best you've felt for twenty to thirty years. Now you break the fast. You eat one egg and within one hour you are crabby and depressed. You have a fight with your husband. You call your daughter long-distance and call her a "bitch" because she forgot your anniversary. Then in a flash of insight you realize that the egg is doing all this. It's enough to make you depressed again, because eggs are a favorite food. Your trouble is allergy, and you are walking proof of the rule: *If you love something, it is probably bad for you.*

Now ADD YOURSELF to this gallery of "average," "normal" people. You should be able to correlate historical information about your family genes, your environment in the uterus, and the stresses that have acted upon you since your mother delivered you. With your present symptoms, signs, tendencies, weaknesses, cravings, susceptibilities, and moods, you should be able to make a working diagnosis of your present needs. I would still insist, however, on a good checkup by a medical doctor to see what light he or she can throw on your more enigmatic body functions.

4

WHAT THE
LAB REPORTS TELL

I LIKE THE CONCEPT that each of us is responsible for most of our own health needs. But sometimes we need assistance. When confusion, overwhelming conditions, or extreme debilitation are obvious, we must get professional help. I also believe it is worthwhile to have a regular doctor to do a checkup on occasion. Children need one every year to monitor growth and weight and to detect conditions that might have slipped by domestic surveillance. Adults between the ages of eighteen and forty need to see the doctor only for sickness, childbirth, lumps, persistent pains. After forty a good checkup every two to five years with blood tests (anemia and chemical screening), a blood-pressure check, an occasional chest x-ray and electroencephalogram, pap smear, breast exam, and possible stress electrocardiogram seem prudent. Checkups after fifty should be spaced every one to three years and become yearly after sixty. There *are* a few sneaky illnesses that can be detected early with these sophisticated tests.

If all results are within normal limits, the doctor may say, "Well, the exams and the tests show everything is really OK. I realize you have stress and your body is getting older. I could give you a prescription for Valium® [or antihistamines or cortisone or a painkiller, or whatever is appropriate to relieve the symptoms], and if you like, I could refer you to a psychiatrist who might be able to help you handle your problems better." If you are quite incapacitated by your symptoms, the advice and the prescription should be followed. They might give you temporary relief and some time to sort out your life. You might also want to search elsewhere. A health professional with a degree other than the M.D. may be worthwhile. A chiropractor usually can find something out of place and get it back in place. A clergyman may help with guilt. A naturopath could discover a food/nutrition/biochemical malfunction and suggest nutritional approaches that may help the body correct itself. You do have some choices.

Very often patients and doctors fail to take full advantage of the tests that have been made. Once the tests show that everything is "within the normal range," they usually are filed away and forgotten. But if you are not feeling the way you think you should, the tests should be scrutinized for further clues to your state of being. You can do this yourself once you have some understanding of the terminology and of what constitutes the normal range for each type of test. This chapter is designed to guide you in reading your own lab reports. Maybe you didn't know you had a right to this information, but you do, so ask for them. It's *your* body, isn't it?

Some common measurements:

g =	gram =	about ⅕ teaspoon
mg =	milligram =	0.001 gram
mcg = μg =	microgram =	0.001 mg
ng =	nanogram =	0.001 mcg
pg =	picogram =	0.001 ng

Some common abbreviations:

% = percent

/ = per

For example, "IgM: 18–280 mg/100 ml" means that the measure of immunoglobulin M is 18 to 280 milligrams per 100 milliliters of blood. May be stated as 18 to 280 mg%.

Blood Tests (See Anemia)

Hemoglobin (iron-containing protein):
females 13.5 to 14.5 grams/100 ml
males 14.5 to 16.0 grams/100 ml
Hematocrit (percent of blood that is redblood cells):
females 39 to 45%
males 52 to 55%
Red blood cells:
females 4 million to 4.5 million/cubic millimeter
males 4.3 million to 4.9 million/cubic millimeter

The *white blood cells* (leukocytes) in the bloodstream traditionally are used to determine the body's response to infection, whether due to germ, virus, or parasite. When the white-blood-cell count rises, it suggests that the body is busy fighting a bacterial infection. Normal range is 5000 to 7000 cells per cu mm; Dr. Emanuel Cheraskin found these levels to be associated with the least number of symptoms.

Appendicitis usually causes a rise to 12,000. Pneumonia might show a 20,000 to 40,000 count. Strep throat may be 15,000.

The type of cell that increases in response to the infection often tells us what is invading the body. The "polys" (*polymorphonucleated,* that is, the nucleus has two or more lobules) usually increase from 55–65 to 80–90 percent if a bacterial infection is in progress. The numbers of immature forms of the cells increase.

The percent of *lymphocytes* is high in childhood, then

settles at 25 to 35 percent in adulthood. The percent of lymphocytes may rise in tubercular infections and mononucleosis. Lymphocyte counts below 1000 per cubic mm indicate moderate malnutrition.

In virus infections the total white-blood-cell count may remain at the preinfection level, because the fight against viruses is waged by *interferon* inside the body cells. (See Virus Infections for a description of the interferon effect.)

Eosinophils, like the white blood cells, have phagocytic (invasion-fighting) activity. They increase in the blood in response to allergies and parasites. They are attracted by histamine and play a role in the destruction of parasites. The usual level is less than 4 percent. (See Infections.)

Monocytes are cells that may increase in special conditions such as cancer. Normal is less than 3 percent.

Basophils carry histamine, and a high percent of these cells indicates an allergic condition. Normal is less than 2 percent.

Sedimentation rate is a measure of how fast the red blood cells fall when the blood is placed in an upright tube. A rapid fall indicates a bacterial infection, especially if pus is trapped somewhere in the body. (A fall greater than 20 mm in an hour is pathological.)

Reticulocytes are early forms of red blood cells, and the percent would rise from a normal of less than 1 percent to a high of 5 percent or so if blood cells are being formed rapidly, a good sign when anemia is being treated.

Platelets are little particles that float about in the blood, ready to plug up leaks in vessels. The level should be "adequate" as estimated by an experienced technician, or at 400,000/cu mm if actually counted. If it falls to levels of under 40,000 or so, dangerous bleeding may appear with a minimal trauma.

USUALLY OTHER blood tests are done at the same time as the above tests. In each case, the level in the blood tells only what was happening in the body at that moment.

The normal *glucose* level in the fasting state—at six hours from the last meal—would be at the 70–110 mg/100 ml of blood. Some doctors prefer to get a level two hours after a meal to help indicate how the patient is absorbing and metabolizing food. A fasting level of over 120–130 suggests diabetes. The five- or six-hour glucose tolerance test would be the follow-up if symptoms of diabetes or hypoglycemia are present (q.v.). A glycohemoglobin level would help.

The BUN, or *blood urea nitrogen,* is a reflection of protein food ingestion balanced by its conversion into urea and of the kidneys' ability to excrete the urea. The level is usually 10–15 mg/100 ml of serum. A very low level would suggest a poor protein diet or poor absorption. A high level suggests the need for kidney studies. (Glomerulonephritis, prostate hypertrophy, or pyelonephritis might explain a high level.)

The *creatinine* in the blood is a breakdown product of muscles, and the kidneys clear this easily. It is normally under 2 mg/100 ml of serum. Its elevation would suggest kidney pathology.

The *fats* or *lipids* are insoluble in the blood but are able to circulate if complexed with proteins called *lipoproteins.* Cholesterol, triglycerides, and phosphololipids are all lipids.

The *cholesterol* level is often—erroneously—considered the most important test done on the blood. Most labs figure 150 to 250 mg/100 ml of serum as normal because the majority of the cholesterol levels are within these two values. It is true that values exceeding 250 or 300 mg are associated with an increased risk of heart attack, stroke, and vascular problems, but many persons have these problems with low or normal cholesterol levels. The lab test should include the amounts of high- and low-density lipoproteins. The high-density form of lipoprotein apparently carries the cholesterol about more safely; an increased amount of low-density lipoprotein is associated with increased risk of vascular disease. (See Coronary Artery Disease.)

The *triglycerides* are the fats being carried about for energy; 50–125 mg/100 ml serum is considered normal. We need some, but a low level is deemed safer.

Uric acid should be maintained within 2–7 mg/100 ml of serum. Diet does have an effect on uric acid levels and should be attended to in anyone with gout in the family and a high level of uric acid in the blood. Foods containing hypoxanthine have the most effect on the uric acid level in the blood. Adenine and xanthine have an intermediate effect. Liver has xanthine and hypoxanthine and should be restricted in the diet. Allopurinol is a useful drug, because it inhibits the enzyme xanthine oxidase, and cuts down the reaction of hypoxanthine to xanthine to uric acid. Ten percent of kidney stones are formed from uric acid. (See Gout.)

Inorganic phosphorus usually is maintained at 2.5–4.5 mg/100 ml of serum. Meat eaters usually have a high level.

Calcium levels are 6.7–11 mg/100 ml of serum; most are at the 9–10 range. The body will attempt to keep it at this level to supply the brain, the blood (for clotting), and the muscles, and to keep the level at this optimum amount, will secrete various hormones to draw calcium from the bones if the diet is not supplying enough. Hair tests and x-rays may give clues to the amount of calcium the body has in storage. (See Osteoporosis.)

Bilirubin should be less than 1 mg/100 ml of serum. It is a reflection of the liver's ability to convert broken-down red blood cells to bile and to excrete the bile. The test measures the spillover into the circulation.

Alkaline phosphatase is present in the liver, bone, kidney, and intestine. If elevated (normal is 35 to 148 units), it suggests liver or bone pathology. If cells are damaged, this enzyme leaks out into the bloodstream and can be measured. Other tests would tell what organ is sick. An adult should get x-rays of the wrist bones to check for bone loss if the blood shows a high alkaline phosphatase level.

Serum glutamic–oxalacetic transaminase (SGOT) level is usually 13 to 55 units. This enzyme is widely distributed in the body, and high concentrations are found in the heart, liver, and skeletal muscle. The SGOT will rise four to six hours after a myocardial infarction because the anoxia of the muscle kills the cells which then release the enzyme. In twenty-four hours the level may range from 2 to 20 times the upper limits of normal. The degree of rise is roughly proportional to the extent of the heart-muscle infarction. The serum level of the enzyme is usually back to normal in four or five days. Blood samples usually are drawn daily to follow the course of the heart attack.

SGOT levels will rise to as high as 100 times normal when the liver cells are damaged and the enzyme reaches the blood (as in viral hepatitis and chemical poisonings). Infectious mononucleosis, cirrhosis, obstructive jaundice, and some tumors will cause a moderate elevation of SGOT. Other diseases that will cause a rise in SGOT are pulmonary embolism, pancreatitis, and muscle damage from any cause.

Serum glutamic–pyruvic transaminase (SGPT) is released into the blood with liver disease (as mentioned in SGOT) and less so with myocardial damage. The normal range is 10 to 50 units.

Lactic dehydrogenase (LDH) is most abundant in the heart muscle. A heart attack damages the cells and releases this enzyme. Normal levels are 62 to 131 (females) and up to 155 units for males. After a heart attack, the level may rise to 2 to 10 times the normal level in forty-eight to seventy-two hours and may stay elevated for five to ten days.

Creatine phosphokinase (CPK), another enzyme, is found in nervous tissue, heart muscle, and skeletal muscle. An elevation above 2.5 units for females or 4.3 units for males suggests myocardial infarction or muscular dystrophy.

Levels of other enzymes, called *isoenzymes*, help to differentiate which organ has been damaged.

Estrogenic hormone levels are measured to evaluate ovarian function. Estradiol is more active than the others, estrone and estriol. The levels of the hormones vary daily depending on the phase of the menstrual cycle, rising rapidly a few days after the flow stops and dropping off at ovulation.

Estrogens rise slowly in the first few months of pregnancy, then rapidly in the last trimester. Measuring the estriol levels in the urine of a pregnant woman is a method of following the high-risk patient. From micrograms the levels in pregnancy rise to milligram quantities. If the values then fall, it suggests the placenta is deteriorating and a miscarriage may occur.

The *thyroid gland* interacts with the ovaries. If there is no obvious reason for disturbed ovarian function, the thyroid should be evaluated. A consistent low morning temperature would suggest hypothyroidism.

Progesterone is secreted by the corpus luteum of the ovary right after ovulation. Its function is to prepare the endometrium for implantation of the fertilized egg. It is found in minute amounts in the serum: less than 150 ng/100 ml before ovulation and 300 to 2000 ng/100 ml during the luteal phase (last two weeks of the period; just before the menstrual flow). The test is used to determine the day of ovulation and assess placental function during the pregnancy.

The adrenal gland produces three *steroid hormones:* (1) Glucocorticoids are compounds which influence protein and carbohydrate metabolism and are necessary in stress conditions (pregnancy, severe hypertension, infectious diseases, surgery, burns, pancreatitis). They regulate the production of sugar from protein (levels rise when blood sugar drops), control loss of potassium from tissues, create insulin resistance and enhance effects of white blood cells. (2) Mineralocorticoids influence sodium and potassium balance. (3) Androgens are hormones that stimulate male secondary sexual characteristics. They have the identical effect as testosterone, and indeed, some of the adrenal androgens are converted to testosterone.

The adrenal gland cortex is controlled by a hormone from the pituitary gland, which in turn is affected by cortisol from the adrenals and by psychic events in the brain.

Protein levels of the blood have to be assessed when a number of diseases are being considered. These levels are affected by diet, metabolic rate, and the ability of the liver to synthesize amino acids. The *albumin* fraction in the blood is related more to diet. If it is low, and if liver and kidney diseases are ruled out, a protein diet of improved quality and quantity should solve the problem. If the level remains below 3.5 grams per 100 ml of serum despite adequate intake, it suggests protein malabsorption. *Globulin,* the heavier fraction, should be about 2.2 grams per 100 ml of serum. Special tests for A, G, M, and E globulins are often necessary for the evaluation of patients with allergies or susceptibility to infections.

Total protein:	6.6–8.3 g/100 ml of serum
Albumin:	3.5–5.0 g/100 ml
Immune globulin A:	100–400 mg/100 ml
Immune globulin E:	Under 300 units/ml
Immune globulin M:	18–280 mg/100 ml
Immune globulin G:	650–1600 mg/100 ml
Alpha 1 globulin:	100–400 mg/100 ml
Alpha 2 globulin:	500–1100 mg/100 ml
Beta globulin:	600–1200 mg/100 ml

MANY nutritionally oriented doctors will order the following additional blood tests depending on the symptoms:

Vitamin A:	65–275 international units/100 ml of serum
Carotene:	50–300 μg/100 ml
Vitamin B_1:	1.6–4.0 μg/100 ml
Vitamin C:	0.2–2.0 mg/100 ml
Folate (serum):	5–21 ng/ml
B_{12}:	330–1025 pg/ml
Vitamin E:	5–20 μg/ml

Lead: 5–40 μg/100 ml
Arsenic (urine): less than 20 μg/liter
Mercury (urine): less than 20 μg/liter
Glycohemoglobin (checks on recent blood-sugar fluctuations)
Transferrin: if below 150 mg/100 ml of serum suggests malnutrition.

Urinalysis

The urine should be tested for concentration ability. The aged kidney cannot concentrate the urine very well, and the need to get up during the night to urinate (nocturia) is one of the ways we have of knowing we are getting older. The cells lining the tubules in the kidneys cannot reabsorb the water as well, so the urine is more dilute.

The urine is tested for bile, glucose, blood, casts (discharged matter), pus, bacteria, protein, ketones, and calcium. New tests can detect abnormal amounts of metabolized hormones and brain chemicals that give clues about the enzyme systems.

Hair Analysis for Minerals

Some years ago chemists discovered that heavy toxic metals were being stored in the hair. An analysis gave a reasonably reliable indication that some exposure to lead, arsenic, mercury, cadmium, and aluminum had occurred to the owner of the hair. What is found in the hair gives an indication of the concentrations of the elements in the body tissue.

These toxins (lead, mercury, cadmium, arsenic, aluminum) float about in the body until the liver and kidneys are able to detoxify and dump them; they have no use and will poison or block the function of many enzyme systems. The hair is one way we excrete minerals; a strand of hair is a virtual printout of past nutritional events in our lives.

Each mineral in the hair produces a characteristic wave-length when burned. In the test, the hair is washed and then burned. The minerals are identified and measured. Many doctors find the hair test necessary to support evidence of the examination and the patient's history.

For example, if the calcium and magnesium are very low in the hair test of a child, the child is usually hyperactive and would respond to calcium and magnesium. B vitamins often act as a stimulant to that particular child because they release histamine from the basophils. Calcium counteracts the rest-lessness.

Calcium deposited in the hair rises in direct relation to the loss of bone calcium. A rise might be seen in the elderly osteoporotic person (q.v.), or in those consuming a lot of meat (phosphorus) and soft drinks (phosphoric acid) and small amounts of dairy products. In those cases, a secondary hyper-parathyroidism results, which pulls calcium out of the bones. Calcium and magnesium in the hair will rise.

In the hair of diabetics the ratio of calcium to zinc is frequently too high. Zinc is needed for insulin activity, and high calcium often suppresses that action. If the magnesium-to-calcium proportion is greater than usual, insulin activity is severely reduced. Manganese is often low.

If all the minerals are below the normal concentration in the hair, it suggests poor absorption (intestinal lining mal-function, food allergies, low hydrochloric acid in stomach, excess phytates in diet, pancreatic enzyme deficiency) or a hypothyroid condition. Many of these patients have been tak-ing more than the usual amounts of vitamins and minerals by mouth, but nothing good happens to them until they have had a few intravenous or intramuscular injections of B com-plex to act as a starter. I use this I.V.: vitamin C, 5 grams; calcium gluconate, 1 gram; magnesium sulfate, 0.5 grams; B complex, 1 cc; folic acid, 1 to 2 mg; B_{12}, 1000 mcg; B_6, 100 mg (or more, if dream recall is poor). Once body functions have been restored, the intestines are able to absorb the nutrients that are needed to facilitate absorption. Sometimes thyroid function returns after the shots, suggesting that the gland was malfunctioning because it was malnourished. Folic acid could upset the histadelic (see p. 359).

If sodium and potassium levels are high, allergies are often present. If the levels are low, the adrenals are often exhausted and the victim needs the adrenal-gland support nutrients (C, A, B_6, pantothenic acid, calcium, and zinc). The normal ratio of sodium to potassium is 2:1. If the ratio is down to 1:1, it suggests a malabsorption.

Arteriosclerosis usually is associated with a high calcium-to-zinc ratio. Zinc should be added to the diet of those with hardened arteries. Calcium may be low in hypertensive patients.

The calcium-to-magnesium ratio is higher than normal in arthritis. Magnesium helps to make calcium soluble; it also inhibits the action of hyalouronidase, which breaks down synovial (joint) fluid. High calcium depresses the activity of magnesium. Manganese is often low in arthritis.

In a number of cancer victims high copper and low zinc are combined. Some schizophrenia is associated with high copper, calcium, and iron, and low zinc and magnesium. High copper is frequently associated with excitability. High cadmium may be seen with hypertension. Copper may be up and magnesium down. Dental caries is noted in those with high calcium and low phosphorus and magnesium in the hair. A high zinc-to-copper ratio may be seen in the hypothyroid patient.

High or low zinc levels are associated with dysmenorrhea, white spots on the nails, and atopic dermatitis (eczema). If zinc is high, B_6 is added; if zinc is low with those complaints, then zinc and B_6 are taken. Low zinc is associated with alopecia.

The zinc-to-manganese ratio is ideally about 50:1. Low stomach acid, low bile acid, and low manganese in foods lead to a manganese deficiency. Manganese can help control diabetes (as do zinc and chromium). Those who eat large amounts of sugar usually have depressed calcium.

An irregular trace-mineral pattern (some higher than average, some lower) is typical of hypoglycemia. Manganese, sodium, and potassium are extremely low and the calcium and magnesium levels are 2 to 10 times the mean.

My experience coincides with that of other prevention-oriented doctors in that the nutrient availability of minerals is limited. The soil is becoming depleted, thus there is decreased mineral content in the plants we are eating.

Absorption is another problem for many people. Just swallowing the vitamins and minerals does not mean that they are sure to arrive inside the cell walls, ready to work. For a mineral to be bioavailable to the body cells and to act as a coenzyme, it must be in the ionic or free state, that is, soluble. Many people get nothing from calcium-magnesium carbonate (dolomite); it is a rock. Some dolomite swallowers find the tablets later in their cesspools. Some dolomite has lead in it. (See Lead Poisoning.) Natural iron is ferric, and digestion must change it to the absorbable ferrous form. Genetic factors, intestinal length, anything that speeds or slows intestinal motility (sympathetic or parasympathetic nerve activity), celiac disease or sprue, food poisoning, chemicals in the food, parasites, drugs, low stomach acid, too little bile, inadequate pancreatic enzyme, food allergies, lactose intolerance, and emotional factors all determine the absorption of minerals.

You might think it wise to include all foods in the world in the diet and then let the stomach and intestines pick out what the body will use. This almost works. But the presence or absence of one mineral may affect the use of another. For example, large amounts of calcium will tend to prevent the intake of several trace minerals. Cadmium and mercury make some minerals less available. Lowered pH levels (higher acid) will improve calcium and iron absorption, which is why it is recommended to take the ascorbic acid with these minerals. Chelated minerals (the mineral ion is attached to a bit of protein) are absorbed best.

The high-vegetable diet consumed in some parts of the world has a sufficiently high amount of phytate to precipitate all the available calcium, but most of these people do not have a calcium deficiency, because enzymes in their complete foods hydrolyze the phytate. The vitamin D these people typically receive also tends to counteract the effect of phytic acid in binding calcium.

The iron in beans is absorbed better if a small amount of meat is consumed at the same time. The abundant oxalates and phytates in a vegetarian diet make it difficult for iron to enter the body. More than twice as much iron is needed by vegetarians as by those whose diet includes some animal protein.

Hair analysis might give the doctor and the patient some clues about disease tendencies, absorption problems, and whether a toxic heavy metal is poisoning the enzyme system. It has been used for over sixty years by veterinarians to determine the need for trace minerals in the diets of animals. Animals usually eat just the fodder from the back pasture. If that soil is deficient—or poisoned—there is nothing to mitigate the effects. The testing of the soil and the animals' hair is very important here.

The human, however, is eating food from all over the state or country, so he or she is more likely to get a full complement of minerals. But there is no guarantee that three meals a day will give you all the minerals you need.

Hair analysis is an adjunctive procedure. I find it useful if I cannot "read the body" well enough to determine the patient's needs. If it points to malabsorption as the culprit, a few vitamin B complex shots may be necessary to get the enzymes, the thyroid, and the absorptive mechanisms in the gut going again.

The U.S. Environmental Protection Agency (Bulletin 600/3–80–089) has summarized the role of the laboratory tests as follows:

> The milk, urine, saliva, and sweat measure the component that is absorbed but excreted. The blood measures the component absorbed and temporarily in circulation before excretion and/or storage. . . . The hair, nails and teeth are tissues in which trace metals are sequestered and/or stored.

Remember, however, that "normal" laboratory results do not necessarily mean you are well. Your feelings about your body (weak, tired, cramps, headache, irritable, memory loss, et cetera) are more real and persuasive (to you) than are the test results. The doctor may be reluctant to treat you until a palpable disease appears, complete with abnormal laboratory findings. But it makes no sense to wait for that eventuality.

We can be thankful if the laboratory tells us we are in pretty good condition. Meanwhile, the signs and symptoms described in Chapter 6 may give us ideas of where to look next for *improved* health.

5

MAKING IT TO 120

OUR NUTRITIONAL PROGRAM should be right not only for our own personal combination of stresses and genetic predisposition, but also for our time in life. The teenager, for example, may be expending so much energy that he or she does not have to count calories. But the seventy-year-old has to pare down intake and stay with foods that are nutrient-rich. The ages in between—of child-bearing, career building, male and female menopause—all put special demands on the body that can be helped with the right diet and supplementation.

Somewhere in the pages that follow, you will find the stage of life that applies to you. Do you think your problems are yours alone? Read on.

Adolescence

Adolescence is supposed to start when puberty puts an end to the relatively carefree stage of childhood. Most young children don't know what is happening to them. They have never been through anything like *this* before. Voices crack, organs grow, moods swing violently, friends become enemies, and overwhelming fatigue alternates with joyful exuberance.

Parents recognizing the signs want to help, but they remember how furious it made them when their *own* parents tried to help. Any suggestions one generation has for the other are usually met with noncompliance or overt antagonism. The survival of the adolescent seems to be related more to luck than to parenting skills.

It is hard to know where to draw the line between a normal passage from one age to another and an abnormal, pathological condition. If the latter is suspected, then somehow you must drag the reluctant, surly youth into a doctor's office for a medical evaluation. To begin with, height and weight should be measured and plotted on a graph with previous measurements to assure that the child is fulfilling his or her genetic potential. A checklist of other questions might be appropriate. Don't be too obvious in pursuing these; the indirect approach is best. For example, if you want his ears checked, you might say, "Sometimes he doesn't hear me. Is it domestic deafness? Or wax? Or something to do with the ear infection he had when he was three years old?"

His throat clearing is irritating you like a dripping faucet, so you say, "Are the tonsils OK? They were large when he was five."

Heart and lungs OK? "My dad had high blood pressure and a stroke. Would you take his blood pressure for me and tell him not to salt everything?"

"If he had mono, would his spleen always be enlarged? He seems so tired and draggy all the time. Does he need a blood test? Could anemia make him feel this way?"

Of course, the doctor may develop a case of "office deafness" if you overdo the questions. He must be stimulated just enough to know your concerns and be free to respond to the patient and the exam and to feel that he is the leader of the team.

If you are not satisfied with your son's or daughter's appearance or behavior, do not leave until a complete exam has been done. That is, not until the doctor has at least *looked* at the genitalia (the best way to measure the completeness of maturity), ordered a blood test (complete blood count, hemoglobin, white and red cells, and sedimentation rate), a thyroid test, and urinalysis.

If everything checks out all right but you are still concerned, you may be overreacting to the child, or your child may be overreacting to the hormonal surge. Usually, with time and love, it all passes. The best way to find out if an adolescent is functioning adequately is to evaluate social relations. Do friends call? Does he call friends? Does she want her friends to stay overnight? Does your child laugh more than he cries?

Schoolwork may suffer during the years of rapid growth, but special interests and the right kind of parental pressure should help the child maintain the expected grade point. A conference with teachers is worthwhile, since they may be the first to notice subtle changes in work habits, attitude, and even handwriting.

Most parents feel guilty (and angry, too) if their child becomes depressed, or starts smoking cigarettes or pot or using drugs or alcohol while under their roof and getting the best of care. They have to understand that a variety of strong pressures work together to waylay adolescents. The desire for peer-group acceptance can lead even the most confident among them into trying the "other" way.

Many adolescents "act out" just to see if their parents are aware or caring. Part of this is a show of independence, but many behave this way *because they do not feel good.*

Sometimes the clues are all there for anyone to notice: the restlessness, foot jiggling, pencil biting, hair twisting. Insomnia, mood swings that have little to do with environmental events, bizarre food cravings, all suggest biochemical imbalances that can be helped by diet.

The problem with intervention is that these delicate eleven- to eighteen-year-olds don't want to be manipulated. They need to feel independent and to see that they are making a few decisions on their own. The trick is to get them to make the right decisions. Some of this is related to the foundation that was laid at age three to six months, when parents should have been instilling a good self-image in their child. With a sense of self-esteem they seem to be able to get through the rough teen years intact.

When parents bring their adolescent in to see me and say, "I want a good checkup," it means they are not satisfied with the young person's health habits or attitude. They are hoping I can find something logical so they won't have to go to the psychologist. The exam usually reveals a few pimples, a normal blood test, and negative urinalysis. In private, they tell me that the boy or girl is sullen, tired, skipping school, and probably on drugs.

I can sense some hostility because the young person is sitting sullenly staring at me with arms folded across the chest. Defiance. I am the enemy because I am an adult and probably on his parents' side. "They won't let me stay out past ten on weekdays and eleven on Friday and Saturday. It's not fair. All my friends get to stay out until midnight!" wails the fourteen-year-old. It's going to be a long session. I feel like an arbiter in a labor-management dispute. Compromise, compromise.

"We would give Dora a lot of privileges if she would keep her grades up." That's a clue. I ask Dora if school is too tough, whether she thinks she should change schools, go to summer school, do the year over again, or what. It makes her feel I am trying to find a solution. Then I ask her if there are any problems with her health or brain or body that she would like to get better.

"Nothing. I'm fine," Dora responds curtly.

"What about being tired in the morning and those head-aches?" asks Mom, a little miffed.

"I can handle it. Lay off."

I get the parents out of the room at this point, and try to remember how I wanted adults to speak to me when I was an adolescent. Not as if I were a kid, not demanding; giving some sympathy, but mainly giving choices I could live with.

"To a certain extent, you are trapped," I say. "You can't run away and survive. But if you keep on the way you are, they will just get more angry with you. You might have to repeat the year at school. If I can help you be less tired and make school a little easier so your grades come up, then I can get them to relax their tight hold on your curfew. You have to show somehow by word or deed—or being a good actress—that you are following the rules.

"I have known your parents for fourteen years and be-lieve them to be fairly bright and reasonably fair. But I'm asking you to do a few things for me. Leave them out of it. If you do what I suggest, you should be able to handle the hassle of living with your old-fashioned parents. You'll have more energy and be able to get your schoolwork done."

Now, I know I can't make her do too many things, but at least these essentials:

"Will you, for me, go without sugar, ice cream, colas, and fries for a month or two? They can make you tired and a little fat. And take these B-complex vitamins with 50 mg each of the Bs. The calcium [500 mg] is for bedtime. I'll call in a week or so to see if you are OK."

She reluctantly agrees and so do the parents. They prom-ise to get off her back and let me make the rules. It isn't perfect, but we all hold together and years from now we will all still be friends.

THE POINT IS that adolescence is an age of stress, or at least is perceived as such, by adolescents and the way they eat compounds the stress. If they eat well and stay away from the junk that seems to be the adolescent lifestyle, they usually feel well enough to handle, with humor, the surges of dependency alternating with joyous maturity and hope.

The "typical" adolescent diet may be appropriate once every two weeks, but is seriously lacking in vitamins A, D, C, and folate. It has too much salt and too much fat. Dr. Laurence Finberg (professor of pediatrics at Albert Einstein College of Medicine in New York) analyzed the content of this exaggeration (but you get the idea):

Cheeseburgers, french fries, milk shake—four times a day—would certainly provide the calories (4000), the protein (17 percent), and the carbohydrates (44 percent), but would be heavy on the fat, albeit the American average (39 percent). A McDonald's Big Mac has more than 500 calories, about one-quarter to one-fifth of the daily calorie requirement for an average adult. It also has 1 gram of sodium, about half the daily requirement. Most of this fat is saturated, and fiber is nonexistent. The Kentucky Fried Chicken Original Recipe Dinner has 2 grams of sodium and about 900 calories. The protein is certainly more than adequate, but with the phosphoric acid in the soft drink, all that phosphate could imbalance the calcium.

We know they will eat sugar and junk with their friends, but we can make sure that every speck of food they eat at home is as nutritious as possible. Extra vitamins and minerals are a necessity to undo the negative effects of sugar and soft drinks and to help them handle the stresses of adolescence, which deplete them further.

"If your adolescent will accept the idea of a daily supplement, use one with the following amounts, more or less: B_1, B_2, B_6, at about 25 to 50 mg each; B_3 and pantothenic acid at about 50 to 100 mg; folic acid, 0.4 mg; B_{12} 100 mcg; inositol and choline, 1 gram each."

Then, if another supplement can be urged or sneaked into their bodies, the next choice would be calcium and magnesium—usually given at bedtime for their calming effect. Rapidly growing adolescent athletes will welcome the lessening of the muscle aches, pains, joint stiffness, and tense backs that plague them. Many females find the calcium/magnesium superior to Midol® for their menstrual cramps. It also helps those who struggle to fall asleep. Calcium, 1000 to 1500 mg per day, and magnesium, 500 mg per day, are about right.

After about a month or two of these supplements, the parents should notice a calmness and evenness in their adolescent. The adolescent should notice that he feels better, more in control, and more cheerful. He even begins to suspect that his parents aren't too mean after all. (He will never say it out loud until he is twenty-five, though.)

The trick of parenting is to survive until your children get to their twenties and become a little thoughtful and maybe even ask if they can do something for you. But they have to be fed so that they feel good. Otherwise it may be hard for you to say, "Hey, you're OK. You're a nice daughter [or son]."

We feel that adolescents are more likely to be pulled into drugs, alcohol, and deviancy if they don't feel good. And one reason for feeling poorly is the lack of a good diet and adequate supplements.

Once the adolescent feels and acts better, the parents can begin working on other symptoms with other supplements—the fine tuning. Acne can be controlled with diet, vitamin A, and zinc. Obesity responds if the appropriate diet and supplements are used. Depression may be a biochemical problem that will improve with a biochemical approach. Not every adolescent gets mono (a virus), but vitamin C can ward it off.

I've often wondered, if we told adolescents that vitamin C is an illicit drug, would they shoot that into their veins instead of other things?

Every adolescent has to be indoctrinated into the basics of nutrition before he or she goes off to the service, college, or marriage. Remember, vitamin C and the B complex are the ones most easily lost when food is cooked or processed, and are the ones most needed whenever there is a stressful situation. A bottle of C and one of the B complex won't crowd their luggage or cause them embarrassment.

The Twenties

Most of us in this decade have pretty well figured out our strengths and weaknesses, but we are not sure what to do about them or whom to ask. You notice how much fun your friends are having at a party, while you are miserable, shy, sweaty-palmed, self-conscious about your (imagined) bad breath, oily skin, greasy hair. No wonder no one notices you or talks to you. You get depressed and have a stiff drink and then either you pass out ("one-beer girl") or become overly loud with a lampshade on your head. The next day you are *really* depressed. You thought all this would pass after you turned nineteen.

You can't seem to get a job you like or one where the people like you. Do I want to be a busboy or waitress all my life? If I am supposed to be a computer programmer, why am I teaching kindergarten? Am I too fat, too thin, too nervous, too stupid, too klutzy?

You are recently married and your partner is a delight most of the time but the honeymoon is over for sure. Is divorce possible this early in the marriage or is annulment best? Why all the fights? Should premenstrual tension last two weeks? Does she really enjoy sex or is she faking it to make me think I'm good in bed? Does he have to have sex three times a day? I thought the male was supposed to peak out at eighteen. Why does she get so mad when I go with my buddies hunting, fishing, playing cards, bowling, drinking a few beers? He could make an effort to be cheerful and talk to my friends at dinner parties; I talk to *his* friends. Why does she have so much gas? We eat the same stuff.

Some young people in college or graduate school, close to a career goal, are devastated by some chronic disease that necessarily alters their entire life: multiple sclerosis, lupus erythematosis, glomerulonephritis, schizophrenia, eczema, asthma, tuberculosis, obesity, alcoholism—there are a thousand of them. Each had warning clues, and most of the diseases could have been attenuated or even controlled if a nutrition program had been launched in time.

Many of these conditions can be traced to the stresses and excesses of high-school and college life, the frequently unbalanced diet of the adolescent, and the disregard of early warning signs. (Adelle Davis believed that the bone tumor that took her at age sixty-eight was the result of the dorm food in college.) But who can get a youth to change by using scare tactics? (The army tried that in World War II in its venereal disease control campaign: "There are no nice girls").

One of the common questions I am asked by people of every age group is, "Why am I so tired in the morning?" We were taught in medical school that early-morning fatigue after a seven- to eight-hour sleep *had* to mean a psychological problem (success neurosis; hate for job, mother, or spouse) that required some long-term, expensive therapy. Most of us know now that it is due to eating the wrong food at or near bedtime the night before. The low blood sugar that follows the ingestion of a sweet snack or allergy-inducing food at bedtime prevents the body and the brain from responding to the sun or the alarm.

It is true, the majority of the workers of the world hate, dislike, or at least are bored with their jobs. But there are many equally turned-off people who are able to leap out of bed in the morning, sing, tap dance, jog, shower—flaunt their cheerfulness and drive their families under the pillows to escape. It is also true that much behavior is genetically determined, and it may well be that a unique circadian rhythm (morning-type, evening-type) is stamped on us at conception. But that is not to say we are stuck with an unalterable genetic pattern of behavior. We all have some ability to preprogram ourselves for the next day. Say you are to go fishing and must awaken at 5 A.M. You may find yourself awake at 4:58 A.M., because your mental alarm was set.

Yes, we are genetically controlled, and to some degree our thoughts, perceptions, and behaviors are predetermined in much the way that growth, eye color, and a tendency to different illnesses are predetermined. We can, however, strengthen our strengths and modify our weaknesses with superb nutrition, training, faith, and some professional help.

If you are a surly monster in the morning, try altering your diet from supper to bedtime just for one or two evenings. No sugar, no white flour, no coffee, pie, or favorite dessert. For your evening meal have meat, or fish, a vegetable, and a salad. Then at bedtime eat a piece of leftover meat or fish or a handful of nuts or seeds. A cube of cheese would be OK. No fruit (sugar). Go to bed at the usual time and see if you or your spouse can tell that you are in any way different—other than your having gas or elephant breath from the nuts.

This is the first step in reading your body, and it is important that you learn how to do it in this third decade of life; you might as well have a few good mornings if you are going to live to be eighty. For you to want to get up and go to work, your brain has to be functioning well enough that you know your own name. If you are eating the wrong foods, your level of cerebral functioning may be somewhere down near your medulla oblongata. You are at the porpoise level. Better than a snake, but not acceptable for a human, humane existence.

Part of longevity is wanting to get up and go to work in the morning, and that is a function of the recent diet. Therefore, longevity is related to diet.

Longevity is also related to a happy marriage. The interpersonal relationship a couple establishes has to do with handling stress: being thoughtful, responding to needs, accepting criticism, passing out good strokes and being able to laugh at one's own peculiarities. How well the partners hold together depends more on each one's good self-image than on the promises made during the wedding ceremony. Many young couples live together to see if they have the potential for making it work. They do not want to repeat the types of marriages they saw at home.

These years are difficult times for many young homemakers: finishing school, establishing a job or profession, getting pregnant, buying a house. These stresses lead to arguments, often centered around finances. Police are aware of domestic violence. Counselors try to arbitrate. Ministers can intervene. But these helpers are often talking to the wrong part of the brain.

Nutrition has more than a little to do with depression, anxiety, mood swings, aggression, exhaustion. If the cortex of the brain is not nourished, then subcortical, animal, selfish responses are the only ones available. This lower brain has no insight; it just seems to act reflexively.

Young couples are often unable to see the connection between the doughnut for breakfast and the slap in the face at mid-morning. Older couples have finally figured it out because their children were their teachers. (Give a kid a Twinkie and watch him pull a knife or walk on the ceiling.)

It is quite important to establish certain eating rules early in one's life, and especially so for young homemakers who have a large emotional—and financial—investment in each other.

Basic rules for college and postgraduate students, single men and women, young couples—well, I guess for everybody:

1. No sugar in the house (includes white, brown, corn, maple syrup, and molasses, though one small jar of pure raw honey is OK). No white-flour products. No boxed cereals; no packaged or processed foods, if possible. Limited salt. Beef only two times a month.

2. Allow for nibbling on raw vegetables, seeds, nuts, fruits. Serve salads daily. Fish, fowl, legumes, eggs, cheese in rotation. Whole-grain bread and cereal. Sprinkle brewer's yeast and wheat germ on things.

3. Vitamin C, 1000 to 5000 mg daily, or more depending on bowel tolerance. If allergies and infections are present, use more. B complex, as listed on page 40. Folic acid should be in there (0.4 mg). Calcium, 500 to 1000 mg at bedtime; this dose would vary depending on dairy intake. Magnesium, 300 to 500 mg at bedtime. Trace minerals in a tablet (like kelp). Vitamin A, 10,000 to 20,000 units, depending on skin clues. Vitamin D, 500 to 1000 units, depending on sun exposure. Vitamin E, 400 units, depending on condition of blood vessels.

After a month on the above, you should notice that you feel better, can handle stress better, have fewer infections. Your allergies are minimal, you are more cheerful, and you make love better. Then comes the fine tuning. Maybe it is muscle cramps or bad breath or a persistent rash you would like to eliminate. You can take a few appropriate nutritional supplements and find that your body knows how to use them to eliminate that specific problem.

You should also feel better about yourself because you can to a large extent take charge of your body. Instead of the body being in charge, your brain can think of what it wants the body to do and the body responds. It should only be at this time that you consider starting a child. The mother's good health for years prior to conception and her excellent nutrition during the pregnancy are necessary to assure healthy, well-formed children.

This is the ideal time to find out about the health and disease patterns of your parents, aunts, uncles, and grandparents—before they all get too forgetful. Some conditions are so strong in families that no child will miss being tainted. Other problems "run" in families but can be avoided by eating a nutritious diet, keeping stress to a minimum, and having a little luck. Genetic counseling may be needed.

Here is an example: If both your parents are overweight, you have an 80 percent chance of being heavy, especially if you have short, tapering fingers and thick lips. Dr. William Sheldon correlated those external clues with an internal characteristic, namely, that these people had 40 feet of bowel. (Thin people have 20 feet.) With this extra acreage for absorption, those people genetically predisposed for obesity must be forever vigilant to avoid calorically loaded foods.

Another worthwhile enterprise is to get your own specific history from your mother—not what the doctors said about her health or her pregnancies or what the pediatrician has in his records, but how she perceived her health and her comfort during the time she was carrying you. How close was the pregnancy to some stressful physical or emotional event? How many months or years between pregnancies? Was there a miscarriage in between? Did she really want to be pregnant with you? (How can a mother answer that and maintain eye contact?) Was it a stressful pregnancy? Could she nurse you and for how long? Many milk changes? Colic? Ear infections?

There is significance to all of this. If, for instance, you are a nice person but have to sniff, snort, hock, and spit every twenty to forty minutes, it may be driving your spouse up the wall. Your doctor will give you an antihistamine, and the ear, nose, and throat doctor will suck out your sinuses, but the trouble is still there. All you have to do, really, is ask your mother if you had phlegm as a baby, or ear infections, or a tonsillectomy, or milk changes. You have a milk allergy and you probably love milk and drink a quart or more daily.

That's how milk can cause divorce!

The Thirties

When I turned thirty-five years old I got a birthday card from a "friend." The message was "Congratulations! You are half way home."

That old biblical saying about three score and ten years has done too much damage and should be eliminated. It was, however, better than what I expected of myself. My father, with whom I have closely identified over the years, died at age sixty. At least my friend let me have another big ten.

But too many of us are giving up as we grow and mature. It's retirement at age sixty to sixty-five, and after that fishing, visiting the grandchildren, and waiting for death. Sounds shortsighted and cruel.

Try another programming technique; this *does* work. Aim for age 120 right now and file it into your computer brain. But to do this it has to be fun, or you have to feel needed, or someone has to say something nice to you at least two to three times a day. You have to be laughing and smiling at least 50 to 60 percent of the time.

What is the point of going on forever if it is all a boring drag? "Live as though you would die tomorrow and learn as though you would live forever." It has to be fun and a challenge. Age thirty to forty is the decade to figure out if the balance is about right. Can you handle these stresses for the next fifty to ninety years? If you don't change your lifestyle, your job, your spouse, and your friends now, you will find it harder in the next decade. Your body—you may not want to believe this—is already aging. It has been measured. You are not the fantastic machine you were at age twenty.

The point right now is that you may be eating or inhaling something dangerous, or getting little exercise, or having some stress that has tilted your biochemistry. But you don't show any symptoms, and your doctor says you are fit, and the lab tests confirm it.

When you are ninety years old and in constant pain with your back because you didn't think calcium was important, you will hate yourself for not following the advice of us health nuts, or you will be embittered because you did not plan to live that long.

You must review your habits and reorganize your priorities based on the facts of life. You need fewer calories because your metabolism is slowing down. Even by following the same good exercise program you are used to, you cannot use up the same number of calories that you did ten short years ago. Smoking or breathing air crud in traffic is taking its toll. The dessert habit is making your liver work harder. The amount of reserve tissue in all your organs is less now.

It is difficult to motivate anyone with scare tactics. A person must be suffering a little bit to want to change. Often I hear people tell me that their loved ones are sick, and we both know that it is due to some junk they are eating. But the sick ones won't change, because they are addicted and they can't be talked out of their cravings.

If you find that the reserve capacity of any of your organs is down, you can resurrect the previous function by super nourishment. This is the gray, borderline area that orthodox medicine does not like to fool with because the tests are not sophisticated enough to tell the doctor what is slipping and by how much. Almost every disease starts someplace, but the orthodox doctor wants to have a positive finding on the physical exam and confirmation from the laboratory. Nutrition-oriented doctors are able to trace symptoms—very subjective complaints or observations that the patient presents—and to connect these subtle deviations to diet, lifestyle, lack of exercise, and stress.

You should be your own expert for your own body. When you had your appendix out, your doctor probably did not ask about bowel movement consistency for the years prior to the surgery. Almost all appendicitis patients have had a long history of constipation; people with sloppy stools just don't have the problem. As you strained to pass a hard, golf-ball-like stool, you should have said: "Something's wrong; I need fiber." See how easy it is?

I had an anal ulcer fixed after two years of eating a lot of hospital food (sugar, white flour, and red gelatine). The only thing the diet did was save me from going to the bathroom once or twice daily; what was there was not worth passing. The inspissated ball must have eroded the lining. I should have figured it out. But when you're busy . . .

Sit down at least once a year and figure out if you should be where you are and if you are going in the right direction. Do you need to change anything? Do you have any symptoms at all? Do you know what it is like to feel great? Have you ever felt well? Don't assume everyone gets the flu or has an allergy. These are clues. Your body is trying to tell you to change something. Simple, cheap, and minor changes or supplements now should save you some expensive, painful medical or surgical intervention later on.

I talked to a health-and-nutrition-oriented woman today. She had had the flu, which usually means three days of fever and headache and then seven days of cough. With her it lasted only four to six hours and never got beyond the tickle in the throat, a slight creepiness to the skin, and muscle aches. She read her body and figured it was the flu and took 2 grams of vitamin C hourly.

Don't think that because you only have the "average" number (four) of colds a year that you are normal. "The kids brought it home from school." If you are in good shape, you shouldn't get sick at all.

The usual first and most common clue that people notice at any age is fatigue. Trouble getting out of bed in the morning after a good eight or nine hours' sleep. Maybe a little reluctance to volunteer to do something for the P.T.A. or your local service club. Drifting off in a movie or while reading a book or when your spouse is talking to you. Some subtle indifference to a sexual overture.

Fatigue has to do with energy. Energy requires oxygen and glucose. You are breathing and you eat sugar, so what is the problem? Enzymes require B vitamins and trace minerals to function. Our bodies are equipped to eat Mother Nature's foods. As we age and the reserve in our organs contracts, we have to eat foods with high concentrations of these vitamins and minerals. If you have ever eaten a piece of white bread or one dish or ice cream, you are behind. Without changing any other part of your life or diet, add the B-complex vitamins (50 mg of each) daily—enough so your urine is yellow consistently.

You may be amazed at how your fatigue disappears, but some other subtle things may change as well. You can lose weight because the responsible enzymes now have the wherewithal to do their job. Your spouse may notice a cheerfulness, an eagerness, a better sense of humor. A new spring to the step and attitude about the job ("I can handle it"). It takes a month. If nothing happens, you haven't hurt anyone, but it does mean you should have seen the doctor and had anemia and thyroid malfunction ruled out first.

People on a weight reduction diet, especially a crash program, often develop subtle symptoms of fatigue, irritability, and indifference, because a diet of less than 1800 calories a day is too meager to provide even the feeble doses of the Recommended Daily Allowances. Supplements are required.

All the following should be attended to now, because they mean the body has slipped: hay fever, muscle cramps, not rested after seven to nine hours of sleep, headaches, straining to pass stools, insomnia, menstrual cramps, irritability at the time of menses, skin rashes, forgetfulness.

The appearance of these symptoms means your body is off, and if they have been plaguing you only recently, nutritional changes usually are enough to reverse the trend away from something more serious.

You owe it to yourself to see that you are ingesting at least the minimum to keep your body running:

- Vitamin C, at least 1000 to 5000 mg a day, and more if allergies or sickness are a common problem. If cancer is in your family, you would be smart to take 10 grams of vitamin C daily, depending on your bowel tolerance.

- B complex, as listed on page 40, once or twice a day; the urine should be noticeably yellow.
- Calcium: we all need 1000 mg a day. Dairy products may not be the best thing for you because of the salt and fat in them and the lack of iron and the constipating effect. Calcium deficiency is common.
- Magnesium controls irritability, keeps the muscles working, may prevent a fatal heart attack, and cuts down on body odor. Take 500 mg per day.
- Folic acid and B_{12} frequently are lacking in diets, and are needed especially by those prone to depression.
- Iron is poorly absorbed; women usually need a supplement. (See Anemia.)
- Vitamins E (400–1200 u), A (10,000–20,000 u), and D (400–1000 u) are needed by most of us as supplements, since the diet and sunshine are not sufficient sources.

The above program is basic if the machinery of the body is to work adequately. Other additions will be necessary depending on special stresses or inherited conditions.

Many people find that their cravings for sugar, booze, and cigarettes disappear, as well as their dependence on Valium and other drugs.

You could still become an ideal person. Don't screw up your potential with a bad diet. Your mother and father still want to be proud of you.

The Forties

Can you remember how when you were twenty you thought someone age forty was really ancient, over the hill? Now that you are in the forties, your life should make some sense. By now you have probably arrived—but maybe you haven't. At least, the fact that you are awake and aware enough to read this means that you are alive. I have discovered that if someone is alive, his condition can be improved.

If your machinery has lasted this long, it suggests that it may go on for several more decades. The trick of your lifetime is to keep all parts functioning as well and as equally as possible, to have a good brain and a body that can keep up. So these middle years are a very important time to take stock of the remains and to see what needs shoring up. Remember, cells have been dying for the past twenty years, and the ones still working have to be nourished optimally.

It is usually in this decade that laboratory evidence begins to appear that reflects your previous neglect of your body. The blood pressure is up a little (130/85); not much, but something is happening. The urine does not concentrate as well. Cholesterol has moved from 200 to 230; not bad, but going in the wrong direction. The doctor can find no signs of disease and pats you on the back and says you're in good shape. Which means you have not taxed your physiology sufficiently to give palpable evidence that your body has slipped. But if you are honest with yourself you can tell from the inside that you don't have the reserve of just a few years ago. You need only two drinks to get a high instead of three or four. You need seven and a half to eight hours of sleep to feel refreshed, instead of bounding out after seven hours. You are noticing more gas. The kids wear you out faster, and you cannot play ball with them over the weekend without feeling stiff on Monday. Muscle soreness takes two or three days to go away instead of just overnight.

You are curt and occasionally short-tempered about requests to go to the store or take the garbage out. You are forgetting names of old friends, although people you see every day or every week are easy to remember still. You have an occasional crying spell for no good reason. You used to be able to drop off to sleep easily, but now you lie awake for thirty minutes occasionally, trying to relax. Persistent and negative thoughts surface: "Is this the life I want to lead until the old folks' home?" "Am I married to the right person?" "The kids are adolescents now and moving away from us. Should I have an affair before it is too late to have an affair?" "Shall we dump the whole thing, sell the house, quit the job, and move to a better climate?"

As a woman you tend to blame some of your difficulties on your husband, who could be more thoughtful. You also are being launched into your menopause and occasionally get mad at your body for playing tricks on you: irregular periods, hot flashes, depression.

As a man you are sometimes relieved when your wife "has a headache"; you didn't have the energy to perform anyway. "Would a younger woman make a difference?" You awake with an erection almost every morning. It suggests you are still holding together. But it does take a little longer to urinate and the stream seems a little narrower and a few drops always seem to come later in your shorts.

Most of us in this decade become more conservative, complacent, and somewhat accepting. But with politics, religion, and lifestyle we are usually fixed and unyielding. We know what would work if the government would see it our way. We are not so sure we will like our prospective sons- or daughters-in-law, but we go with the flow. We remember some lack of enthusiasm in our own parents when we announced our engagement.

We don't mind the frequent put-downs of daily living as long as no one changes our habits of eating, drinking, going to the bathroom, reading the paper, watching TV, exercising (or not exercising), going to church, talking on the phone, and so forth. Interruptions or attempts to change these personal, comfortable ways of doing things usually are met with sullen negativism and sometimes angry outbursts. Have you tried to tell your spouse that he (or she) is drinking too much?

Changing unhealthy habits is what this book is all about.

But if a checkup with the doctor reveals only borderline lab tests and a normal exam and x-ray and electrocardiogram, how does a family motivate a loved one to do healthy things? Reading a list of statistics never works. The sugar lover says, "My whole family ate sugar and they did OK!" Or, "I've heard of people who never smoked and they still got lung cancer." Motivation seems to wait for a painful symptom or a body change that interferes with the daily ritual.

A nagging backache is a good signal sent by the body to the brain to do something. The doctor's exam and x-ray reveal nothing, which is reassuring, but the pain remains. Pain pills help but they are only relieving the symptoms. The doctor tries to be helpful: "Stress. Take a day off occasionally. Get a back brace for the car or office." Sympathy can relieve symptoms, so we were taught. Did the doctor ever once ask what the patient is eating? Where one is getting calcium and magnesium? What is the ratio of phosphorus (meat and soft drinks) to calcium (dairy products and leafy vegetables)? Sympathy *plus* 1000 mg of calcium (and 500 mg of magnesium) will work better to relieve the pain.

Perhaps, like many of us in this decade, you are disappointed, discouraged, and depressed. You didn't get to the top in your field. The kids didn't turn out exactly the way you wanted them to. Your spouse is not exactly what you thought you married. The dollar is not worth even fifty cents. Traffic is awful. You want to sock people who tell you, "Have a good day!"

As a doctor, I have had an opportunity to see and probe a great number of lifestyles. Some people should be terribly depressed about what life has dealt them—death of close relatives, sickness, cancer, rape, financial losses—but they are reasonably sane and cheerful. Life is a great and exciting adventure to them. Others have had the silver spoon and life for them should be a breeze, but they are afraid to move because of what they are sure will happen.

These differences are largely nutritional. I believe that

distortions of reality—dysperceptions—are responsible for different lifestyles. *Anything to avoid anxiety* is the touchstone of behavior. If you believe a car might jump the sidewalk and kill you, you will be reluctant to walk outside. Talk will not change it. Reducing anxiety by psychotherapy will help, but the reduction cannot be complete unless nutrition is involved.

The anxiety that we try to avoid can be minimized by nutrition. Blood sugar fluctuations act as a stress to the brain, the pancreas, the liver, and, most importantly, the adrenals. The adrenalin secreted creates the anxious feeling. It is the *chemical* that we are trying to avoid. We drink alcohol and rationalize that we had a bad day at the office or with the children. We are really drinking to raise the blood sugar that dropped because we had a Coke and a doughnut at 3 P.M.

The anxiety and worrisome thoughts that prevent you from dropping off to sleep may be due to the adrenalin your system produced to offset the drop in blood sugar that followed the rise in blood sugar from the ice cream you ate an hour before bedtime. Your doctor does not believe that hypoglycemia can create this response, but he does believe in drugs. Rx: Valium.

Surely you have at least one symptom you would like to alter. Backache, phlegm, rash, dandruff, insomnia, hay fever, gas, drowsiness when spouse is talking, or headaches. Look them up in this book—or in other books, if they work better for you—and try the suggestions for that symptom for four weeks. (I am assuming you have had a complete checkup with your doctor recently and that he gave you the old "Well, you're not eighteen anymore.") If those suggestions produce improvement, go on to the next symptom.

We work on the theory that if the body is provided with the proper nutrition (and poisons are kept at a minimum), it will heal itself. As we get older we have to get our nutrients in more concentrated form; if we eat enough food to get them, we will get fat from the calories. And you don't have to broad-cast your intentions. If you tell everyone you are going to get healthy by eating twenty tablets of brewer's yeast every day, and all you do is get a lot of gas, your family and friends will giggle and make fun of you.

Example: Your low back pain is always nagging you. You go to the health store and get calcium and magnesium tablets. You take enough to get 1000 mg of calcium and about 500 mg of magnesium every night at bedtime. In a week your back is less painful and more limber. At the same time you notice that you fall asleep more easily and awaken more rested and cheerful. Your body odor is reduced. You tell a friend who has muscle cramps about your discovery. You are now a health nut.

Suggested nutrition for this decade:

- Three or four small meals a day.
- If you have to drink, use wine only. Two glasses maximum.
- No sugar or white flour in the house.
- Sweets limited to fruit.
- Beef only once or twice a month.
- Brewer's yeast daily or liver biweekly.
- Vitamin C, at least 1000 mg per day. Up to 10 grams a day, depending on bowel tolerance, cancer tendencies in family, and incidence of infections or allergies.
- B complex (25 to 100 mg of each), one to four times daily, depending on your stress levels and the color of your urine; if it is pale, take more. Find a supplement that includes folic acid.
- Enough bran to give you one to three easy-to-pass, mushy stools a day.
- Calcium: if a quart of milk per day does not make you sick or constipated, that's enough calcium. If you have muscle cramps or backache, you are not absorbing the

calcium from the milk. Use calcium orotate (or gluconate, lactate, or oyster shell).
- Magnesium, 500 mg.
- Vitamin A, 10,000 units; more if your skin clues indicate.
- Vitamin D, 500 units is about right.
- Vitamin E, 400 units, unless you have a problem that calls for more.
- Multipurpose mineral tablet with trace minerals including zinc, chromium, selenium, iodine, molybdenum, manganese.
- Lecithin, 1200 mg daily.

The Fifties

You are now a mature adult. You are old enough to give advice but too old to set a bad example. The kids are grown and out—or almost—and you try not to worry about them, but you do. You would like to get back to whatever it was you were having fun with when you were twenty years old and the family interrupted you. You may have even forgotten what it was. I wanted to be an actor, but I have discovered since then that I cannot remember lines. You've read enough about retirement to know that if you don't have some consuming hobby, another job, or a coveted skill, you will be a goner because there will be nothing to get out of bed for.

We are really sick of these smiley, never-complaining, perfect people who advise us from the TV talk shows that love is the answer, or being nice to one another. Or that God will do it. Sure, easy for you to say, celebrity; you're an anomaly. What about the rest of us? My wife says to me, "You, Lendon, have a wife. *I* hold you together. Who's *my* wife? Who holds *me* together?" I have no answer.

Many of us, in our tunnel-vision drive for self-aggrandizement, forget that we are social human beings and need to give along with the getting. We do a lot of things hoping for applause, self-fulfillment. Those things make us feel good.

But if you don't feel good, it's hard to be open, friendly, and giving. Hungry people are more likely to go to war or fight or steal. You are eating, but are you eating the proper foods to supply all the needs? Most North Americans get enough calories, but in the past fifty to one hundred years, the vitamins and minerals have been slowly disappearing from our food. Three meals a day is no longer the golden rule of nutrition; it is probably even hazardous to your health.

My problem in dealing with surly, glumpy people is to decide if fifty years of bad or inappropriate diet is the chief factor, or whether surly, glumpy parents have produced this misanthrope either genetically or environmentally. I am sanguine enough to assume that some brain chemicals are not being produced in sufficient quantity to allow the patient to minimize the bad in the environment and to notice some of the fun and beauty in life.

Again, what is needed is motivation. Try explaining to a cola lover that his poor sense of humor is related to soft drinks. He knows that the world and its evils are the cause. Now, I cannot deny that the world is messed up, but I can't be depressed about it *all* the time.

The difficulty in changing the diet and exercise habits of the slightly paranoid grown-up is reminiscent of the struggle we have with the negative adolescent. "Change the world, change the school; don't change me." These people have no insight into their own problem because the only part of the brain available for thought is somewhere below the neo-cortex.

I have a few contingency plans when working with the recalcitrant fifties. Sometimes they succeed. I search for a symptom or sign that the patient would be willing to get rid of. A backache, some impotency, tiredness, an allergy, or an eczematoid rash. These are insignificant deviations from "normal" that a doctor would tend to ignore, but they are clues indicating a nutritional imbalance. At age fifty or so, a good diet is almost never enough to get rid of a symptom; supplements are usually required. But because the stomach and intestines are not digesting food properly, we have no guarantee that the goodies will be absorbed if swallowed. You have to be healthy to be healthy.

I try to work around the malfunctioning intestines by giving an intravenous or intramuscular shot or two. The intravenous injection has 5 grams of C, 1 gram of calcium, ½ gram of magnesium, 1 cc of a B complex. I may put in some extra B_6, B_{12}, and folic acid if the patient is particularly depressed. It totals about 25 cc and takes ten minutes to mix and inject into the vein. The patient tastes the B complex and feels the heat of the dilated blood vessels from the calcium.

I tell them that the backache or drippy nose or tiredness should be lessened overnight, with the improvement lasting for five to sixty minutes—just enough to signal that those ingredients are good for the body. I say nothing about the surliness because there I am looking for a real difference, not a placebo effect, which is possible in any doctor-patient interaction.

If I have been accurate in reading the patient's body complaints and if I feel confident that the patient's regular doctor has ruled out the major diseases, I get improvement in 80 percent of those so treated. When I talk to them the next day, some say, "It's no good; it didn't last. I was great for about two hours this morning, but the ache and drip are back."

"Hold it right there," I say, "that's the point. If you are even temporarily improved, it means that the ingredients in that I.V. are good for your body. Your cells are crying out for those nutrients." Then, by treating the more obvious symptoms, we often get the mental attitude to improve.

Often a spouse's work is needed. "Wow, she was her old

self there for a day. She walked more spritely, she awakened more cheerfully, and her color was better. A cloud lifted for a while."

The reason most people and doctors have so little faith in nutritional support, or actual nutrition or megavitamin therapy, is that it is so slow and often the results are inconsistent because of the poor absorption via the oral route.

Vitamin B shots in the muscle are painful but endurable, and most patients will stick themselves or have a friend or spouse do it. I suggest two shots a week for three weeks. Improvement should be noted. If not, I may have missed some sneaky condition—food allergy, yeast infection, low thyroid condition, heavy-metal poisoning. These can be tested for later.

The vitamin shots, I.V. or I.M., usually are sufficient to tell the patient that his body is worth servicing, that his condition is remediable, and that he can begin to feel good about living again. Sort of like Scrooge on Christmas morning: it's never too late. The patient gains insight because his brain chemicals are starting to flow and make connections between the areas of his brain that govern how he perceives and responds. Then he becomes cheerful and optimistic because he *is* cheerful and optimistic. Friends notice and respond appropriately, and their responses reinforce his.

Prisoners of war who had a lifetime of nutrition undone by four years of malnutrition were never able to feel good again unless they took megadoses of vitamins and appropriate amounts of minerals. So it is with us too as we move past age forty to fifty years and more. At a time when the body organs need fewer calories because the metabolism needs less energy, vitamin and mineral requirements of those organs remain the same, or even rise because of the loss in efficiency in the absorptive cells that line the intestines. And, to repeat, once these cells become malfunctioning they lose some of their ability to absorb the vitamins and minerals they need to activate the enzymes that pick up the vitamins and minerals they need . . . et cetera, et cetera.

Folic acid deficiency is common. It is necessary for adequate absorption. Evidently we need folic acid to help in the absorption of folic acid. The juices should start flowing again with a few shots of the B complex plus B_{12} and folic acid. Many patients—even youthful ones—tell me that they are taking all the proper vitamins and minerals but are still feeling tired and uncomfortable. Nothing happens until they get a few shots. Then the absorptive cells begin to work and the shots are less necessary.

The point seems to be that we are all in trouble with our bodies. Actually our organs are very honest. If we abuse them in our youth, they answer back later on and remind us of our past neglect. Too much booze, sugar, and white flour all add up. These are nonfoods; their use has a negative effect in that the body actually uses up vitamins and minerals in the process of detoxifying them. If you have ever eaten an ice cream cone, or if your mother did when she was carrying you, then you are behind. And you will get *more* behind because you *are* behind and less efficient—otherwise you wouldn't have symptoms.

Try the supplements mentioned at the end of decade forty to fifty, but with more emphasis on niacinamide if you have lost your sense of humor (try 500 to 1000 mg for a few weeks); B_6 if you cannot remember dreams (50 to 200 mg should do it); vitamin C, if you are getting sick too much (up to 5 to 10 grams daily); vitamin E if you have angina or pain in the muscles with exercise (400 units, gradually increased to 800 or 1200); more bran if your stools are getting dry and firm; calcium and magnesium at the 1000- and 500-mg doses, unless you are having symptoms suggesting a calcium deficiency, in which case increase the dose or try another brand.

Before the next dinner party, eat some protein and take 1000 mg of C, a B complex, and some calcium (500 mg). You should notice that you are as bright, clever, and wakeful as the young, callow, immature brats there.

The Sixties

Just as you are getting all set to retire or buy a condominium or sell the business and sail around the world, you are hit with a heart attack, a stroke, diabetes, a cancer, hepatitis, or a car. It was your day to get it. You are still alive, recovering in the hospital. Your spouse is at your bedside offering love, encouragement, and sips of water. You feel foolish, alone, naked, angry, puzzled. This has happened to some of your friends, people "in your age group." But you thought you were doing OK; you had even taken some vitamin C. So why were you struck down? Your insurance will cover some of the cost of all this, but there goes the life savings you had set aside for the grand tour to look for your retirement home.

There is another way to look on this disaster. Perhaps it is a sign that you should change your lifestyle, the way you exercise, your eating practices, and the supplements you take—Mother Nature is telling you that your diet has been faulty. She assumes you will take the hint and change. She sometimes overreacts and teaches with some fatal disease. Warning clues suggesting the approach of one of the biggies are sometimes too subtle for the victim to perceive. Most cancer victims are taken unaware, although the actual lesion may have begun twenty years before any symptom or sign gave a whisper of trouble.

So the doctor treats you now because it is a verifiable disease that can be described and codified. He is not dealing with your vague aches and pains; he has pathology to treat. Drugs work, surgery works, x-ray works. You are on your feet now, weak and trembling, with the doctor's instructions, the bill, and some resolve to fight the problem and win.

The name of the disease helps to identify the organ system that is your particular weakness. A stroke or heart attack or diabetic gangrene would indicate that your vascular system needs attention. Countermeasures here would include weight loss, extra vitamin E, C, selenium, and lecithin, and perhaps the Pritikin program.

Pneumonia, hepatitis, sinusitis, or blood poisoning would direct the attention to the immune system. Vitamins C, A, and E, zinc, and thymus gland may all be needed.

Cancer surgery may require some special psychological programming as well as megadoses of C, A, E, and selenium.

Bones that break easily need evaluation and some effective treatment to slow the osteoporosis and the periodontal disease.

Anemia may require not just iron, but vitamin C, E, folic acid, B_{12}, and molybdenum as well.

The skin heals better with good doses of vitamin A, C, and zinc.

If thinking, mood, perception, and behavior are altered, then hair and blood tests for heavy metals might help. Large doses of B_3, B_6, B_{12}, and folic acid might straighten out that department before the victim is labeled senile or arteriosclerotic and left off at the nursing home.

It is too bad that people must get seriously sick before they do something about their health. It is too bad that doctors do not look their patients in the eye and pound some preventive measures into them. Maybe a lawsuit would help. The patient should sue the doctor for not being more insistent about losing weight. At the trial the doctor would only say, "I tried."

The patient's attorney would then respond, "Doctor, you didn't try hard enough." (Remember when you were twenty and told your mother she hadn't tried hard enough to make you stick to your piano lessons?)

At least you are alive, which means your heart is pumping blood around to the organs and you are remediable. So follow the doctor's orders, but take some supplements to enhance the body's efforts. The stress of the disease and of hospitalization has depleted the C and B-complex vitamins in your body, and you lost calcium because you were lying in bed. And if you ate a few hospital meals or got glucose I.V., you are really behind. You've lost protein also.

In addition, your devastating disease means that you have been neglecting your body for a long time, so there is some making up to do. The water-soluble vitamins C and B complex are the most quickly lost and should be taken intravenously and intramuscularly while you are still hospitalized. When you get out, I would think it wise of you to ask your doctor to OK some vitamin B complex shots at your local drugstore. When you ask for the syringes the druggist will assume you are a junkie, but you tell him you are a diabetic, or better, tell him you have a malabsorption problem and are not absorbing oral vitamins adequately.

Your doctor should monitor your progress and push you slowly, steadily, firmly into an exercise program you can live with. It will help you live. (Betty Kamen says that our lives are lengthened by the time we devote to exercise from adolescence onward.) Exercise is very boring to many people, but it makes all the organs work better because of the increased flow of blood and consequent oxygenation. Many now use the mini-trampoline. The bouncing around they get is easier than jogging on the organs and the feet, and because it's done at home, one does not get mugged and/or breathe exhaust fumes.

In this decade you may be faced with another stress: the company you have worked for has a mandatory retirement age of sixty-five, and you have mixed feelings about your life without the company or your business. Any stress depletes the body of nutrients. This depletion could trigger a depression, a sickness, a vascular collapse—something in the patient's particular area of vulnerability. The trouble is that crisis situations are so distracting, we tend to forget to take the extra nutrients we need to handle the pressure.

It is probably best for you to take all those vitamins and

minerals recommended at the end of forty to fifty. In addition, knowing your family background, your own past illnesses, and your susceptibilities, you should be taking the nutrients compatible with those conditions.

The Seventies On

People who reach their hundredth birthday always have a reason to offer for their hardiness. It may be religion, heredity, bourbon, sex, cold showers, running naked through the woods, doing pushups, eating a steak daily, being a vegetarian, sleeping with the window open (or shut), drinking eight glasses of water every day, eating the salad last, never eating sugar, always eating sugar, and/or—the most telling of all— never seeing a doctor. And who are we to argue? After a hundred years, these people are experts at knowing what is best for their bodies.

But a thread of consistency runs through all the life stories these people tell. It is that *they always wanted to get up and go to work in the morning.* Take away motivation, take away the feeling of being wanted or needed, and it is, essentially, the end of that person's life. Nutrition-oriented therapists speak as if what you eat and what you breathe and how you exercise will detemine how long you live. Those things are important, but if they are not connected to the spiritual and emotional parts of living, meaning and purpose are lost and the adventure is overshadowed by the enormity of the depression and boredom that is always waiting close by.

The game plan for longevity is to keep all the organs going at an optimal level of functioning until the end of our time span, and then have them all go at once at age 90 to 110. If you are driving a team of twelve horses and one goes down, the others are handicapped. If your liver goes because you had too much alcohol for your particular liver, your lungs or your joints don't know how to take over the 500 or more enzyme functions that are the unique job of the liver. Your mental attitude is no less important in programming the body for longevity. If you *believe* you will die at age seventy, you probably will die at age sixty-nine to seventy-one. Animals have a characteristic time span, often about 10 times the age at which puberty appears. Should we carry on until age 120? The fact that some of our brothers and sisters have made it until well over one hundred suggests that we all have the potential to live at least a little more than that "three score and ten." Careful autopsies of the very old indicate that they died of worn-out tissues; no specific disease was clearly responsible.

Young folk, the forty- to seventy-year-olds, usually succumb to cirrhosis, heart attacks, stroke, cancer, kidney failure, emphysema, or some specific organ disease that *could* have been prevented. That disease dragged the rest of the body down with it. Really quite unfair. Doctors try to replace the damaged tissue with a transplant, but transplants just don't work as well, and they are terribly expensive.

At age twenty to thirty, all our organs have a reserve capacity, perhaps 4 to 10 times the amount of tissue required to sustain life. When an organ is stressed—by pollution, climate, emotion, poor nutrition, and the aging process—its capacity to maintain the status quo, or to function up to its warranty, becomes progressively less. "As organ reserve decreases, so does the ability to restore homeostasis, and eventually, even the smallest perturbation can prevent homeostasis from being maintained."* When the pathologist cannot find the "cause of death," it usually is due to this homeostatic tilt. "We don't know" means we have limited ability to get to the basic cause. A lot of cells in one organ or in several organs just gave up. It could be that their collective nutrition was compromised to the point that cellular metabolism could not be maintained. Their tiny little lights went out.

The problem with this slow and sneaky loss of organ

* Bland, *"Aging and the Reduction of Illness."*

reserve is that detection is difficult. The bridge stays up until the last support beam is removed, then the whole thing goes with an obvious thud. We get the doctor involved at this final collapse stage, but we, the occupants of our own bodies, must be more responsible for our own maintenance. We should have known.

The advanced medical technology of our time is a patchwork mechanical exercise. It's like mopping up the floor while the faucet is running. The major breakthroughs in health care in the last hundred years have been related to sanitation, nutrition, and changes in lifestyle. Maybe we are ready to accept certain connections. I mean, those older folk who wanted to get up and go to work probably felt well enough to be able to want to get up and go to work. And wanting to get up and go to work may be a function of what was eaten the night before.

Everyone should be able to read his or her own body and—with the help of the doctor, laboratory, electrocardiogram, x-ray, dentist, chiropractor, and spouse—figure out a program to hold these tissues together in one cooperative body. Most of the following are inevitable functions of the aging process, but lifestyle and supplements may slow the rate of change: hair and skin become thinner; hair grays; "age spots" appear; tissues dehydrate and lose pliancy; muscles lose tone; cartilage is more easily damaged; joints stiffen; nerve conduction lessens; sight and hearing become less acute; general metabolism, kidney function, sexual performance, and breathing capacity lessen.

All of these symptoms and signs are related to the aging process. Our tissue juices just don't flow as well. What the gerontologists have not been able to tell us is, how much is normal? Are there some absolute limits that separate normal from abnormal kidney functions or visual acuity at age eighty? We really have very few guidelines.

Dr. Hans Kugler has done surveys concerning nutrition and lifestyles. He has come up with the disturbing statistic that a mere 3 percent of our population comes close to doing things right. The following questions are those he has found valuable in assessing one's own chances of enjoying a long and relatively disease-free life. They should be a part of the Q-and-A that every health professional puts to his clients:

1. *Do you smoke?* We all know the suicidal aspects of smoking. One pack a day cuts eight years off the lifespan; two packs a day, ten years. We must understand that smokers have a nutritional problem *and* an addiction problem. Their addiction allows them to rationalize: "I can quit anytime." "Not everyone who smokes gets cancer." Addicts can be helped with nutrition.

2. *Do you eat unadulterated foods,* fresh from the soil, low in animal fats; minimal sugar and white flour; foods high in complex carbohydrates (fruits, vegetables, whole grains); and just an adequate amount of low-fat protein? Eating properly seems to be the key to preventing or delaying the onset of degenerative diseases (q.v.). How much alcohol?

3. *Do some of your foods come from organic gardens?* The more you eat that is free of chemicals and pesticides, the better.

4. *Do you exercise at least three times a week,* strenuously enough to get your pulse up to 130 to 160 beats per minute (depending on age and training and cardiovascular status, of course)?

5. *Do you take a vitamin and mineral supplement?* None of us can get all we need from the standard three meals a day. Depending on age, genetics, stress, and absorption, some of us need more than the Recommended Daily Allowances.

6. *Do you drink and cook in purified water?* Very few water supplies in our country are free of some of the 600,000 tons of toxic waste buried around us. Chemicals in the air are

washed out to produce an acid rainfall. This acid dissolves lead and copper from pipes coming into our homes.

7. *Are you living or working in polluted air?* Choosing to smoke is bad enough, but many of us have no choice about breathing what comes out of the exhaust pipes of all those cars. Until our government takes steps to stop the noxious emissions, our options are to take extra E and C, move elsewhere, or hold our breath.

8. *Do you have stress?* A little stress makes our lives interesting, but unresolved stress is frustrating and usually leads to a psychosomatic illness.

9. *Are you financially ready for retirement?* An obvious stress if you're not. You will have to do something more than rely on the government. A job, a lover, a pet, a hobby, some interest to get you out of bed, will help.

10. *Do you take medicines?* Some prescription drugs are obviously necessary, but good nutrition and a stress-free life may preclude the need for mood elevators.

Even as children, we should start asking ourselves these questions; doctors should put them to their younger patients. Those who live past seventy usually have found what "works" for them, however, and some young whippersnapper of a doctor is not going to get them to make any big changes. Most of the elderly I see have been doing the things that Dr. Kugler suggests in his questionnaire for some time, which explains why they are over seventy and doing so well.

Research has proven what we all suspected, that nutritional adequacy early in life equates with health and well-being later in life. Nutrition and lifestyle improvements should be made in adolescence and early adulthood so that people may enter old age with fewer chronic diseases and be better prepared to withstand the onslaught of acute illness if and when it does occur.

You should have been reducing the number of calories consumed daily from age thirty years on, even if you were maintaining a consistent exercise program. The basic metabolic rate lowers slowly over the decades, and because lean muscle mass is disappearing, calories do not get burned up and fat accumulates. A person could follow the same diet and get the same amount of exercise as he did when younger but still gain weight as a result of the reduction of the basal metabolic rate. The reduction of food energy requirements from age thirty to sixty-five amounts to about 20 percent. The muscle loss is replaced with fat tissue. Muscle loss in males amounts to about one-third by age sixty-five; in females the loss can be one-half. Overfeeding after maturity increases the incidence of degenerative diseases common in later life. After age seventy, the calorie or energy requirements are reduced another 10 percent. Tough on the dessert lovers; eat a grape instead of the slice of apple pie.

In mice at least, by cutting calories (sugar and fat) to a minimum, and feeding them just enough to maintain life and growth, experimenters were able to reduce the incidence of cancer and degenerative disease to almost zero in previously susceptible animals.

Protein, vitamins, and minerals must be maintained at previous healthy levels, so the foods consumed at this time must have a high nutrient density. It is impossible to get enough B complex, folic acid, calcium, iron, zinc, and magnesium on 1400 calories a day; supplements are required. This is all the more urgent for the senior citizens who have lost their teeth and who cannot eat more than Cheerios, applesauce, cottage cheese, and white bread.

Even if elderly persons are eating well, chewing thoroughly, and watching Kugler's ten problem areas, their stomach and intestines may not know what to do with the ingested foods because of atrophic intestinal lining and insufficient enzyme and acid production. Despite oral supplementation with the B complex, folic acid, B_{12}, and iron, many of these poor absorbers need injections of these nutrients in order to prime the pump. The B vitamins are needed to help the B vitamins absorb the B vitamins that are needed to help the B vitamins absorb. I discovered that the first clue to slow intestinal absorption is nocturia—nighttime calls to empty the bladder. The fluid the poor absorber drinks during the day may not present itself to the kidneys until after midnight.

Many older people find that the dairy products they eat to satisfy their calcium needs result in obstinate constipation. Calcium and magnesium mixtures usually are absorbed better. There is no need to fear arthritis and kidney-stone formation if magnesium and B_6 accompany the calcium.

Kidney function deteriorates slowly throughout our lives, but we have so much in reserve that clinical signs become noticeable only in old age. Old kidneys do not concentrate the urine as well. Excess protein (more than just adequate amounts) might stress the kidneys to the point where they could not excrete all the urea (a breakdown product of protein). Pay attention to the BUN blood test (q.v.).

A quart and a half of water per day is about right for the elderly person, depending on ambient temperature and frequency and amount of urine. Water in soups and juices is considered part of this, as is the water in foods.

The problem of lowered organ reserve makes the connection between food and physical and mental health more crucial now than at any other time of life. A happy outlook affects the digestive juices, and what is absorbed affects the brain, and if the brain is depressed the family and the world may want to put the "old one" outside the city gates for the wolves.

Attributing mental and physical problems to "old age" is unacceptable medical practice. Various surveys have indicated that special nutritional deficiencies are involved. The elderly need fewer calories, but they may need more of certain vitamins and minerals.

Iron deficiency is common.

Vitamin A deficiency is equally omnipresent. Riboflavin and vitamin C are often below the tiny Recommended Daily Allowance. Calcium deficiency is widespread.

Loss of muscle tissue is related to the decreasing ability of the body to synthesize body proteins. The stomach lining atrophies just when we need all the acid we can get to digest the food we need to keep going. B_{12} and iron are poorly absorbed. The transit time through the intestines is slowed, leading to constipation and diverticulosis. We need more fiber just when our teeth are falling out and we cannot chew. We need more calcium just when we find out that dairy products are constipating. We have to get up to go to the bathroom in the middle of the night, but we weren't sleeping too well anyway. Some parts of our bodies are getting larger and some parts are getting smaller.

Many experts speak of a general "latent nutritional deficiency disease," an inadequate nutritional state among many of the elderly which manifests ifself as degenerative and acute disease but not as obvious nutrition-related entities (scurvy, pellagra, beri-beri, rickets).

Some experimenters believe that the immune system is responsible for the effects we call aging. If the immune system were competent, the body could handle emotional and environmental (food, air, climate) stresses without suffering cellular loss. Animal experiments bear this out. Animals fed only enough food to keep them adequately nourished lived 50 to 100 percent longer than those fed to satiety. The barely fed ones had *less* cancer and degenerative disease. Some feel that the loss of immunity to degenerative diseases is due to the atrophy of the thymus gland (big in infants). The thymus manufactures T cells, which are necessary for fighting infection. It also produces a hormone, thymosin, which somehow directs the activity of the T cells. If thymosin is given to these well-fed and susceptible animals, they achieve a long life uninterrupted by degenerative diseases.

Many diseases of humans are called autoimmune; some change in the biochemistry allows the normally protective immune cells to attack their own body parts (as in nephrosis and lupus). Vitamin E has been helpful in the management of these illnesses because it prevents peroxidation of polyunsaturated fats. (Sugar and fats are the excess calories we don't need if we are to be "just adequately fed.")

Vitamin E is said to slow the aging process by helping to maintain the integrity of the phospholipids in the cell walls, which are vulnerable to peroxidation. As the cell wall goes, so goes the cell. Control cell death and you may control rapid aging.

What to do? Let us say you are seventy years old and in reasonable health. You are 2 inches shorter than when you were twenty-five. You are 5 pounds over your perfect weight at age eighteen. Your stomach is a little paunchy, but you can suck it in when walking on the beach in a swimsuit. When lying flat on your back, a ruler resting on your ribs and your pubic bone barely grazes your navel.

Your walk is a little hunched over. You can turn your head from side to side but there is a little sound in your neck like filing your nails. The muscles in your neck and back get tight and achy if you do too much. You notice your joints more than you did ten years ago. The joints of your jaw bone pop occasionally. You have lost 30 percent of your teeth, so your bite is a little off.

Your hair is gray. You can find the TV schedule but you need glasses to read it. Road signs are a blur, so you miss a turn once in a while. Your spouse notices that your hearing is weakening; you have trouble at parties when all seem to be speaking at once, but you smile and nod, as if you got the joke.

You are noticeably short of breath but still jog a mile or two a week, and your pulse gets to 130 or 140 beats per minute. Tennis makes you sweat, and you sleep better after exercise. You are trying to eat four to five meals a day; you eat beef only once a month; you get some sugar occasionally, coffee and tea or cola three times a week; you love steamed vegetables, keep eggs to six a week (two servings of three); you aim for a rotation diet (particular foods every three or four days), but don't quite make it. Bowel movements are infrequent and pebbly if you eat cheese, loose and frequent if you gorge on nuts, raisins, and dates.

If a man, you notice your urinary stream is narrower and you are more likely to lose a few drops in your underwear. Sex is satisfactory if you can arrange for it during a nocturnal erection. If a woman, you are more relaxed about sex and even willing to initiate the foreplay that leads to the act. You need more lubricant than before.

Your skin is dry and thin in some places and oily and scaly in others; your doctor calls it senile keratosis.

Your checkups with the doctor are fine because you are in better shape than he or she is. Your blood pressure is 140–150 over 85–90. Your heart and ECG are OK, your cholesterol is 200 mg, your triglycerides 100 mg, and you're not anemic. Your BUN is 20, up a little. Your urine only concentrates to 1.020. The doctor asks if you want a flu vaccine shot and you say you'll take your chances. You are taking Dr. Carl Pfeiffer's recommendations:

- Vitamin C, 3000 mg per day, increased when ill.
- Vitamin B complex, 100 mg of each of the Bs per day.
- Brewer's yeast, 5 to 20 tablets daily.
- Safflower oil, 1 tablespoon, as salad oil.
- Calcium (orotate is best), 1000 mg at bedtime.
- Magnesium (magnesium oxide), 500 mg at bedtime.
- Zinc (gluconate), 30 mg per day.
- Vitamin A, 25,000 units per day.
- Vitamin E, 400 to 800 units per day.
- Vitamin B_{12}, 1000 mcg as injection every three to four weeks, or 100 mcg daily.
- Folic acid, 0.4 mg per day.
- Inositol, A.M. and P.M., 250 mg.
- Lecithin, A.M. and P.M., 1200 mg.

- Vitamin D, 400 units per day.
- Drink pure, copper-free water, as far as possible.

The above are just to hold you on an even course. Many of those over seventy have special needs (see below), and the nutrients have to be increased or given intramuscularly or intravenously.

Too many infections and allergies: Add more vitamin C; increase the dose until the bowels are a little loose.

Too many aches and pains, tight muscles, cramps, insomnia: Add more calcium and magnesium. Do not rise above 3000 mg of calcium per day for more than a week or so. Have your doctor give you an I.V. of calcium gluconate (1 gram); if it really helps, albeit temporarily, it suggests you have an absorption problem.

Anemia persists: Add iron with vitamin C and try folic acid and B_{12} intramuscularly. Folic acid was found to be low in aged psychiatric patients. Folate needs C to convert it to usable form. B_{12} often is present in the tissues of the elderly without being used.

Depression: B_3 up to 1000 to 3000 mg per day. B_6 (25 mg), folic acid (1 mg), and B_{12} (1 mg) in the muscle daily for three days.

Memory failing: Up the B_6 (100 to 400 mg a day) until dream recall occurs. Manganese, 5 to 20 mg, helps.

Any symptoms suggestive of lack of oxygen: Add vitamin E (careful if you have high blood pressure). Try 400 units a day for a week, then twice a day for a week, then three times a day for a week.

Poor nutrition prevents one from seeking out interests and exercise, which are the other keys to successful aging. Poor food leads to apathy and fatigue. People in this bind turn in upon themselves, become selfish and mean. If we are to enjoy life, the brain has to perceive the world as a fun, exciting place. The well-fed body and brain like to work, and they know how to rest.

PART
2

6

FIND YOURSELF (OR SKIP THIS IF YOU ARE IN PERFECT HEALTH)

FIND YOUR SYMPTOM, find your disease, find yourself.

This chapter is a dictionary of symptoms, signs, and conditions which could be the result of nutritional deficiencies. The reader is invited to find his or her own unique complaints and try to remedy them before they increase in severity, combine, and become a palpable diagnosable disease.

The more common, obvious diseases are also discussed; the nutritional supports they require are listed. (Appropriate medical references are found at the back of this book.) Doctors and health professionals should now be comfortable recommending these supplements because of their usefulness in the preventive approach, which has been documented.

Most chest pains are *not* due to heart attacks but may be the body's way of saying it needs calcium and magnesium. A runny nose and sneeze should be an indication that an allergen is nearby, but it may or may not mean that asthma is down the road. One can become tired before the laboratory shows anemia.

Listings like Bed Confinement, Diet, Dreams, Exercise, Eyes, Fasting, Female Hormones, Growth, Hair, Heart Rate, Heat, Male Hormones, Nails, Pregnancy, Reflexes, Surgery, Taste, Tongue, and Vision are obviously not diseases; read the entries if you have disorders that would fit those departments. We must be more aware of what our bodies are telling us. Every symptom is urging us to take some remedial action.

A

ABDOMINAL DISCOMFORT: Gas, Bloat, Cramps, Diarrhea, Constipation, Nausea □ Gas is Mother Nature's way of telling you that you are alive. Breast-fed babies have gas and stools with a not unpleasant, yeasty, bread-baking-in-the-oven odor, and a baby who smells good is more likely to get the cuddling he or she needs.

Babies are generally either complaining about hunger or are cramped from the distension caused by eating. Their growth needs are so great in the first few months that they must eat the equivalent of six spaghetti dinners a day to control their hunger. And they notice gas going around a corner in the abdomen more acutely than adults do.

As we age and our growth slows, we should be aware only of the emptiness of hunger and the slight distress in the lower left side (plus a rectal signal) meaning that we need to have a bowel movement. Other pains, aches, cramps, and distentions are due to food allergies, inadequate enzyme function, swallowed air, constipation, ulcers, diverticulitis, appendicitis, heart failure, kidney disease, gallbladder stones, pancreatitis, liver malfunction, and gun-shot wounds.

Some things are pretty obvious. If you get sick after eating a chocolate cake, for example, then don't eat chocolate cake. You will need the doctor's attention, however, to diagnose persistent or incapacitating abdominal distress. But if you don't have any of the biggies (ulcers, cancer, appendicitis, obstruction), the doctor may not know what to do, because he had no course in gasology in school.

Many of us complain of bloat high up in the abdomen just after a meal, which is sometimes relieved by a burp. We assume it is a reaction to the food we have just swallowed. Usually it is the air swallowed prior to the meal that gets displaced downwards (causing intestinal gas) or upwards (burp). "Everything I eat turns to gas" is wrong. It should be, "When I eat, the gas moves up or down." The volume of gas from stomach to small bowel has been measured at about 4 ounces, which doesn't seem to be much. The patient's problem may be that the gas is running through too fast; or he perceives that he has a lot of it, especially in the intestines.

In the old days when we used to fluoroscope infants, looking for the thymus, I was always amazed at how unrelated the amount of observed gas was to a baby's symptoms. Some babies were loaded and yet were content and slept through the night. Others, who might have one small dollop of air in the abdomen, complained as if they'd been stuck with a knife. Since then I have come to realize that there are sensitive, ticklish people who notice everything. They may become shy and withdrawn, or else outgoing, hyperactive, and excessively responsive. They are often low in calcium, magnesium, and the B-complex vitamins, especially B_6. Low calcium in the intestinal musculature would allow more severe cramping when the gas bubble gets sequestered (gas going sideways?). A flaccid gut would hold a large amount of gas before distension would be perceived as discomfort by the owner, but in a tense gut, a small amount of gas would be sufficient to cause a cramp.

Understanding the physiology of the cramp is important, so that it may be differentiated from a condition which has similar symptoms but is not present in the patient. Gas and pressure in the stomach may mimic a heart attack, but the distress is felt in the left chest, not under the lower end of the breastbone. The patient may panic, swallow more air, and so perpetuate the problem. Sometimes the gas is in the colon under the right rib edge, just where the gall bladder is. If an x-ray shows gallstones, the assumption is made that the stones are causing the pain, so the gall bladder is removed, but the pain recurs. New diagnosis: irritable colon. Surgery should be just about the last resort.

Hiatal hernia (a part of stomach pushing up into the chest) and peptic ulcers may produce pain high up in the abdomen just below the rib edge. Upper gastrointestinal x-rays would be the most important diagnostic test for these nasty conditions.

Dr. Dennis Burkitt has found that hiatal hernia is due to straining at stool. He has rarely seen it in those eating enough roughage, bran, and fiber, because little pushing is needed. One more Western disease. According to Dr. Burkitt, the larger the stools the people of a country produce, the smaller the hospitals needed. Small bowel movements create big problems.

The nonsurgical treatment of hiatal hernia is to drink a glass of water first thing in the morning. This is to be followed by standing erect on the toes and letting the full weight of the body drop down on the heels twenty times. The whiplash effect is supposed to slide the errant stomach back down below the diaphragm where it belongs. Weight loss helps. Coffee and alcohol are forbidden.

Gas, distention, and discomfort occurring at the end of the day or in the lower part of the abdomen suggest swallowed air and fermentation of food particles remaining in the intestines. The gaseous products of bacterial action on undigested foods account for one-third or more of the intestinal gas (one-half to two-thirds is swallowed—nitrogen and oxygen). Fermentation produces hydrogen, methane, carbon dioxide, and a few other really smelly ones. Fats become rancid, proteins become putrid, and starches are fermented. Controlling the swallowed air may be enough to make the patient comfortable.

Chewing starches until they become a soupy fluid will decrease the amount of swallowed air and also get the digestion started properly. Ptyalin from the salivary glands begins the digestion of starches, which is finished by amylase from the pancreas.

An old, dear friend of mine took his residency training in intestinal medicine at the Mayo Clinic, hoping to see some exotic, rare, and challenging diseases. People came from all over the world to the famous health center for help. He learned to say "gas" in sixteen languages. Evidently the condition—distension, flatus, bloat, belching, cramps with and without diarrhea or constipation—is universal.

Most of us have an idea about our own problems—what foods or stresses are likely to precipitate a gas attack—but few of us realize that most intestinal gas comes from swallowed air. We all take in some air just swallowing saliva. Chewing gum, sucking on a mint, smoking a cigarette, all contribute to intestinal gas. Drinking a can of pop will release about a pint of carbon dioxide. Canker sores, ill-fitting dentures, and emotions like worry, grief, tension, and excitement all increase the intake. Some people swallow air and belch but only release about one-third of that swallowed. Eating more slowly and sipping the fluids will help. Eating and talking are best done separately.

If the results are not obvious in a few days, a trial of pancreatic digestive enzymes might solve the problem and diagnose it at the same time. If the gas problem is increasing after age forty to fifty and is really getting offensive, it suggests a pancreatic gland dysfunction.

The patient who has chronic pancreatitis is usually sick enough to need a doctor's care because he is unable to digest fat and protein adequately. He will have weight loss and steatorrhea (greasy diarrhea). Special tests are necessary to measure the amount of undigested fat coming through. It is estimated that this does not occur until the digestive juices of the pancreas have been reduced by 90 percent. These people really need capsules of pancreatic enzymes. B_{12} is a common deficiency, so this would be an important adjunct—along with folic acid—to the therapy. A low-fat diet would be used. If the patient is eating well but losing weight, a serious investigation must be organized. If the stools are bulky, frequent, pale, shiny, and tend to float, the patient probably has steatorrhea (sprue) and needs the diagnostic workup. Tests for xylose tolerance, serum carotene level, and B_{12} absorption all produce abnormal results if malabsorption is occurring.

There are gradations of pancreatic insufficiency from slight to severe. Sugar has an inhibiting effect on the production of pancreatic enzymes. Do not eat sugar with a protein meal. The fructose half of sucrose (table sugar) has an inhibiting effect on the mitochondria in all cells; the work of the cells is impaired. Many people assume their gas is due to the meat in the diet. Actually it may be the ingestion of grains and fruits that prevents the complete digestion of the meat. Putrefaction sets in. Friends leave the room. If pancreatic granules work, the cause of the problem is obvious. If the gas and distress are still obvious after just a few days, a few other specific maldigestions may be occurring.

Lactase deficiency afflicts 70 to 90 percent of blacks, Indians, Orientals, and a small percentage of others. After infancy the amount of lactase produced in their intestines decreases. This digestive enzyme splits the milk sugar, lactose, into simple sugars that can be absorbed. If lactase is insufficient, bacteria will ferment the sugar, and cramps, gas, and diarrhea will appear. No deficiency is ever complete, however, so most of these people learn how many ounces of milk they can drink and how often. Fermented milks and some cheeses can be tolerated. These people have to find some way to get sufficient calcium.

Instead of being actively digested, food simply sits in the intestinal tract of a person with these malabsorption problems. There the food mass attracts an upward growth of bacteria from the lower intestines. The encroaching bacteria growth may further impede vitamin and mineral absorption. Those nutrients are necessary to manufacture enzymes to absorb nutrients to manufacture . . . and so on. You must be healthy to be healthy.

Celiac disease is a not uncommon malabsorption illness usually diagnosed in infancy when solid foods are begun. The lining cells of these children cannot tolerate a protein in gluten, which is found in most flour. These mucosal cells are injured to the point that all the small bowel is involved and all nutrients are unable to be absorbed—not just the gluten. Most of these people find as they mature that they can ingest some of the forbidden gluten intermittently. Some have found that vitamin B complex injections that include B_{12} and folic acid will almost normalize, temporarily, their digestive functions. It is important to delay the introduction of solids until the baby is over seven to nine months of age. (See Celiac Disease.)

Experts will try to diagnose the cause of the cramps, gas, and diarrhea that are severe enough to bring the patient into the office, but they don't know what to do when all the "diseases" are ruled out and both doctor and patient are still faced with the original problem. "Just live with it," or "Try this Pro-Banthine." Is the patient oversensitive? Is he a navel gazer? Many people do not realize how common—or universal—flatus is in the human. We don't talk about it, but every doctor hears about it. The amount passed per day may reach close to 2 liters, half swallowed, half manufactured by the colon bacteria. The oxygen, nitrogen, hydrogen, carbon dioxide, and methane have no odor (some of these gases are flammable; try a match). Some—less than 1 percent of the released gases—are malodorous, including hydrogen sulfide (rotten egg smell), volatile amino acids, fatty acids, and the revolting indole and skatole. Our noses can tell but machines cannot. Wives can tell, and they complain about their husbands. But husbands don't complain about their wives, or they don't care, or maybe women really do have less gas. Some people produce methane which is absorbed and exhaled. This is no problem unless it is set afire.

Because breast-fed babies have such inoffensive-smelling stools, attempts have been made to imitate the bacteria in their intestines. *Lactobacillus acidophilus* (L-acidophilus) is the predominate bacterium in breast-fed babies. Capsules with the live bacteria can be swallowed in the hope that these good bacteria will set up housekeeping. They help produce an acid stool with a buffering ability (acetic acid and acetate), and with low counts of *E. coli* and putrefactive bacteria. Enthusiastic users of L-acidophilus say that gas is less, canker sores disappear, and energy improves. It's cheap and safe, but may have to be reswallowed periodically. Those with diarrhea that is unresponsive to antibiotics often improve with L-acidophilus.

We all have bacteria, viruses, fungi, and yeasts growing in and on us. When our immunity is compromised, these nasties invade us. Antibiotics do not improve our immune systems, so we are likely to get the stupid thing again. Since antibiotics have been used for everything in the last thirty years, yeasts have been overgrowing in many of us and can produce almost any symptom. (See Yeast Infections.)

Nausea, queasiness, bloat, and a moldy smell may be the only clues that *Candida albicans* is living inside.

Sometimes specific foods are responsible. Beans, broccoli, cabbage, cauliflower, brussels sprouts, onions, garlic, turnips—anything can do anything. One of the worst is apple juice. Allergies explain gas in some people. The allergen is recognized by the intestinal lining, which secretes mucus, increases peristalsis, and pushes the undigested food down to where the bacteria can get ahold of it and turn it into gas.

If a person has had cramping all her life and her mother confirms that she was colicky, with many formula changes and use of soybean milk, it would seem logical to abandon the use of all dairy products (and even beef) for at least three weeks; it usually takes that long to be a fair test. It is amazing how many people notice that other departments of the body also improve—no more sinus trouble or popping in the ears, sleeping better without snoring, muscle cramps gone, less itchiness about the anal area, constipation gone, and headaches minimal. Milk is the most common food to cause allergies, and food allergies can cause symptoms anywhere in the body.

One of the quickest ways to find out if foods are causing the gas is to go on a four-day fast. The gas should be gone on the fourth day. When eating is resumed and gas returns, most find that the allergen causing gas is their favorite food. (See Allergies.)

Gas can back up behind constipation. Obviously the idea is to loosen the bowels with fiber foods, vitamin C, Oregon prunes, while avoiding white foods and dairy products. Humans should have an easy bowel movement one to three times a day. Lead and aluminum poisoning will make the bowel sluggish; a hair test might be helpful. Most people can find their dose of vitamin C by increasing the dose by 1000 mg per day until the stools become a little softer. That or slightly under that dose would be the daily dose. Bran, wheat germ, alfalfa tablets, should all help. (See Fiber.) B_6 seems to help cut down gas.

If protein foods seem to cause distress and bloat immediately upon swallowing or within two hours, it implies that the stomach juices, especially hydrochloric acid, are not sufficient, or that the sugar and grains in the diet are suppressing enzyme function. Betaine hydrochloride, 300 mg, with the first bite of food, should help. (May be labeled 5 grains.) A glutamic acid hydrochloride will serve as well. The dose is regulated depending on the sensation of heartburn. Two cayenne capsules five minutes before meals will help the stomach make acid. Pepsin, 30 to 130 mg, should make digestion easier. Testing for stomach acidity would seem worthwhile. Low acid secretion explains poor absorption of minerals. Some find that eating all the protein on the plate first, without fluids, will utilize acid stomach digestion most efficiently. Starchy foods should be chewed and mixed (in the mouth) with saliva until the bolus is thoroughly ground up—no pieces—then swallowed.

Pancreatic granules and papain would be helpful for the poor digestion and gas that appears two hours after a meal. For a special occasion (wedding, recital, anniversary, speech), three capsules of activated charcoal immediately after a meal and three capsules two hours later significantly reduce the "flatus events."

If the adrenal glands are hypofunctional due to stress or allergy or sugar ingestion, digestion is usually faulty. Vitamin C, pantothenic acid, B_6, vitamin A, and zinc would help. I see many patients who seem to be doing all the proper things and yet are gaseous and apparently not absorbing the foods and supplements. I give them two or three muscle injections of vitamin B complex and the change is obvious. More energy and less gas. The vitamins are needed to help the enzyme systems in the intestinal lining function. These enzymes need the vitamins (B complex, C, folic acid, and B_{12}) to function well enough to pick up the vitamins to help the enzymes . . . and so on. Folic acid deficiency interferes with synthesis of cells and the absorptive function of the bowel.

Fifty percent of infants on whole cow's milk lose blood due to microscopic bleeding. Iron deficiency can lead to fat malabsorption and steatorrhea. Food allergies, chemical ingestion, pica (eating nonfoods), consumption of sugar and processed food, all tend to hurt the lining cells of the intestines needed to absorb the nutrients needed to protect the lining cells from damage. (See also Colitis; Diverticulosis; Gallstones; Heartburn; Hemorrhoids; Ulcers.)

If you have some new abdominal symptom, you should get an examination to rule out the possibility of some nasty condition. Pinworms are a most common and usual cause of nocturnal abdominal distress and anal itching. If you live with children it is easy to get them. A standard medicine rapidly eliminates them.

If diet is the problem, you might begin by eliminating

the foods you eat daily—milk, wheat, eggs, soy, booze, chocolate, corn. It usually takes four days of abstaining to tell the difference.

Next, try either hydrochloric acid tablets or pancreatic granules.

Add vitamin C, B complex, B_{12}, folic acid, zinc, and vitamin A. It all takes about three to four weeks.

Comfrey, 225 mg; bromelain, 10 mg; papain, 97 mg; lipase, 65 mg; bile salts, 50 mg—all help digestion at different levels of the intestines. Belchers eructate less if they use ammonium chloride, pepsin, and betaine hydrochloride.

If your gas is really smelly, try the acidophilus next. Get some vitamin B complex shots with folic acid and B_{12}. Get a prescription for nystatin and stop talking while eating.

ABORTION □ Most spontaneous abortions represent Mother Nature's way of ridding the world of an abnormally formed fetus. However, a healthy, well-nourished couple can be expected to have a healthy baby growing in a healthy uterus. If an OB-GYN doctor can find nothing structural to account for a miscarriage, and if no obvious anemia or low thyroid function is present, then vitamin B complex (50 mg of each of the Bs), vitamin C (at least 1000 to 5000 mg), vitamin E (400 to 800 units), vitamin A (10,000 to 20,000 units), calcium (1000 mg), and magnesium (500 mg), all daily, would be a place to start. A high-protein diet should help prevent future miscarriages.

ACHALASIA □ Achalasia, or "failure to relax," is a term applied to the obstruction at the junction of the esophagus with the stomach. The muscles at the lower end of the esophagus fail to relax when food is swallowed. The esophagus expands, mealtime is prolonged, and regurgitation is frequent. The returned food appears the same as when swallowed. X-rays confirm the diagnosis.

Large doses of calcium and B vitamins may relax the spasm, but usually drugs are necessary.

ACHES □ The accumulation of lactic acid in the muscle is the major cause of aches following muscle strain or exertion. In a resting muscle, lactate and pyruvate exist in a standard ratio. The chemical reaction from lactate to pyruvate requires oxygen (aerobic). In heavy exercise the lactate builds because the reaction is anaerobic; the pH goes down and lactic acidosis occurs, which encourages cramps, usually accompanied by generalized fatigue.

Regular exercise to increase the aerobic efficiency will reduce the acidosis. Ingesting B-complex vitamins and correcting the diet should help. Alkaline-ash foods—vegetables, sprouted grains, fruits, and cultured milk—should be included. Any thyroid deficiency should be treated.

Muscle aches and cramps that have no relation to strain or injury usually are due to low levels of calcium in the body. We all need calcium daily, and for Americans, who are a nation of milk drinkers, this shouldn't be a problem. Yet many of us, even those who drink several glasses of milk daily, do not get enough calcium. The desire for milk in these people suggests poor calcium absorption. (A blood test usually does not reveal a low level of calcium.) A deficiency can be helped by taking 1000 mg of calcium daily together with magnesium at the 500-mg level. They are best taken at bedtime because of the sedative effect. The cramping tendency should be gone after ten days of calcium intake. (See Arthritis; Pregnancy.)

Aching in the shoulder, arm, or hand, usually at night, is a type of neuritis and frequently is solved with 100 to 300 mg of B_6 daily. (See Carpal Tunnel Syndrome.)

In an old person muscle distress, tightness, and a cramplike sensation when the muscle is used suggest the narrowing of blood vessels and oxygen deprivation. Vitamin E is very helpful. Beginning at 400 units and building up over a few days' time (400 to 600 to 800 to 1200 units) should cause the distress to disappear in seven to ten days.

Muscle aches in the back and neck that are longstanding, nonradiating (in one spot), and nontender usually are due to the collapse of vertebrae, which causes impingement on nerves and consequent muscle spasm.

Disc symptoms result when nerves coming from the spinal cord suffer pressure from material that is being pushed out from between the vertebral bones. This herniation of soft material from inside the disc means that the support structures holding the disc in place have weakened. These support structures are made of collagen. Vitamin C is needed to make collagen. If the symptoms are detected early (pain running down the leg; numbness on outside of foot made worse with coughing or straining), the use of a good diet and vitamin C might correct the problem and obviate the need for surgery. The surgery in these cases is extensive, and several of the vertebral bones must be fused to prevent a recurrence. This forever limits the flexibility of the back. A nutritional approach should be the first choice. If it is unsuccessful, it might at least prevent other discs from weakening. It will also help the patient to handle the stress of surgery.

Get a diagnosis from a doctor, orthopedic surgeon, or neurologist; the therapy may vary from aspirin to muscle relaxants to surgery. If it is a strain, a sprain, a torn ligament, or tension in the muscles, then try the doctor's recommendation for physiotherapy, but you might wait to fill the prescription he hands you and give the nutritional program some time to work.

A chiropractor or osteopath may be better skilled at diagnosing the deficiency by feeling the muscles. Some use a "therapeutic thrust" to get the spine back in alignment. If it works, but only temporarily, I have found that this means calcium is low and that the repeated spasms and constant ache will recur until enough calcium and usually magnesium are given, occasionally intravenously. Without these minerals the muscles will pull the spine out of alignment and the nerves will again be pinched.

It doesn't take long for these nutrients to work, so you will not jeopardize your health by trying nutrition first. Allow ten days for the following program. If you do not become more flexible or in less pain, be reevaluated or acquiesce to surgery. Supplementation should include calcium, 1000 mg; magnesium, 500 mg; vitamin C, 3000 to 10,000 mg (enough to soften the stools); B complex, 50 mg of each of the B's, 2 times a day; zinc, 30 mg; manganese, 5 to 10 mg; vitamin E, 400 to 800 units.

I have been amazed at how pantothenic acid, all by itself (at 100 to 500 mg per day), works for muscle strain or tense muscles. This B-complex vitamin seems to act as a cortisol precursor and to promote adrenal function. It has been reported that degenerated discs have 90 percent less manganese than normal discs.

Because the disc problem may be in the nature of an emergency, your doctor would do well to try the following I.V.: vitamin C, 5000 to 10,000 mg; calcium gluconate, 1000 mg; magnesium sulfate, 500 mg; B complex, 1 cc.

If this really helps for a day or two, then you know your dysfunction is remediable with nutrition, but that you may have an absorption problem. Vitamin B complex intramuscular shots two times a week may help the intestines work more efficiently. (See Chest Pain.)

ACHLORHYDRIA ☐ Achlorhydria is the condition of lack of hydrochloric acid in the stomach. This acid is necessary for protein digestion and to help put most minerals in a soluble and absorbable form. Most of us produce less of it after age thirty-five, and hydrochloric acid tablets would be more appropriate than antacids in most cases. (See Abdominal Discomfort; Heartburn.)

ACNE ☐ Acne is a discouraging problem to the victim, a source of merriment to those who have outgrown it, and an indication to the ignorant of how bad thoughts and sexual self-abuse can change the skin. The answer to the problem involves more than just cheering up the afflicted person or suggesting that he or she stop masturbating. When the physiology is understood, the nutritional treatment seems obvious and logical.

At or shortly after puberty the adolescent's hormones cause many changes all over the body and in the skin as well. The outer layer of skin becomes thicker and obstructs the free flow of the oils out of the follicles. Comedones (blackheads) are formed. This irritates the surrounding skin, inflammation follows (red pimple), and frequently a pustule appears (with yellow or white pus inside). The owner picks it, the pus is evacuated, the sore quiets down, but another one soon appears.

The treatment should be directed at unplugging the follicles and controlling the infection. Soap-and-water washing is not the basic treatment, since the surface accumulation of dirt has nothing to do with the acne. The impatient adolescent frequently uses an abrasive washcloth to rub the skin off and start afresh. This is dangerous and solves nothing.

The topical application of a benzol peroxide gel product helps remove the outer layers of skin faster; Cetaphil lotion is a safe application if inflammation occurs. Dermatologists are taught that food has nothing to do with acne, but many of them and all the rest of the world knows that you "eat it today and wear it tomorrow." Acne is aggravated by foods. Some believe that blood sugar fluctuation (see Hypoglycemia) will aggravate acne because the excess sugar in the diet and in the bloodstream will feed the germs that cause the infected pustules. It would seem reasonable to cut out the quick sugars, the pies, cakes, pastries, and soft drinks. Chocolate seems to be a trigger for many acne sufferers; if pimples show up on the buttocks as well as the face, it is surely a food-caused rash. Iodine in kelp and some cough syrups might be a factor. Seafood contains much iodine. If these are responsible, a month's abstinence would prove the connection.

Some adults get an acnelike rash from the B_{12} they are taking for fatigue or depression. Our old friend milk may be causing the problem because of an allergy (colic or respiratory trouble as an infant would be the clue) and also because of the progesterone in cow's milk. Stop the milk for at least a month and take another pimple count. Sexually active women may find the contraceptive pill is the cause of the eruption. If the acne occurs close to the menses, extra B_6 (pyridoxine) at about 50 to 200 mg per day will control these flare-ups. It is known that B_6 is necessary to activate the liver enzyme that metabolizes female hormones.

Decreased absorption due to low hydrochloric acid in the stomach will prevent minerals (especially zinc) from moving into the body. Many of us forget to ask the patient about bowel movements (should be easy and soft), about soap (mild and no scrubbing), and cosmetics. An infrared lamp for just a minute or two daily, along with 100 mg of niacin, are measures that may help by dilating the blood vessels and nourishing the defective skin.

If none of the above is sufficiently helpful and the dermatologist is reaching for a prescription blank to fix you up with tetracycline or erythromycin—antibiotics used to control the infection of the severe nodular type of acne—maybe you ought to say "No thanks" and try, with the doctor's support and interest, of course, the vitamin A therapy described below. Topical clindamycin appears to be a safe method of controlling the damaging secondary skin infection without upsetting the balance of bacteria-to-yeast-growth in the intestines. (See Yeast Infections.)

Water-soluble vitamin A (Aquasol A) has been used with some success with patients with tough acne (acne conglobata) and a desire to stay away from antibiotics. Many people are afraid to use high doses of A (greater than 50,000 u); like anything in excess (water, food, air), there are side effects. High doses shouldn't be taken during pregnancy, and if taken for prolonged periods by children, they can retard growth. But in comparison to antibiotics and other powerful medicines, the margin of safety with vitamins is so great that they should be used first if there is a chance of controlling a condition. The toxic effects are reversible, which is not true of many medicines. If the patient is aware and reasonably alert to the messages from his body he can simply stop the huge doses and back off to a lower controlling amount.

I have used 100,000 units of vitamin A on a number of patients with acne, hyperkeratosis, psoriasis, and warts. It works. Vitamin E at 800 units per day enhances the benefits of the A. A recent report suggested that 300,000 units of Aquasol A (water-soluble) daily for two to three months brought the acne under control. The dose was reduced as improvement was attained. The skin becomes dried out at this dose, and that response suggests the patient is on the proper dose. Apparently when the skin is dried out, the follicles do not get plugged up and comedones do not form. Vitamin A has been effective in controlling infections; its use in acne may reduce the need for the antibiotics.

There are few toxic effects when large doses of water-soluble vitamin A are given, but one must be aware of headaches, which suggest a swollen brain—a condition mimicking a brain tumor. Dry skin, hair loss, and muscle stiffness would be clues that the therapeutic dose has been exceeded; but if the skin is dry, the acne should be improving.

The new vitamin A-analogue has been recommended for treatment of the cystic type of acne. Called 13-cis retinoic acid (isotretinoin), it reduces sebum production and shrinks the sebaceous glands—thus there is less debris to plug the ducts. It has a short life in the body and is not stored as is the usual vitamin A. It can, however, raise the triglyceride level in the blood. It does sound safer, but its use should be restricted to the cystic type that often leads to scars.

Many of us have found that zinc helps the skin stay healthy. Zinc is necessary to activate the enzyme that puts protein into the skin, so it is important in any skin deterioration. Surgeons know that the burn patient will get out of the hospital in half the time if given zinc. It is probably good to give zinc with the vitamin A; they work together. Zinc therapy would be especially important if white spots are noted in the nails.

The dose of zinc is at least 50 to 100 mg of the element. Some doctors report success only at the 130- to 150-mg level. Some increase the dose of zinc sulfate until nausea sets in. That's the daily dose until control of the acne is achieved (usually after eight weeks of treatment), when the dose is cut back to 50 or 60 mg daily. Zinc in large doses may inhibit absorption of copper and cause anemia.

Dr. David Shefrin suggests dandelion root, chaparral, chickweed, yellow dock root, and alfalfa tablets as natural sources of zinc. The point of naturopathic healing is to supply the body with what it needs, and it will do the rest.

All authorities recommend the avoidance of sugar, cola, chocolate, and processed foods. We recommend large doses of vitamins and minerals because we believe that sufferers have a genetic dependency on these nutrients and because the adolescent is at his or her most vulnerable time, struggling to adjust to changes in lifestyle, diet, stress, hormone balance, and growth.

If nothing changes for the better, thyroid function may be faulty (q.v.). Some doctors try dead bacterial vaccine shots in the hope that some immunity to the invading bacteria may be built up.

ADDICTION □ Ohio has had some terrible winters lately. In 1977/78 the snow was piled up for two or three months and travel was paralyzed. Supply trucks could not get to the thousands of local stores in the blanketed area. A manager of one of these small country grocery stores told me that his patrons accepted the hardship. No one complained as he sold out the fruit, vegetables, milk, bread, and other perishables and many of the boxed foods that get replenished every four months. But when he ran out of Pepsi-Cola, his customers threatened and swore at him. "You should have thought ahead!" People can get hooked on anything. We are talking about food and drugs—not sex or night baseball. (See Allergies.)

Sugar, honey, alcohol, coffee, corn, milk—any food has the potential of setting up the addictive criteria: A craving for the substance becomes the daily reason for existing. It has first priority. Sudden withdrawal produces uncomfortable symptoms, the severity of which is determined by the strength of the addicting substance. Morphine and heroin must be the strongest, since addicts will kill to get them. But coffee must be right up there on the hard-to-get-off list. I know, because I have been on the floor getting unhooked from the brown stuff myself.

A couple of decades ago, when China was reopened to us, along came acupuncture. Because of its quite evident ability to change the body's reception of pain, neurologists searched for a reason and found that acupuncture is capable of releasing endorphins into the body. These chemicals are our own narcotic. We make them daily. When people take narcotics—heroin, morphine, codeine, methadone, cocaine—a little-understood feedback mechanism causes the body to reduce its production of endorphins. Then, when the addict quits his use of the narcotic, the body cannot manufacture endorphins rapidly enough to replace the exogenous variety. Terrible—almost unbearable—pain, cramps, feelings of misery and depression, restlessness, and sweating overwhelm the victim, strongly suggesting that he get more of the addictive substance. Crime is often needed to supply the cash to buy the fix; the motivation is really powerful.

Acupuncture is now an accepted technique to help get the addict off his junk, whether it is narcotics, alcohol, cigarettes—or cola drinks. The patient has to want to get off his addiction; that is paramount, although some have noticed less craving when they had acupuncture for some other unrelated problem.

Some use a solution of calcium, B complex, B_{12}, and a local anesthetic injected into the stomach and lung and points in the ear and at the wing of the nose. This perhaps stimulates the production of the person's own narcotic.

Drs. A. E. Stone and Irwin Libby worked out a fairly easy and inexpensive method of controlling addiction using vitamin C. Big doses are given, amounting to 40,000 to 60,000 mg, depending on the severity of the addiction. These people are so far in the nutritional hole that the huge doses of C do not cause the diarrhea usually associated with such large amounts. It is thought that the endorphins are manufactured by the adrenal glands, which store large amounts of vitamin C. Perhaps the painkilling effect of megadoses of vitamin C can be attributed to its enhancing effect on the production of endorphins.

For a few of my patients I have given the vitamins and minerals intravenously (20 grams of C, 2 ml of B-complex vitamins, 1 gram of calcium gluconate, and 0.5 grams of magnesium sulfate). The next day they report they do not need their fix. In a few days they are getting tense and anxious and another I.V. is worthwhile. Some psychotherapy and a good diet plus vitamin and mineral supplements do help.

These people really do feel better, and because they now make their own endorphins they do not need to use an outside source. But they never forget how wonderful they felt when they got the first hit. Our society must become better skilled at keeping us all feeling fairly good with diet and supplements so we won't need to try to feel better with drugs (or coffee or colas or chocolate).

ADRENAL GLAND FAILURE □ "Adrenal gland failure" is a phrase used erroneously to account for a variety of symptoms: fatigue, weakness, weight loss, somnolence. We were taught that adrenal failure meant death and was an endocrine emergency. An overwhelming infection, invasion by the tuberculosis germ, and massive hemorrhage could destroy the adrenals and their life-giving hormones. But inadequate adrenal gland secretions could explain the above symptoms and a few other problems as well, including allergies, depression, and digestive and elimination malfunctions.

The adrenal glands are called upon to produce whenever the brain perceives stress. If they cannot recover due to lack of rest or poor replacement nutrients, a disease could appear. Vitamins A, C, and B_6, as well as pantothenic acid, calcium, and zinc are needed.

AGGRESSIVE BEHAVIOR □ Antisocial, surly, mean, selfish, terrible-tempered, hyperirritable, touchy, noncompliant, unpredictable, jerk. I don't need to list more symptoms and signs for this type of person, because if you are married to one you have a few adjectives of your own. We all know people like this, especially if we do police work, social work, probation work, battered-parent counseling, or disciplinary work in school. Teachers and pediatricians who see these aggressive types when they are still children often wonder what becomes of the antisocial child. The answer is that 50 percent of antisocial children become antisocial adults. Most of the rest become alcoholics (q.v.), have mental illness, or have marital or job problems or both. About 5 percent of those naughty children grow up to be OK adults.

Because so many of these people end up in the hands of some social agency, psychiatrists have been consulted to render an opinion. In the last century it was all blamed on "bad seed" ("just like his grandfather"). Freud was able to sidetrack that unscientific notion and find evidence that these children *may* (please note, *may*) have been influenced in the first few weeks or months of life to think that they are "bad"; they developed a bad self-image. The kind of behavior described above often goes along with a bad self-image.

The classic work of Dr. T. Berry Brazelton has indicated how thoughtful and perceptive newborn babies are. A baby apparently can feel the indifference and apathy or even antipathy of its mother (and father) in those first few hours, days, and weeks of life. Those feelings can affect the behavior of a person for *all* of his or her life.

In the half-century since psychiatry made its first contributions in explaining unacceptable behavior, parents have shouldered much guilt. If anyone is to blame for the child's (and subsequent adult's) rotten behavior, it was said, then the mother must be the culprit. This stigma forced many women to leave home and seek employment so they would not be blamed ("We had a bad babysitter in those days").

In 1966 Dr. Lee Robins, a psychologist, tried to bring some order into the chaotic thinking by publishing some fascinating and revealing statistics on the follow-up of "disturbed" children. Most of the shy, withdrawn, thumb-sucking, touchy children grew up to marry and have children who seemed frightened and who had to suck, twist, or rock. But the delinquent children, as a group, had only a 50 percent chance of winding up in crime. Where the father (not the mother) had been an alcoholic or a criminal, 80 percent of *his* children ended up on the police blotter. So heredity has a role—but not the total role.

We are now confronted with a multifactorial explanation of unacceptable behavior. Many of these children do not feel good, so they act the way they feel—grouchy, surly, touchy, noncompliant, excessively shy. As small infants they had colic, were wakeful and uncuddleable; they stiff-armed their loving parents and arched away from caresses. Parents discovered that the child made them nervous or mad, and they fought back (became battering parents), or they turned their backs and indicated indifference or nonacceptance.

Many of the children in these homes grew up to have a bad self-image. A bad self-image is a prerequisite for a neurosis, a depression, a life of crime, or for an aggressive, touchy personality who all his life feels gypped and cheated. Everything must go his way.

Two types of personality must be defined further within this basically touchy, mean, and aggressive general group. One is the person who is always sour and uncooperative, has no friends, and is a surly loner. He may be a little paranoid too. As long as he is left alone, he is able to function. But he cannot be investigated or treated if he is not brought to the authorities or to a doctor.

By far the most common type is the terrible-tempered Mr. Bang, a reasonable person until he is stressed or challenged. He has mood swings; he is a child-batterer or wife-beater only if he has had three drinks; he is the Jekyll-and-Hyde with really high ups and low downs. A battered wife (or husband) may stick with and by this person because of the good days or hours that come between the aggressive, hostile explosions.

The on-again-off-again nature of the problem is the give-away clue that it is basically a nutrition-based defect. When the blood sugar drops from the overproduction of insulin following the ingestion of refined sugar or a food allergen, the part of the brain that is responsible for self-control, the neocortex, is unable to function. The circuits that say "I'm a nice person; you're a nice person" are simply nonenergized, and lower, more animal responses take over. Selfish, aggressive, antisocial attitudes predominate.

In a recently reported study of university students, the incidence of mood swings, depression, paranoia, desire to do violence or run, was *not* correlated with exercise, sleep, age, genetics, or coffee ingestion. The feelings were positively correlated with the intake of allergens, sugar, and the lack of vitamins and minerals in the diet.

Dr. José Yaryura-Tobias found that people with explosive, uncontrollable aggression loved to eat carbohydrate foods. The hostility could be turned toward themselves, but it was usually externally directed. The acts were associated with dizziness, tremor, insomnia, headaches, fatigue, and sweating. After an episode a sense of relief would appear, but in a few subjects guilt would take over. All in his study had hypoglycemia and abnormal brain waves. (See Hyperinsulinism.)

The difficulty in dealing with these people is that they have no insight into the cause and nature of their behavior. Because they are living down at their hypothalamic level they believe that someone said some "evil" thing or made some provocative gesture, so they were forced to take some appropriate action. They do not realize that their "appropriate" action was judged inappropriate by the rest of the world.

Alexander Schauss, a criminologist, quotes Dr. William Lederer, whose study of couples with marital crises revealed that in 57 percent of these cases at least one spouse had a treatable biochemical imbalance that when activated provoked negative behavior. Cerebral allergies to foods and inhalants, vitamin and mineral deficiencies, and hypoglycemic reactions caused a wide variety of symptoms: fatigue, depression, temper outbursts, headaches, anxiety, sensitivity to light, and irritability.

Those of us who live with these people are so swept away by the suddenness and strangeness of the behavior that we can't see the relationship between the diet and the animal action. They drink a beer, have a piece of pie or an egg (to which they are allergic), and the blood sugar bounces up and then down. They frequently go into acidosis or hypoglycemia and social controls are lost; the inappropriate behavior follows. As observers, we must be more alert to these changes and ask, "What did you eat and when?" When you are shouted at, mugged, raped, hijacked, or whatever nonhuman indignity you are subjected to by some fellow human, try to remember to ask, "Have you had breakfast?"

An ex-patient of mine is in prison now because he robbed a bank on an empty stomach. It is a stressful occupation. He was so nervous and shaky he accidentally shot his uncle. If he had eaten a satisfactory meal he might either not have robbed the bank because the social part of his brain would have been in control enough to say "That's not right," or he would have been so well fed that he would have pulled it off smoothly and adroitly.

Schauss has seen the relationship of diet, bad self-image, and crime. Stress and sugary meals give me a headache. Someone else would have asthma; another, diarrhea. Barbara Reed, a probation officer in Cuyahoga Falls, Ohio, knows that a prisoner who is on probation *and* on a nutritious diet rarely returns to crime. She states in her new book that *"no one who stays on the diet returns to crime"* [italics mine].

Someone has pointed out that in countries where corn consumption is high, there is a high rate of aggression. A study of murderers in the last few decades revealed that one-third were suffering from pellagra. Many of these corn eaters are not getting sufficient tryptophan, which is converted to serotonin in the brain. Serotonin has a calming effect on the emotions. A deficiency can give rise to alarming hallucinations, and these can lead to paranoia and aggressive behavior, as well as to insomnia.

Niacinamide (vitamin B_3) in large doses helps some schizophrenics. It helps the brain make serotonin, and brings the blood sugar up in twenty to thirty minutes. The dose should range from 500 to 3000 mg per day, depending on how severe the surliness is. If the iron-to-copper ratio is $1:2$ in the hair, that person is often more volatile.

Magnesium is a calming mineral and, like calcium, will calm the tense and hyperactive insomniac. (Usually calcium and magnesium are taken together.) Magnesium, in doses of 500 mg per day, is especially valuable for those who are easily aroused to anger. (See Allergies; Hypoglycemia.)

ALCOHOLISM □ People who need to drink alcohol have a biochemical need to drink alcohol and an inability to disregard that need. "One drink is too many and a thousand are not enough," the saying goes. For years psychiatrists and psychologists have tried to nail some pervasive psychopathological trait onto these people.

Some felt that the alcoholic had been deprived at the breast and was trying to make up for it by sucking on the whiskey bottle. Others felt that the dependent needs of the alcoholic had never been fulfilled in childhood and that he was acting out this frustration. Some alcoholics seemed to drink because of depression and still others drank because of anxiety. The lists of psychiatric motivations were almost as numerous as the alcoholics—now estimated at about 10 to 15 million in the United States alone.

Every study that has been done has only determined that there are numerous reasons for *starting* to drink, but most of these studies have not told us why the drinker *continues* to drink until his life is ruined. The common denominator seems to be that people who like to drink are people who drink. It's as simple as that.

Biochemical testing indicates that alcoholics have hypoglycemia. Some are hypoglycemic before they take up the bottle in earnest; these are more likely the restless, sensitive ones who find that a drink calms their anxiety. Glycogen is depleted from the liver; there are no stores of available energy except the alcohol. The blood alcohol rises and falls; the rapid fall triggers the release of adrenalin which creates a feeling of intolerable anxiety and the victim is forced to take another drink. In some the explanation is as easy as that. As the blood alcohol level rises, they feel good about themselves—usually convivial and with renewed energy. They are rewarded for drinking. The stress of the world closing in when the blood alcohol level falls reminds them to have another drink. From a delightful, energetic interlude (a good time—the response most people have with a few drinks), these biochemically vulnerable people find that drinking becomes a way of life. Even if sobered up and dry for years because of Alcoholics Anonymous intervention or substance-abuse counseling or nutritional support systems, these ex-alcoholics can never forget how good they felt when they had a drink.

The progress is often slow and sneaky. Most of those who become alcoholics start as ordinary social drinkers. But soon their unique biochemistry separates them from the majority. They begin to gulp drinks, getting a second when their peers are still nursing their first. They go on to doubles; this fools them into believing they are having the same amount as before.

Blackouts appear next. No one but the drinker suspects because the drinker acts in a perfectly normal fashion. "Where did I leave the car?" "Why am I in Kansas City?" These amnesia periods indicate the brain cortex was not functioning adequately—not enough energy to light up the memory cells. Nerve cells were put to sleep by the alcohol and the low blood sugar. Blackouts are the best clue that the drinker is on the road to alcoholism.

Loss of control follows quickly. Fewer drinks produce inebriation. He promised he would have but one drink, well, maybe two at the most, but the alcohol in the bloodstream and the falling blood sugar combine to anesthetize the brain cells that were trying to abide by the promise. The low-blood-sugar effects are the chief reason why alcoholics try to sober up by consuming candy, doughnuts, coffee with 5 tea-spoons of sugar—anything to quickly raise the blood sugar. (I met a man who said that he sobers up by drinking a cup of honey every two hours for three days.)

All employers know what "Monday morning flu" is. It is not a virus, but an attack of liver and brain exhaustion combined with hypoglycemia and manifested by weakness, headache, shakes, nausea. A couple of drinks will often cure this flu, the result of weekend bouts of drinking.

At this stage the now-confirmed alcoholic is hiding bottles about the house or car, so he will never have to face several hours of abstinence. There are arguments with his (or her) spouse about what is really happening. "I can stop any time I want" is a common self-deception. His life becomes dedicated to the central theme of where is the next drink? Drinking before breakfast is pretty much the giveaway to confirm the diagnosis. The "hair of the dog" first thing in the morning settles the queasy stomach and the shakes which are the result of the low blood sugar and withdrawal effects on the brain.

He is now a solitary drinker. That bothers him, so he drinks in the bar. He deludes himself again. He *couldn't* be an alcoholic because he is surrounded with people; he is, however, a solitary drinker who happens to be in a crowd.

Gross tremors of arms, head, and neck may follow. He loses his tolerance for the alcohol; a small amount now may produce intoxication. Brain cells have actually been destroyed by this time, and it takes little to anesthetize the remaining. Deterioration has set in. Delirium tremens, brain damage, fears, and insomnia all combine with a severe nutritional deficiency to put these people close to death unless some medical support is initiated.

Alcoholics die ten to twenty years earlier than their non-drinking peers. Pneumonia, cirrhosis, cancer, stomach ulcers, tuberculosis, brain damage, accidents, are all much more common in alcoholics, and because of their severe nutritional deficits, these illnesses are more likely fatal. Heavy smoking combined with alcoholism really makes them pushovers for illness.

Alcoholism is the most common chronic illness encountered by surgeons and may account for poor results, postoperative complications, infections, and wound disruptions. Surgeons would be well advised to deal with the well-known serious vitamin, mineral, and protein deficiencies before and during surgery. One-fourth of patients in metropolitan hospitals have alcoholism.

Police officers all know about the slaughter on the high-

PROGRESSION OF DRINKING SYMPTOMS

Social drinking
Once a week
Drinking faster than associates
Drinking more than associates } **Developmental Zone**
Drinking doubles
Memory blackouts
More drunk than associates

Loss of control
Weekends lost
Protects supply
Before breakfast } **Zone of Overt Alcoholism**
Solitary drinking
Tremors
Decreased tolerance

Delirium tremens
Vague fears
Sleeplessness } **Zone of Deterioration**
Avitaminosis
Death

ways related to the impaired perceptions of the drinker. Judgment deteriorates although driving skills are not seriously affected. Unfortunately many use the roads as a suicide tool.

Despite societal controls, our "children" are drinking earlier and earlier. One out of seven to ten high-school seniors gets drunk every weekend. Are our homes and lives so anxiety-producing or so boring that so many of us need a recreational drug as well as recreation?

When I was actively treating hyperactive children, I discovered that there was a high incidence of alcoholism, diabetes, and obesity in their families. It helped me realize the biochemical connection. Indeed, many hyper kids are hooked on sugar. I have followed enough of them to know that it is an easy step from sugar craving to alcoholism. Not all, but enough to help give away the concept that hypoglycemia is the compelling force behind alcoholism.

In a little study I did on some real skid-row alcoholics, I found a high incidence (60 to 80 percent) of the following:

1. Nordic, Irish, American Indian background; no Jews or Orientals.

2. Alcoholism in family; craved sugar as a child.

3. Blue or green eyes, brown in Indians.

4. Ticklishness as a child, hyperactivity in school, poor academic performance, discipline problems.

5. Frightened in new situations, shyness, many bodily complaints.

6. Strong need to win or achieve, never satisfied, boredom.

7. Poor self-control, temper outbursts, Jekyll and Hyde.

8. Poor self-image, often called "bad."

9. Drinking began before age sixteen; passed out a few times before age thirty; arrested because of drinking; lost job, spouse, or friend because of drinking; drank because of insomina; drank in morning to get going, and once started couldn't stop.

A study published in 1974 by Drs. Hague and Howard reported that alcoholics perceived stress differently than did a control group of nondrinkers. The alcoholic perceived more stress from changes in eating and sleeping habits and from vacations and holidays than from divorce, a death in the family, or job loss. The authors' treatment involved teaching the alcoholic new ways of looking at life's events. I see in the study the rather obvious nutrition connection.*

An alcoholic's perception of the world is that it is close,

* Hague and Howard, *Alcoholics.*

threatening, and anxiety-producing. These scary feelings disappear when the blood alcohol rises and the self-denigrating
circuits of the brain are anesthetized. A similar dysperception of the world is happening to little children who must
suck, rock, or twist their hair, who seem shy, have difficulty
in going to sleep, and love sugary foods.*

It is well established that many children have school
phobia only on days when they eat a sugary cereal and a glass
of chocolate milk for breakfast. It is equally obvious to most
observers that the 2 A.M. night terror is related to the bowl of
ice cream at bedtime. The common denominator here is the
adrenalin that makes the victim perceive his environment as
frightening. His heart pounds; he is drenched in sweat. (See
Anxiety.)

When blood sugar falls because of the high output of
insulin caused by the ingestion of quick sugar, adrenalin
pours out and mobilizes the body for flight or fight: pupils
open and ready, heart racing, sugar coming out of the liver,
palms sweating. It is these perceptions that the alcoholic
finds horrendous: feelings of anxiety and impending doom.
The drink covers them up. The blood sugar fluctuations and
the vitamin and mineral deficiencies force repetition on him.
(Valium is often used for these symptoms.)

We believe alcoholics drink because they don't feel
good. The hereditary influence manifests itself in several
ways: overproduction of insulin in response to sugar ingestion, a different way of metabolizing alcohol in the liver, and
some temperamental factor that prevents the person from
perceiving that a couple of convivial drinks are enough.

An allergy/addictive response to the food from which the
alcohol is derived may explain the craving the alcoholic
shows. Allergic reactions may act as a driving force in the
desire to drink.

The message any reader should receive from the above

* Hague and Howard, *Alcoholics.*

paragraphs is that good nutrition may help a social drinker from slipping into alcoholism, or it might slow the rate of progress, or might allow for the pickup of a fallen brother or sister. Therapists who deal with alcoholism only—and they know whereof they speak, since fully half of them have been diagnosed in that category themselves—know that the toughest part of the treatment is for the patient to accept the fact that alcohol is running his life.

Maybe if an incipient alcoholic who is reading these words can see that he is not a bad person but is only trapped by his grandparents' genes, he might be able to alter his nutrition just enough to see if this helps him control his intake.

Some background family stresses that may predispose one to alcoholism:

1. Received little guidance or supervision in accepting responsibility.

2. Rejecting, punitive, alcoholic father (gives rise to role confusion).

3. Indifferent, inconsistent (in discipline and affection) mother (gives rise to dependency conflicts).

4. Parental conflict, deviancy, or crime (parents who are inconsistent with discipline are often hypoglycemic too).

5. Some behavioral problems that would indicate a tendency to drink more than that required for conviviality; Jekyll-and-Hyde behavior, love or craving for sugar, insomnia, hyperactivity, little inhibitory control, unrestrained aggression.

If any of the following situations apply to you, it suggests a real problem: lose time from work due to drinking; drinking making your home life unhappy; financial difficulties because of drinking; ambition decreased because of drinking;

craving a drink at the same time every day; a drink needed in the morning; difficulty sleeping because of drinking; drinking to escape anxiety and worry and to aid self-confidence; panic when faced with nondrinking days; carrying bottle in purse, pocket, or glove compartment; defensive when someone asks you about your drinking.

The treatment or the control of the intake of alcohol requires a team effort. Nutrition can contribute to the abstinence by maintaining an adequate blood sugar level. Once that slips, the alcoholic needs a drink. A pretty good rule synthesized by one many times on and off the sauce: "If I don't drink, I don't get drunk."

Abstinence is the goal. Most alcoholics cannot become social drinkers again; they continue to slip back into the heavy drinking. I am hoping to catch a few social drinkers before they fall. All people who drink must remember that alcohol is a biochemical stress, and each swallow must be accompanied with B vitamins, some nourishing food, and, at least sometime that day or week, the minerals known to be lost.

Alcoholism counselors should learn that biochemical adjustments are mandatory in addition to the counseling:

1. Small amounts of protein—meat, cheese, fish, fowl, legumes, nuts, seeds—every two hours to maintain the blood sugar at a level that usually prevents the intense craving. No sugar. No white flour.

2. A good strong multivitamin and mineral supplement that has all the recommended daily requirements and is generally higher in the B-complex department, especially B_1, B_3, and B_6.

3. L-glutamine, 2 grams a day, has proven helpful.

4. Pangamic acid (B_{15}, called dimethylglycine) somehow seems almost a specific for alcoholism. Many become indif-

ferent to alcohol after three weeks of this; 50 to 100 mg a day is about right.

5. Vitamin C increased by 1000 mg daily until the stools are a little sloppy; that's the saturation dose. The dose is then cut back to a submessy dose—the daily dose. This would be increased if a disease appears.

6. Niacin—vitamin B_3—is necessary for glucose metabolism and helps prevent dips in the blood level of glucose. It helps some people handle anxiety; it seems to keep the world at a safe distance. Some cannot tolerate the flushed, hot skin that appears within a few minutes after ingestion. We suggest 100 mg per day, then increase by 100 mg daily until 1000 or 2000 mg, and even up to 5000–6000 mg is reached. If the burning skin is too much, niacinamide should be used. The high doses can be reduced after a month or two when the condition is stable and the craving minimal.

7. Magnesium is lost from the body when alcohol is ingested and can account for some of the restlessness, irritability, and insomnia that contributes to the craving. We all need about 300 to 500 mg a day, and it is usually taken with calcium at about the 800- to 1000-mg level. If taken at bedtime with vitamin C, it controls insomnia to a considerable extent.

8. Zinc is excreted in the urine in high amounts during alcohol ingestion and must be replaced; 30 mg of elemental zinc daily is about right.

9. Some therapists find that cystine, an amino acid, will help the alcoholic need less alcohol.

Exercise is an important part of the treatment for the alcoholic. It improves the circulation—and health in general—and seems to help normalize the appetite center in the hypothalamus.

Vegetable juice (2 to 4 ounces of carrot juice every hour or so) cuts the alcohol craving better than fruit juice. A cup of coffee added to 2 quarts of water as an enema has been recommended by natural therapists. Chronanthus virginicus helps the liver. Nux vomica, capsicum, and hydrostis will control some cravings for alcohol, promote the appetite, and improve digestion.

Other liver aids: cheledonium majus, chelone glabra, and podophyllum peltatum. A restorative diet should include vegetable soups, beets, steamed potatoes, boiled brown rice, brewer's yeast, and sprouted seeds and grains.

Even though a reader may not feel he is an alcoholic, if he is having a drink or two every night, then his liver needs some or all of the above. The reader should try to go without the alcohol, then see if he is miserable—that would suggest more than a craving. Habituation can slip into addiction. Almost all of us have some favorite—cola, chocolate, coffee, sugar; we are victims of our body chemistry. Booze is just a little more destructive than the others.

Remember, a good diet and vitamins are not sufficient to prevent the cirrhosis that is caused by ethyl alcohol and its breakdown product, acetaldehyde. These poisons inhibit the activation of the vitamins inside the liver cells. The nutritious diet and the vitamins are supposed to cut down the need to drink.

ALLERGIES, SENSITIVITIES, and **INTOLERANCES** □ "Allergy cannot cause everything, but may be the cause of anything." So said Dr. James Breneman at a meeting of the American College of Allergy in 1980. It really summarized what I had been suspecting after thirty years of trying to understand my patients' problems. As a pediatrician I was witness to a host of problems stemming from milk intolerance: face rashes, bottom rashes, gas, diarrhea, constipation, ear infections, croup, asthma, susceptibility to infection, insomnia, pallor, bowel bleeding, anemia; it went on and on. Even hyperactivity, surliness, noncompliance, and a few vague psychiatric problems that we had been trained to send to the psychiatrist were on the list. Bed-wetting is an extremely common problem that is supposed to be a form of aggression aimed at the mother (mother equals bed); by now, however, most pediatricians have discovered that it is the "sneezing" of a sensitized bladder. Headaches and dysperceptions (as in schizophrenia) can be traced to allergies. Hyperactivity and dyslexia can be traced to allergy. We have a rule: if you don't understand a symptom or a sign, it is probably an allergy. The reactions can initiate and imitate every psychic and physical illness known. The incidence is growing and the onset is occurring earlier and earlier in life.

What are allergies? Allergies are the "altered" responses that some bodies manifest when exposed to an antigen for the second or a subsequent time. The human immune mechanisms are supposed to protect the body from foreign substances. Apparently these protective responses are not always beneficial. The clues that indicate that an allergy is responsible for the symptoms are:

1. The cause is obscure.

2. The problem is recurrent or persistent.

3. Close family members have similar disorders.

4. The symptoms seem to be related to change of enviornment or diet.

5. The relief of symptoms follows the removal of the allergen.

The most common type of allergy is that caused by a circulating protein called IgE antibody. These are manufactured by the body when a foreign substance (antigen) gains access to the lungs, intestines, or skin; this antigen can be a pollen, mold spore, animal dander, or food. The IgE antibodies became attached to most basophil cells, and when the antigen is reintroduced, it becomes attached to the antibodies. The cell wall is disrupted and the chemicals that produce

the symptoms are released: histamine, slow-reacting substance of anaphylaxis, and an eosinophil chemotactic factor.
Antihistamines will help, but the side effects are frequently
disturbing. In asthmatic patients drugs like epinephrine and
isoproterenal tend to raise the concentration of a chemical
(cAMP) inside the cell that inhibits the release of the histamine. The search is still on to find drugs that will act to
suppress the allergy without too many side effects;
aminophyllin, theophylline, cortisone, and cromolyn often
are used in varying amounts.

Skin tests are fairly reliable for diagnosing allergies that
operate through the IgE antibodies; they are useful for most
inhalant allergies.

In evaluating the patient, a doctor may not ask enough
questions and so fail to discover some obvious environmental
factor that may be the key to the sneeze, the wheeze, or the
itch. Special attention must be paid to pets, pillows, dust,
carpeting, stuffed toys, the basement for dampness, and the
crawl space for mildew. If the allergic troubles are seasonal,
the skin tests can be confined to the pollens usually blowing
about at that time of the year.

What most doctors and some allergists fail to appreciate
is the childhood history of the patient presenting himself for
the allergic workup at age twenty, thirty, forty. These allergic
people have been allergic all their lives, but they knew they
had outgrown their childhood eczema, so why the asthma
now?

The allergic person is usually allergic all his life—and
probably developed some of the problem while in his mother's uterus. The allergy rather typically moves from one organ to another. I had a patient who had a gastrointestinal
reaction (colic) to milk as a baby, then asthma when he drank
milk at eighteen months, then bed-wetting at age seven
years, and now at twenty-six years he gets a skin rash when
he drinks too much milk.

Frequently a child will outgrow a wheat allergy that was causing gas and diarrhea and then be hit with a grass pollen allergy at age ten that makes him sneeze and rub his nose. Wheat is in the grass family, thus the connection. These people inherit the tendency to manufacture IgE, so they are susceptible all their lives. And there are more of them now, and their ranks are growing yearly. And it just might be that the obstetricians, the Dairy Council, and the pediatricians have promoted our allergic society.

If you have allergies and your mother is still alive, find out what she ate during the pregnancy with you, if she had stress at that time, and if she had symptoms suggesting an allergy. You were sharing her body and if she had an allergy or stress, her adrenals—and yours—would not have been working up to their potential.

If you have an allergic symptom now, you might have a better chance of tracing it when the prenatal and childhood history is revealed. If you had a lot of allergies as a child and you have some oddball symptoms now, there may be a connection. If you had colic as a baby and you now have sinus trouble, milk may be the villain—or wheat, or eggs, or house dust. It is possible that you are mildly allergic to a number of things and will have symptoms if you are exposed to them all at once; the allergic load is too great. This would explain a skin rash that happens only when you visit grandmother's house in the springtime. You can eat corn and pet the cat, but the soap at her house and the grass in her yard are too much.

Dr. Douglas Johnstone, pediatric allergist at the University of Rochester, has found a connection between surgery requiring an anesthetic in the under-two-year-old and the later development of hay fever, eczema, or asthma. It suggests that stress to a young body makes that body susceptible.

The most effective treatment of allergy is the discovery and removal of the allergens. A history of repeated episodes of bronchitis or pneumonia should suggest the possibility of asthma. Repeated "colds" are the giveaway clue that the victim has allergic rhinitis (hay fever). Sneezing, itching, and rubbing of the nose are minor symptoms, but their persistence indicates allergic rhinitis. Coughing at night or on exertion are common symptoms that suggest asthma. These symptoms should alert the prudent victim to do something about the pollens, molds, animals, wool, feathers, and food his body is reacting to. If the problem is allowed to continue it could become devastating.

Most adults should do a little detective work in an effort to rid themselves of irritating, debilitating symptoms. See if you can figure out if your problem is due to a food, contactant or inhalant, or whether you are suffering a vitamin or mineral deficiency. For example, muscle cramps might be due to low calcium, but a food allergy may cause the same spasm. Some people are drinking milk to get their calcium and the milk is the cause of the cramping.

Some discerning people can tell what foods will cause distress while that food is still in the mouth. Subjective sensations of "burning," "rough," "tangy," "soggy," "coated" "wet," "dry," noticed in the mouth are clues to the chewer that if the food is swallowed, gas, bloat, diarrhea, abdominal pain or anal itch will follow. Many hay fever victims notice that the watery nose is worse while chewing some food thought to be innocent.

The minimal workup the doctor should do is the history—touching on the points outlined above—and the physical examination. Pale, boggy, slightly bluish nasal mucous membranes would certainly give away the diagnosis of hay fever. If the patient states that he sneezes every fall when ragweed pollen is active, the evidence is conclusive.

Skin testing is the diagnostic tool of the allergist. But like everything else concerning the body, false tests are common. (Skin tests for foods are unreliable; the patient would do better by testing himself.)

Allergy shots to desensitize the patient would be the standard treatment. The allergy shots "immunize" the patient against the antigens to which he is allergic. The shots increase the production of immunoglobulin G (IgG), a blocking antibody that reacts with the invading antigen before this antigen can attach to the IgE and release the histamine.

If the examination and skin tests are not confirmatory, complete blood counts may reveal an illness masquerading as an allergy. A high eosinophil count in the blood would suggest allergies, but parasite infestation will produce this also. Most asthmatics can be diagnosed over the phone because of the wheeze on expiration, but a chest x-ray is mandatory because anatomical anomalies, vascular rings, or collapsed lobes could produce similar sounds. Pulmonary function tests are valuable to diagnose and to assess progress.

Most hay fever, asthma, and eczema victims have elevated IgE levels; the IgE test would be valuable to see if this is the basic problem. A high level of IgE plus positive skin tests for pollen, dust, or airborne allergens would tend to indicate that desensitizing shots would be helpful. The RAST is a blood test in which the patient's IgE is identified and made to respond to a variety of allergens. It is reasonably accurate and can direct the patient away from the allergens. This is the situation in older children and young adults. IgE-mediated asthma is less important in very young children and older adults. Under age four and over age fifty, most asthmatic attacks are triggered by infection. It appears that asthma control in the young and old might be best aimed at infection control. (See Infections.) It may also be true that the infection exhausted the child's immune system and adrenal glands to the point that the allergy could become manifest. It is felt by some that these infections (or dust, smoke, or cold air) stimulate the vagus nerve and hence cause bronchospasms which would be called asthma. These people have diminished responsiveness of beta-adrenergic receptors and are usually placed on daily doses of theophylline or ephedrine-like medicine that would control the histamine release from the sensitized mast cells.

Food Sensitivities

Some allergists believe that many food allergies can not be classified as allergies because they are not always mediated through the IgE immune system. If, however, we use the common definition of altered response, or changed host reaction, following exposure to agents that the host deems "foreign," we can certainly believe that a person has become sensitive to a food. If one gets a headache every time one eats eggs, it would suggest eggs are causing some biochemical response that produces swelling in the head.

Some allergists prefer to call these *food intolerances* if they are not mediated via the IgE immune mechanism. These are the foods that usually do *not* show positive skin reactions to the pinprick allergy testing done on the skin. (If a reaction occurs on the skin it is usually an IgE-mediated response and is more likely to respond to the allergy desensi-

FOOD ALLERGY REACTIONS

Immediate	Delayed
Not related to the quantity	Dose related
All-or-none reaction	
Immediate or within an hour	May be delayed up to 5 days
IgE-mediated	Faulty digestion and absorption
Skin tests positive (usually)	Skin tests almost never positive
Occasionally fatal	Sick, but not seriously
May have shocklike reaction	Sickness comes and goes; cyclic
Usually hits just one organ	Fatigue and malaise common
Permanently responsive	Avoidance may permit future tolerance
Antihistamine helpful	Antihistamine of no value

tizing shots. These reactions that operate through immunological mechanisms are best called hypersensitivities: a dose
of antigen in a previously immunized host will result in an
immune reaction that causes tissue damage.)

Where it begins: Only recently has the American Academy of Pediatrics made official this sensible standard feeding
rule for infants: breast-feed the baby for a year or two; begin
solid food cautiously after seven to nine months of age; no
citrus, wheat, eggs, corn until the child is over a year old.
(You might ask your mother what she did with you—your
allergies could be based on early and enthusiastic solid food
feedings.) We thought we were helping by urging solid food
down kids' reluctant throats at three weeks of age, as they
were so prone to milk anemia at one year. Then some smart
researcher found out that the infant's intestinal tract was unable to digest the food properly; a piece of protein or carbohydrate would be absorbed whole, and the body would
assume it was a foreign invader and produce antibodies
against it.

Along the intestinal tract the lining cells act as monitors
to prevent the absorption of large particles which may be
allergenic (or sensitizing). Secretory immune globulin A is
the antibody system that aids in the defense against the invaders. Infants up to age six months or so have small amounts
of this material; therefore, delay introducing solid foods until
the last part of the first year. A deficiency of this IgA could
enhance the development of food allergy. The food-absorb-
ing cells lining the intestinal lumen become swollen and
inefficient. Protein—as amino acids—is absorbed if cells are
totally normal.

These antibodies and the uncomfortable responses they
can produce when the offending food is reingested, may last
a lifetime. They could become fixed allergies. When the antigen meets the antibody, and histamine and other chemicals

are released from the sensitized lymphocytes, these are but a few of the reactions that may occur: smooth muscle contractions (stomachaches, bed-wetting), blood vessel dilation (plugged nose, headaches), mucous gland stimulation (runny nose, diarrhea), and tissue edema (puffy eyes, fullness in head and chest, leg aches).

The tension-fatigue syndrome is a common manifestation of a food allergy, most often milk. Oversensitivity and fatigue accompany creases, lines, or dark half moons in the lower eyelids. The cheeks are pale. Headaches and stomachaches are frequent.

Postnasal drip (snorting, sniffing, throat clearing, zonking) is the real giveaway that some food is causing excess phlegm. Loved ones usually go nuts listening to the noises and finally cry out, "Blow your nose!" They do, but it's back in fifteen minutes. It is called a systemic food allergy. A common related sign in food allergy is the pale swelling of the uvula (the bit of tissue hanging down from the soft palate); this appears within a few hours after the ingestion of the allergen. Milk, chocolate, corn, and wheat are the usual foods causing the tension fatigue syndrome.

With some foods—such as milk—it may take twenty-one days of abstinence to allow the symptoms to disappear. With most foods, four to five days is enough. When eliminating foods, all the related family members of that food must be stopped.

The most common allergen is cow's milk. If an infant is sickly, we stop the cow's milk and try something else. One patient would have 104° fever plus chills and backache (kidney infection) the day after drinking but one ounce of milk; no milk, no infection. If your child throws up every time he drinks milk and does not throw up when milk is withheld, it suggests that the child is at least sensitive to milk, if not allergic to it. If the doctor only asks about the incidence of the more common allergy problems (asthma, hay fever, or eczema) in the patient's family, he will easily miss the many real, albeit subtle, manifestations of the allergic response. I just had a father tell me about his daughter, who could not relax and go to sleep at a reasonable bedtime until she stopped drinking milk. We know that calcium has a calming effect, but not if one is allergic to the milk that contains it. The girl's mother loves milk and worries that without it she will turn into a gelatinous blob. Little does the mother realize that *her* chronic bronchitis is due to the same allergy to milk, just operating on a different organ system.

Sources of milk: Milk, buttermilk, ice cream, sherbet, cheese, custard, creamed soups, sauces, gravies, creamed vegetables. Use no milk in cooking. Caseinate, a milk protein, is in Pream, Coffeemate, Cremora. The small amount of milk in butter is usually safe. Processed meats and frankfurters usually contain powdered milk.

Sources of corn: Candies, Karo, canned fruits, nectars (nectars with "cane sugar" on the label are permitted to contain up to 25 percent corn syrup without it appearing on the label), jams, jellies, some peanut butter, cookies, chewing gum, icings, sweetened cereal, catsup, ice cream, beer, mayonnaise, luncheon meats, and many liquid medicines. Corn sweeteners are so much cheaper to make than the sugar from cane or beet that they are found in almost everything that tastes sweet. Most soft drinks that are sweetened are sweetened with corn sweeteners. Most products labeled as "vegetable oil" may contain corn oil. It is also in aspirin, in the glue on the back of envelopes and stamps, and is often found in toothpaste and talcums. No wonder it is such a common allergen.

Sources of soy: Lecithin, margarine, breads, meat extender, salad dressings, cereals, sauces, luncheon meats.

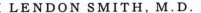
Formaldehyde may be found in milk, shampoo, soap, tea, and cosmetics.

Yeast is usually used to make vitamins. It is also present in beer and wine.

Chlorine is now in almost everything, because it is used in almost all cities' water.

Wheat is very hard to avoid. It is in gravies, soups, beer, almost all breads and crackers, luncheon meats, ice cream, and gin and whiskey.

Eggs are often found in baked goods, wine, hamburger mix, noodles, pretzels, and tartar sauce.

Tetracyline and other antibiotics are often found in chicken, eggs, beef, and seafood.

Be alert to hidden sources of allergens. Watch out for mustard; one of the spices may be monosodium glutamate. Citrus peel may be found in canned meat as a water binder. I can drink European beer but American gives me a headache; it's probably the corn or bisulfide. Green-picked apples, pears, oranges, and tomatoes are stored in ethylene, a petroleum product—a nasty allergen. "Pure chocolate" on the label sometimes means cereal, coffee, honey, and nuts are inside.

What the Patient Can Do

The best plan for the elimination of symptoms is to go on a four-day fast. Only water (distilled is best) is allowed. Most allergic people have weakness, headache, and other with-drawal symptoms on the second and third days, but the fourth brings its reward. The allergic body is rid of the allergen and the cleansed person is supposed to feel good inside and out. Then a new food is ingested daily and when symptoms return, the villains are identified. If an allergen is avoided for ninety days, usually it can be re-eaten once a week or at least no more frequently than every four days.

If one is too much of a coward to get down to just water, the following diet will eliminate the most common allergens.

Breakfast: hamburger patty or oatmeal, banana, apple, pineapple, or prunes.

Lunch: Chicken, almonds, walnuts, raisins.

Supper: Pork, fish, or lamb, rice or sweet potato, carrots and lettuce.

After a few days the allergens or sensitizing foods should be out of the system enough that the victim feels good, or at least better. One must try to differentiate between a sensitivity and a digestive overload. (See Abdominal Discomfort). Many people have gas from onions, cabbage, beans. Some have diarrhea from milk sugar (lactose) because they do not have enough of the enzyme lactase to split this milk sugar. A growing number of us have abdominal distress when yeasty things are consumed, because of an overgrowth of candida. (See Yeast Infections.) These are not allergies.

The foods we love and eat frequently are the ones to which we are usually allergic and addicted. (Orientals are often allergic to rice, and many Mexicans seem to be addicted to corn.) The American College of Allergy has stated that 80 percent of people with food allergies have hypoglycemia. Dr. William Philpott has documented this. When the blood sugar rises and then falls, the hypoglycemia condition triggers a "foraging" response for the food that will correct the low level of blood sugar. The food is eaten, the blood sugar rises,

FOODS ALLOWED ON ELIMINATION DIET

Vegetables		Fruits	
Asparagus	String beans	Apples	Grapefruit
Cauliflower	Lima beans	Blueberries	Pears
Brussels sprouts	Broccoli	Watermelon	Cranberries
Radishes	Cabbage	Plums	Canteloupe
Beets	Sauerkraut	Peaches	Dates
Celery	Lettuce	Nectarines	Cherries
Eggplant	Mushrooms	Raspberries	Apricots
Green peppers	Cucumbers	Dewberries	Blackberries
Onions	Okra	Boysenberries	Loganberries
Turnips	Carrots	Grapes	Bananas
Bean sprouts	Squash	Pineapple	Figs
Kale	Parsnips	Raisins	Persimmons
Avocados	Sweet potatoes	Blueberries	Prunes
Greens (beet,	Collards		
mustard,	Rutabaga		
spinach,			
turnip)			

the symptoms are relieved—temporarily. The hardest job I have when working with children and adults is to get them off these addicting foods. Most do not see the connection between their symptoms and the foods and hence are not motivated to try. Also, the withdrawal symptoms are difficult to ignore (fatigue, irritability, anxiety, headache, upset stomach, muscle cramps). But the appearance of these symptoms helps in making the diagnosis of the allergic-addictive condition, and the victim must realize that his diet is destroying him. He is headed for one of the great levelers: diabetes, alcoholism, arthritis, colitis, and possibly cancer. Vitamin C, B complex, and calcium will help ease the passage through the withdrawal.

I gave up coffee two years, eleven months, three weeks and six hours ago, as I found I was enjoying it so much I was drinking it from the pot. There has to be something wrong with someone who drinks coffee from the pot! The most commonly swallowed foods are the ones more likely to cause the allergies, and they are the ones we usually love: dairy products (sometimes cheese is OK but homogenized-pasteurized milk is not), eggs, soy, wheat, corn, citrus, chocolate, peanuts, cinnamon, buckwheat, food coloring, fish, and shrimp.

The lack of alkalinity in the duodenum and small bowel due to a poorly functioning pancreas not only prevents the digestive juices from working optimally but allows an acidosis to sneak in. This can be demonstrated by testing the saliva pH (acidity/alkalinity). Normal is 6.4 to 6.8. If the pH is low after a meal, acidosis is taking over, and ¼ to ½ teaspoon of sodium bicarbonate in a glass of water might be enough to balance or neutralize the problem temporarily.

If the pH is high (7.0 or more) just before a meal, it suggests that not enough stomach acid is present to digest the protein food about to be swallowed. Hydrochloric acid tablets (1 or 2) can be swallowed (not chewed) to aid the stomach in the acid digestion phase. (See Abdominal Discomfort.)

When an allergen is eaten, the blood sugar falls; the body considers it a stress and releases adrenalin from the adrenal glands. The body is assuming some tiger attack is going on outside or the blood sugar would not fall so fast, so it squirts out adrenalin to get the heart beating faster, to move the sugar out of the liver, and to enlarge the pupils to see the stress.

This rapid heartbeat gives away the fact that something eaten ten to thirty minutes before is an allergen. The rapid heartbeat—up 15 to 20 beats over the resting pulse—is the (Dr.) Coca test, which has been used for a decade as a quick and fairly consistently accurate home method of discovering food allergies (See Heart Rate).

Most of us have tried kinesiology as a quick allergy test. The theory is that if one is allergic to something—food or chemical—and that substance is in contact with the body, it will weaken that body. The patient sits comfortably in a chair with his right arm extended straight out to the side. The investigator pushes down on the arm to estimate the strength required to hold the arm up. Then the patient holds different foods in his other hand and the strength is again estimated. A weakness suggests the patient is allergic to the food being held. Try it. It may work for you.

Many people find themselves allergic to food because the body's immune system is being overloaded with a yeast infection (q.v.). Refined-carbohydrate ingestion (sugar, corn syrup, maple syrup, honey, molasses) makes the blood sugar fluctuate and requires cortisol to control. Cortisol from the adrenal glands will be dissipated in this response, so little is left to counteract histamine and the other chemicals that cause the symptoms. Many have found that without sugar, these allergies disappear. Some find that they can drink milk unless they are sleeping with the cat; too many allergens will overtax the adrenals.

Low thyroid function may be to blame (q.v.). Chemical exposure can make many susceptible to allergies. Gas heat, perfumes, pesticides, formaldehyde (in fabrics), cigarette smoke, car exhaust, preservatives, detergents, household cleaners, solvents, deodorants, furniture polish, antiseptics, mouthwashes—the list is endless. Anything can do anything. All of these can trigger inflammatory diseases such as arthritis, sinusitis, colitis, and headaches.

What the Doctor Might Do:

Most doctors are forced to deal with allergies and sensitivities; it is estimated that 60 percent of illness is directly or indirectly due to allergies. Identifying and controlling the effects of these substances has grown to become a discipline called clinical ecology.

Ecologists study the patient in his total environment. The patient's weaknesses as determined by blood and urine screening, hair analysis for minerals (q.v.), careful history of significant events in the patient's life, diet evaluation, physical examination, are all plotted and correlated with the symptoms the patient describes and his or her contact with air, water, and food-born allergens.

Because the skin tests are so unreliable in tracing these sensitivities, ecologists rely on cytotoxic (how blood cells respond to allergens) and sublingual tests in addition to the RAST. They are helpful in establishing some allergies.

Most of the workers in this field have discovered a few metabolic deficiencies in those people plagued with food allergies. They frequently have a digestion/absorption problem. The digestive enzymes (stomach acid, pepsin, trypsin, amylase, bile) may not be in sufficient quantity. Also these enzymes need the proper acidity (high in the stomach) or alkalinity (high in the small intestine) to activate them properly. If the foods are incompletely broken down before absorption, the body is more likely to perceive these food particles as invaders and produce antibodies against them. The appropriate treatment would be to provide hydrochloric acid for stomach acidity and pancreatic enzymes for small bowel digestion. This poor digestion and faulty absorption probably explains why so many restless, jerky, hyperactive children are low in calcium despite their large ingestion of dairy products.

Thus to aid the body in digesting foods, one to five proteolytic, or protein-digesting, enzyme tablets are taken about thirty minutes prior to a meal, and then one or two hydrochloric acid tablets are taken at the beginning of the meal (best to eat all the protein at the beginning of the meal to get the most out of the acid digestion). Some can tell by the way they feel; others may want to rely on the saliva pH tests before and after the meal. More pancreatic enzymes may be needed thirty minutes after the meal.

We also must remember that these lining-cell enzymes are vitamin and mineral dependent. But they need to work optimally. One must be healthy to be healthy. I have seen many patients who seem to be taking the proper supplements but everything turns to gas or hives until they get a few vitamin B complex plus C shots.

Another factor is the exposure to petroleum byproducts. These are stored in our fatty tissues awaiting detoxification and excretion by the liver. A toxic overload would produce bodily symptoms: queasiness, nausea, fatigue, insomnia, aches, pains, blurred vision, and depression.

Dr. Doris Rapp is one of the leaders in the field of sublingual testing. She has seen all the symptoms and signs that the body is able to produce when food and chemical extracts are dropped under the tongues of sensitized patients. Once the tests verify the sensitivity, the patient is given a bottle of food and chemical concentrates. The patient places the drops under the tongue when he or she is exposed to a sensitizing agent that could not be avoided. It neutralizes the allergy. I have met people who can now drive through traffic if they drop petroleum extract under their tongues ten minutes before they move out of the garage.

Any stress the body receives, whether it is psychic, allergic, physical, climatic, or infectious, will ultimately affect the adrenal glands. When the adrenals are called upon to perform, they secrete cortisol (plus other hormones from the cortex) and epinephrine (adrenalin from the central area of the adrenals). These are the body's chemicals to prepare for fight or flight. If the vitamins, minerals, and amino acids are not supplied in sufficient amounts to help rebuild these glands, a deficiency of adrenal hormones results.

The experts are not entirely sure why cortisone-like

drugs induce remission of asthma, eczema, and hay fever. Cortisone suppresses histadine dicarboxylase, the enzyme that makes histamine from its precursor. Without histamine the symptoms of allergy are minimal. Cortisone decreases the permeability of the blood vessels by restoring the integrity of the cell membranes. This reduces inflammation. It may also make cAMP work better in inhibiting histamine release.

Many allergic people have an impaired response to stress. Normally stress causes a reduction in blood sugar, which in turn causes a release of adrenalin (epinephrine). Asthmatics do not produce the normal amount of epinephrine when the blood sugar level falls.

Since cortisol and cortisone-like drugs will control asthma, hay fever, eczema, and hives, it makes theoretical sense to supply the body with the precursors of the adrenal hormones that suppress the allergic reaction.

EVEN THOUGH IgE-mediated allergies and food sensitivities use different biochemical pathways to produce the symptoms, the nutritional approach seems to minimize both conditions. If the adrenals are supported, if the intestinal tract is made to digest and absorb properly, and if the cells are well oxygenated and not damaged by pollutants, allergies should subside. Allergies are not normal; their presence tells the victim the body has been mismanaged. Don't accept your allergy. It's a signal for you to use the following:

Vitamin C: this would be increased daily by 1000 mg until one's stools are a little loose. That is the bowel tolerance dose. The daily dose is just a little less than this amount; the maintenance dose is usually between 5000 and 15,000 mg for allergic people. Then, when an infection appears or an allergy surfaces, this daily dose is taken every hour or two. Vitamin C has an antihistaminic action; a 1973 Yale study indicated that vitamin C reduced the bronchial tube spasm produced when histamine was blown into the lungs of allergic people. Vitamin C in these big doses would probably work better in those whose allergic symptoms are triggered by virus infections.

Vitamin C is stored in the adrenals, but it seems to be more of an aid in manufacturing endorphins (our own natural pain suppressant) than in manufacturing cortisol. Vitamin C is found in the brain; it may be a nutrient. It may act to suppress some of the incoming stimuli that have to be discharged down the vagus nerve, causing the asthmatic spasm.

Once a patient gets his family disease, the disease condition is sufficiently stressful to further deplete the adrenals, requiring these heroic doses to normalize the tissues. A few nights of sitting on the edge of the bed wheezing would be— or should be—a stress for anyone. And this stress hits already weakened adrenals.

Pantothenic acid, at about the 500- to 1000-mg level, is known to a cortisol precursor.

Vitamin B$_6$ is lost with stress and will help the body rebuild its adrenals (200 to 400 mg).

Calcium seems to have a counterhistaminic action. I remember when I first began to use vitamin B injections on hyperactive children. I gave a B complex shot to a restless two-year-old boy. He went home and promptly tore all the curtains off the walls, threw the cat out of the window, and stepped into the toilet. The mother called and wanted to know if this was OK. Somehow I had the feeling this was not right. I subsequently found out that this hyper response is the result of the release of histamine from the mast and basophil cells; it means that the person so stimulated is low in calcium.

Niacin will help control allergies. (Some believe that the red, itchy, hot skin that follows the ingestion of niacin is due to histamine release; maybe this gets rid of it in some way that doesn't trigger asthma.) One to 3 grams of niacin (niacinamide doesn't work as well) a day will control an allergy. If the person is eating a food to which he is allergic, he will need 6 to 12 grams to control the symptoms.

Vitamin A (from 10,000 to 30,000 units a day) and zinc (30 to 60 mg) are helpful for allergy symptoms and would be especially useful if the allergy affects the skin and mucous membranes. Vitamin E potentiates the A; vitamin D, the calcium absorption. Best to use magnesium with the D and the calcium.

Folic acid is a common deficiency in our country and helps with absorption (10 mg).

An all-purpose *trace mineral* tablet with zinc, chromium, and manganese is good to take. *Selenium*, 50 to 150 mg, may protect the cell walls.

Adrenal gland tablets, two or three a day, are supposed to help the allergic person's adrenal glands make their own cortisol.

The use of the above vitamins and minerals is safer than the standard drugs for hay fever, eczema, and asthma. Antihistamines make most people drowsy. The side effects of rapid heart, wakefulness, and elevated blood pressure from the stimulant ephedrine-like drugs often limit their effectiveness. Cortisone drugs can be lifesaving but are often used too early and for too long. Their use tends to suppress the body's own adrenals by a feedback mechanism. Prolonged use may cause stomach ulcers, psychosis, depression, moon face, and calcium depletion.

Vitamin, mineral, and diet therapy is slow but is not incompatible with allergy desensitization shots or allergy-suppressing medication. Most allergy victims find they need fewer shots and less medication as their bodies become healthier. Some are in such a nutritional hole that they need vitamin C and B muscle shots to "prime the pump," or a few I.V.'s with calcium, magnesium, B complex, and C. The vitamin shots may be necessary to activate the enzymes that are needed to digest and absorb the vitamins that are needed to digest and absorb . . .

Many allergies are more manifest from 2 A.M. to 7 A.M. Research indicates that asthmatics have their highest level of histamine at 4 A.M.; they also have the least amount of epinephrine at this time. Normal, nonallergic people have their lowest levels of cortisol at 8 P.M. and highest at 6 to 8 A.M. Since cortisol can suppress the allergy symptoms, it would seem best to take a long-acting vitamin C (1000 to 5000 mg) plus 1000 mg of calcium and some pantothenic acid at bedtime to allow uninterrupted sleep.

A case here illustrates this. Lea is a bright, vivacious, pretty twenty-two-year-old with chronic eczema. This red, itchy, thick, scaly, stubborn rash was on her neck, in front of her elbows, and behind her knees. She would awaken every night at about 3 A.M. in a pool of blood from scratching. This "itch that rashes" would be triggered by the dilation of the skin capillaries that we all experience in sleep, and possibly by the low levels of protective cortisol.

A variety of doctors, including dermatologists, had worked on her problem and had controlled it to some extent with ointments locally (including cortisone-like creams) and antihistamines orally in an attempt to break the itch-rash cycle. Her somewhat stressful job in a nightclub contributed; part of her work was cutting up the lemons and limes—like salt on a wound.

Eczema, or atopic dermatitis, becomes neurodermatitis in adulthood, because a chronic irritation will make anyone nervous. The reason her skin was involved is genetic; she has a gene or genes for this. But the reason it *occurred* is the fault of her adrenals. One clue is that cortisone creams are helpful in controlling the red, itchy skin. To help the adrenals, I injected intravenously the following:

10 ml of ascorbic acid (5 grams C)
10 ml of calcium gluconate (1 gram calcium)
1 ml of magnesium sulfate (½ gram magnesium)

1 ml of a B complex (10 to 20 mg of each of the Bs: B_1, B_2,
   B_3, B_6, pantothenic acid)
1 ml of B_{12} (1 mg of B_{12})

It all cost about a dollar, including the 30-ml syringe and needle. Pushing it in takes about ten minutes.

The calcium dilates the blood vessels throughout the body, so she felt as if she were in a hot bath. I had her lie down, since some people get a little weak and dizzy for a few moments.

She returned the next day, cheerful and ebullient. The redness had disappeared from all the rash areas. The thick, dry skin was still obvious. "I slept through the night for the first time in ten years! And I have more energy and I am calmer—all at the same time." My delight almost matched hers. Here was a therapeutic situation that combined all the goals we were trained to achieve: do no harm; relieve the symptoms; work toward a cure; use scientific principles; and remember, medicine is an *art*.

She had a rash which was responsive to cortisone. We help her make her own—in the proper amounts—and if she gets better we may get a cure rather than just a control of symptoms. I also wonder if the calcium and magnesium have a calming, sedating effect on the nervous system so that her brain receptors did not have to pay attention to the itch message at 3 A.M. It broke the itch-rash cycle. I am also sure that my confident approach when I injected the mixture helped in a psychotherapeutic way. I am more than a sugar pill.

I told her, "It has to mean that those vitamins and minerals are good for your skin, brain, and your body in general. Maybe you have an absorption problem. Maybe the little lining cells of your intestines don't perform because of a deficiency of vitamins and minerals. Those enzymes in all cells are dependent on the vitamins and minerals. The enzymes have to have those nutrients to help them digest and absorb the nutrients to help the enzymes digest and absorb, and so on. You have to be healthy to be healthy. The I.V. gets the vitamins and minerals into your system without relying on your inefficient intestines.

"Take 1000 mg of calcium, 500 mg of magnesium, increase your vitamin C by 1000 mg daily until your bowels are on the edge of sloppiness, and give yourself an intramuscular shot every other day of about 0.7 to 0.8 ml of this same complex I put in the I.V. I use Darby/Rugby #7. Eventually we can bring your tissues back up to normal function so you won't have to take such unphysiological doses."

She departed with hope and confidence. In a week she called to say her hay fever was under control but she was beginning to awaken scratching again. She came back. I did the same I.V. and she responded. The third I.V. in as many weeks *did not work*. I was crushed. Was it a new stress in her life? Had I not been using some psychic support effectively? I asked her back and did another I.V., leaving out the B_{12} entirely. The results were as dramatic as with the initial triumph. I had remembered reading about the possible rash effect that may occur from too much B_{12}. As with most things on this earth, some amounts are too little, some are too much, and some are just right. The nice thing about vitamins and minerals is that there is a wide margin of safety in contrast to drugs, which might have devastating, crippling, or lethal results if a slight deviation from the standard dose is used—or even if the *right* dose is used.

After six months of some readjustments this young lady has normal-looking skin. She takes her supplements, gives herself a crude liver shot each week, and avoids stress. She can cut up the citrus fruits in the bar without crying.

Dealing with many patients with similar psychosomatic symptoms has taught me that once the symptoms appear, they themselves set up a situation that perpetuates the stress that further fatigues the adrenals that permits more symptoms to appear that act as a further stress. This is the reason for using these massive doses to bail these people out. We, therapists and patients alike, should not be uncomfortable when using megadoses, at least at the beginning of treatment. Once the symptoms are under control and stress is somehow eliminated, doses closer to "normal" amounts usually can maintain health.

Allergists have become aware that their patients are sensitive, touchy, goosey people. Many have fair skin, light-colored hair, and blue or green eyes; they notice things too easily. Sensitive, touchy types can be calmed by the use of calcium and magnesium. These two minerals seem to make the perceptive part of the brain feel the world as less close and threatening. The key to allergic disorders is not always the increased ability to manufacture IgE. These are highly reactive people. Cold weather, virus infections, stress, and life changes tend to set them off. The treatment should include some other modality than just the chemical/nutritional approach. Biofeedback, transcendental meditation, self-hypnosis, reflexology, are all valuable. Being surrounded by supportive friends and loved ones helps everything. The world and its irritants are too close to these people. They have a poorly structured space bubble.

ALOPECIA □ Loss of hair takes several forms. It may occur in small separate patches (alopecia areata) or as a general thinning of scalp hair; in alopecia totalis all body hair drops off—pubic, axillary, facial, eyebrow, and scalp.

If the ends of the hairs that can be easily pulled from the scalp are clubbed and whitish, they are called telogen hairs or resting hairs. About fifty to a hundred of these are lost each day, pushed out at the end of a hair cycle. Women may experience a sudden increase in hair loss about three months after delivering a baby or discontinuing birth control pills. The change of hormone levels converts growing (anagen) hairs into resting (telogen) hairs. This loss is temporary.

Hypothyroidism, iron deficiency, and severe stress can change the hair-growth cycle and cause the loss.

A dermatologist should be consulted to differentiate hereditary factors from acquired factors. Some cases of alopecia areata are now thought to be a type of autoimmune systemic disease (q.v.; a group that includes thyroiditis, pernicious anemia, adrenal gland disease, vitiligo, lupus erythematosis, rheumatoid arthritis, and dermatomyositis; not necessarily associated with hair loss.) Diabetes often occurs in relatives of hair losers.

In some of these patients the immune system has failed. Something has made the body turn on itself. Its own tissue is destroyed as if it were a foreign antigen. This is why many cases of alopecia can be treated successfully with cortisone-like drugs, either injected directly into the bald spots or given orally. Most doctors are understandably nervous about the systemic use of cortisone and use this treatment only for the total type. Local injections of cortisone may bring the hair back for the areata or patchy type.

The male-pattern alopecia is considered impossible to halt or reverse, since it is the manifestation of a strong genetic factor. Some believe it is due to an excess of male sex hormones, which thicken the tissue just under the scalp and reduce circulation. Prolonged mental work and stress possibly could constrict the blood vessels of the scalp and interfere with the nutrition of the hair; digital massage of the scalp could help the circulation in this case. (Someone found out that castration before puberty will prevent baldness—a drastic treatment.)

Nutrition should not be asked to provide a solution to male-pattern baldness. Once the hair follicles are involved, thick, normal hair will never regrow. But the fact that hair will grow as a side effect of the use of some drugs suggests that research someday will find a way.

As an adjunct to whatever the dermatologist would use, the alopecia patient should understand the importance of the nutritional supports.

If diet will help, protein is the mainstay, but silicon-rich plants are also valuable. These include alfalfa, comfrey, young horsetail, common nettle, onions, kelp, oats, buckwheat, and barley.

Zinc should help the skin and hair and would be especially beneficial for those who have ever had acne, white spots in the nails, stress, frequent virus infections, or a history of allergies; 60 to 90 mg of zinc (as in zinc gluconate) might be tried for six to eight weeks and, if effective, should be continued in smaller doses (30 to 60 mg). An occasional blood test would be appropriate because the zinc intake may replace copper, which could lead to anemia.

Vitamin A should help the scalp, but one of the signs of an overdose of A is hair loss. It would be best to keep the A intake at 25,000 units daily.

Vitamin C in doses large enough to control infections might allow the body to recover sufficiently to permit hair to regrow in affected areas.

I have seen hair regrow in the seemingly hopeless alopecia totalis, but it took a course of oral cortisone to do it. Nutrition by itself is usually not enough to reverse the autoimmune mechanism that is probably responsible. But if this treatment is used, it would be smart to use the vitamins and minerals that help the adrenals (C, B_6, pantothenic acid, calcium, zinc, and A).

ALZHEIMER'S DEMENTIA □ Alzheimer's dementia is also called presenile dementia, as it usually appears before age sixty. A hair test would be appropriate for anyone, old or young, who has lost memory function and cognitive skills. Lead poisoning may produce this loss of the nerve cells from the cortex of the brain, but aluminum intoxication, syphilis, brain tumor, drug effects, low thyroid function, and kidney and liver disease must be considered.

Vitamin C, calcium, magnesium, zinc, the B complex, and a healthy diet (see Diet and Hypoglycemia) should help get rid of the aluminum and the lead. Chelation therapy has helped with heavy-metal poisoning. A chemical is injected into the bloodstream and the heavy metals bind with the drug and are harmlessly excreted through the kidneys.

Aluminum is present in pots, pans, and some antacids; it is suggested that we cook in cast-iron pots.

(See Hair Analysis, Chapter 4; see Confusion.)

ANAL FISSURE □ Anal fissure is a crack in the mucous membrane of the anal opening that extends into the skin. Bowel movements, especially if they are large, hard, and dry, make healing difficult, reopening the crack each time. Some oil (vitamin E, A-and-D ointment) or cream or softeners (like Balneol) should make the skin more pliable.

Constipation should be eliminated; any food allergies (milk, chocolate, soy, eggs, etc.) should be discovered and the allergens eliminated.

ANEMIA □ The hemoglobin test is the measure of the iron-containing protein globulin. A low count suggests an inadequate supply of iron-bearing foods in the diet, poor absorption from the intestines, or a loss of blood from the body greater than the gain. Iron-deficiency anemia is seen in children who are growing rapidly on a diet of white foods and much cow's milk. Menstruating women on a low iron or poor protein diet may get blood-loss anemia. However, intestinal allergies, ulcers, chronic illness, and cancer also will cause this, so some investigation should be launched if a leak is suspected.

Doctors will claim your test is normal if it is somewhere within the high and low levels the laboratory uses as standard. But those standards are based on a curve that represents 95 percent of the tests of "normal" people. If your level is at either extreme the figure could mean an abnormality *for your particular physiology.* Thousands of people are suffering today because their lab tests were "within the normal limits"; what is OK for one may represent disease for another.

If your tests are borderline and you do have the symptoms of anemia (pallor, breathlessness, fatigue, weakness), be sure to have cell indices done on your blood to differentiate iron-deficiency anemia (small cells) from megaloblastic anemia (large pale cells). The treatment for each type is different. The degree of saturation of your body's iron-carrying capacity and the amount of iron the body is storing are worth checking.

The treatment for the usual iron-deficiency anemia is to stop the leak, improve absorption, and add iron. Ferrous sulfate is the doctor's favorite form, but it is poorly absorbed (10 percent) and may cause distressing stomachaches and severe constipation. Ferrous gluconate or chelated iron or the iron in liver gets into the system more readily. Food sources of iron are: liver, egg yolk, lean meats, poultry, leafy green vegetables, oysters, wheat germ and whole grains, beans, and peas.

We all need about 10 to 20 mg of elemental iron daily to make up for losses. Menstruating women should be at the 20- to 30-mg level; 50 mg a day for at least two months would be a therapeutic dose for an iron-deficient person. If the hemoglobin is low, the iron stores are down also.

Iron deficiency does not show up consistently in the hair test. Systemic iron is best determined by the serum iron and the total iron-binding capacity. Blood hemoglobin levels are usually maintained at close to normal at the expense of the iron stores in the body. Iron-deficiency anemia suggests the iron stores also are depleted.

If you are really having trouble with absorption, vitamin C will boost the absorption by 200 to 300 percent. The iron in beans is absorbed better if accompanied by a little meat. You may have an anemia that requires B_6. Copper helps absorption of iron. High intake of zinc may depress copper levels and cause anemia, but low zinc diets can lead to iron-deficiency anemia. Too much iron depresses the copper levels in the body and vice versa. Heavy-metal poisoning (lead, cad-

SERUM IRON, IRON-BINDING CAPACITY AND
PERCENT OF SATURATION IN SOME CONDITIONS

	Serum Iron	IBC	% Satur.
Iron-deficiency anemia	low	high	low
Other types of anemia		low	
Pernicious anemia	high		
Chronic infections	low	low	
Hemochromatosis			
(iron intoxication)	high	low	high
Late pregnancy		high	

mium, mercury) may cause iron-deficiency anemia; a hair test may be helpful.

Although folic acid and B_{12} deficiency are associated with pernicious anemia, they both have a hand in putting the red blood cells together, and these two B vitamins might help. The B_{12} converts methyl folate into folate, which is needed for DNA and cellular manufacture. The macrocytosis of red blood cells appears similar in B_{12} and folate deficiencies, but only the B_{12} deficiency produces the central nervous system changes. Vegan vegetarians do not get B_{12}; vegetarians require double the iron intake because of the low availability of iron from their diet. Phytates and oxalates in the diet bind some of the iron ingested, cutting down on absorption. Vitamin E helps the body make hemoglobin. Manganese may be low in those with a macrocytic anemia.

Tests for determining the cause of the anemia:

Serum: B_{12}
Folic acid
Iron
Iron-binding capacity
Bilirubin

Whole blood: Hemoglobin fractionation
Carboxyhemoglobin

Red Cell Enzymes: Glucose-6-phosphate dehydrogenase

ANOREXIA ☐ Loss of appetite is associated with those noncompliant two- to four-year-olds who eat but six peas a day. They gain only two pounds a year, so they need in a year what they ate in a month as little infants. Many adults, too, eat what seem to be small amounts, really insufficient or inadequate nutrition, but seem to survive and even to be quite healthy. Some people have a better absorptive lining in their intestines or more efficient enzyme systems that handle the work of the body.

The appetite mechanism in the brain responds to low blood sugar, empty-stomach clues, visual and olfactory sensations, and even time of day. We expect appetite loss with fever, flu, infections, emotional crises, and physical trauma. If anorexia appears for no good reason, some nasty disease or condition must be considered and searched for. Cancer, hypothyroidism, tuberculosis, anemia, stroke, high blood pressure, kidney failure, and depression are but a few serious illnesses that may begin with anorexia as the only revealing clue. The fifty-year-old who always cleans his plate may begin to feel full when only half finished. He may have suffered a slight heart attack or a minor stroke in the past week. (But it may be a normal response to the lessened need for calories that occurs with aging. Despite an exercise program, if the same amount of food is consumed at age fifty to sixty as was eaten at age twenty to thirty, obesity is likely.)

Intestinal enzyme deficiencies, anemia from any cause, low zinc levels, loss of sufficient stomach acid, and food allergies will all contribute to appetite loss. The culprit may be milk or wheat or eggs or beef or corn or whatever turns to bloat right away, suggesting the next bite might be returned. The four-day fast would reveal the cause of the problem and suggest what to avoid. If the fast is not helpful, and especially if there is a weight loss, a diagnostic effort should reveal the true nature of the symptoms. (See Abdominal Discomfort; Allergies.)

If the doctor's examination reveals nothing, most people will try the B complex (50 mg of each of the Bs) two or three times a day for a ten-day period. Vitamin B_1 (thiamin) has the most dependable action on the appetite, as it nourishes hypothalamic cells related to appetite increase. Biotin helps normalize gastrointestinal motility. Iron tonic could be hazardous over a long period of time if there is no laboratory evidence of its need (that is, hemoglobin, hematrocrit, and iron stores are adequate).

Zinc, 30 to 60 mg, might be tried next; it is good for finicky eaters. If nothing happens in ten days, another review of the history, physical examination, and laboratory reports could be in order, especially if the loss of appetite is associated with gas, bloat, diarrhea, low-grade fever, subnormal temperature (see Thyroid Problems), or odd odors. Some people have a yeast overgrowth in the intestines (see Yeast Infections) and just feel dumpy; the most common symptoms are fatigue and loss of memory.

Some find magnesium helpful. Copper will improve the appetite if it can be shown (hair test) that it is low in the body; usually we get more than enough. A potassium deficiency has been shown to lower the appetite; fruits and vegetables should handle this. Any diuretic may have to be discontinued.

L-histidine combines with zinc in the serum where it is bound to albumin; it is then lost in the urine. Large amounts of L-histidine will cause anorexia (8 grams a day!); if zinc is given, the appetite returns. Many people will adjust their food intake by finding a balance between L-histidine and zinc.

Often, people who have fasted feel so good when they have been off their allergen for four days that they forget to eat anything. They do not realize that the uncomfortable feelings (fatigue, bloat, headache, insomnia) they have when they eat are due only to the ingestion of one or two foods. They may slip into the category of the *anorexia nervosa.*

Anorexia nervosa is assumed to be a psychiatric response that many young women use to shield themselves from the perils and responsibilities of maturity. It usually shows in a previously healthy and well-adjusted female who discovers at age eleven to fifteen or so that she is becoming a woman. She announces that she is fat (she isn't) and launches on a two-peanut-and-one-lettuce-leaf diet. In a few months she is skin and bones, but she still feels that she is fat. She obviously has a dysperception.

She does accomplish her escape from mature womanhood, as her fat stores (breasts and hips) are gone and her menses stop. Apparently, when body fat is reduced below a certain critical level, a control mechanism tells the hypothalamus and pituitary to tell the ovaries to stop ovulating.

Whatever the motivation is to fast—whether an overzealous weight loss program in an obese person, a psychiatric denial of maturity, a sense of wellness when fasting, or loss of the sense of taste due to a zinc or iron deficiency—all fasters eventually lose enough vitamins and minerals to produce secondary symptoms that make the individual unable or unwilling to break the fast.

The brain reaches a point where reality is distorted ("I am too fat," says the 80-pound sixteen-year-old). The taste buds without zinc may tell the brain that this food in the mouth tastes like feces. The thyroid, in response to wasted tissue, slows production in order to conserve what is left. The intestinal lining atrophies, so if food is presented it fails to provide the enzymes necessary for digestion. Everything shuts down; there is slowed peripheral circulation; the appearance of soft, fine body hair; restlessness. Many will become grossly hungry, will eat and then vomit or take a purge. Low blood potassium and dehydration may occur. Many take thyroid and/or amphetamines to lose weight. It is serious; without intervention these people will die.

No matter what type of doctor is in charge of the general care of the anorectic, attention to nutrition is basic. They must be fed. An I.V. with B-complex vitamins and calcium and magnesium would be a start. Sometimes *this* works:

"You must gain four pounds a week or we will tube-feed you."

Psychiatry or insight therapy cannot work if the receptive part of the brain is not nourished.

Anorexia is a symptom of a disease; the primary diagnosis may be depression, schizophrenia, or some organic illness. Treating just the symptom will rarely cure the patient. Hilda Bruch, an obesity expert, feels that anorectics and the obese share common convictions: self-loathing and an inability to estimate their body size. (Many obese people will overdo the weight-loss diet as if they had lost some cerebral control mechanism.) Treatment centers can help these people gain a realistic self-appraisal and become less dependent on manipulating body size through misuse of the eating function.

(See Diet.)

ANXIETY □ Anxiety is the subjective sense that something awful is about to happen. One can appreciate the appropriateness of the emotion when it is connected with a stressful event (being in an earthquake or traffic accident, almost drowning, going into surgery for cancer, asking the boss for a raise); it's logical. The body has perceived a threat to the status quo. The cortex tells the pituitary, which tells the adrenals to pump out cortisol. Nerve stimulation gets the adrenals to excrete adrenalin. The adrenalin makes the pupils enlarge (to see the problem better?), the heart to race (to run or fight better), the stomach and intestines to stop working (energy needed elsewhere), the palms to sweat (better grasp on the weapon?), and the hair on the neck to stand up (so the animal looks more formidable).

But if all these symptoms of impending doom are frequently present, and for no good reason except that the phone rang or you have to get some groceries or you have to write a check, then it is called free-floating anxiety. These are inappropriate sensations and are considered a clue that some neurosis is present. It could help to have a psychotherapist dig about in one's psyche, find the deeply buried conflict, and help to resolve or defuse it.

A doctor can prescribe a tranquilizer (Valium), a sedative (phenobarbital), or a beta-adrenergic blocker (Inderal), so the patient does not notice the symptoms. People on these drugs must remember that they are only treating the symptoms; the *reason* for the symptoms is still present.

The adrenalin could be flowing from a drop in the blood sugar, from quick carbohydrate ingestion, or from a food allergy (q.v.). Many have anxiety because they are low in calcium. Niacin or niacinamide (vitamin B_3) has an antianxiety effect similar to Valium but must be used at the level of 1000 to 4000 mg. B_3 does not get to the brain easily, so these large doses are needed. Some will put a 100- or 200-mg tablet on the back of their tongue when they feel the anxiety of hypoglycemia coming on; this seems to abort the attack. Magnesium has a calming effect. Vitamins B_6 and B_1 are well known for helping the world move back a step or two.

Many hypoglycemics who have anxiety as their chief complaint find that nibbling on good foods—protein and complex carbohydrates—and avoiding sugar and junk in general are all they need to do to control this wasteful condition. One of the most common episodes of inappropriate anxiety occurs between midnight and 4 A.M. The victim, child or adult, awakens suddenly, crying out with all the clues that indicate an adrenalin release: rapid heartbeat, big pupils, sweating. The psychiatrist would say "anxiety"; we would say "adrenalin release" due to falling blood sugar caused by the ingestion of something, say, ice cream (20 percent sugar), at bedtime. Instead of a tranquilizer, a diet change usually solves the problem the first night.

Now that I understand how and why the body releases adrenalin, it is easy for me to see why many psychiatric conditions become established in the first place. Many children develop school phobia because they happen to be entering the building at the precise moment that the adrenalin hits them. And, of course, the adrenalin is pouring out because the blood sugar is falling because these kids overproduce insulin when they eat sugary cereal and chocolate milk for breakfast. They associate this feeling of dread with school. They assume the *school* did it, not the breakfast. They have learned that school is the enemy. Logical persuasion does not work. Even with better breakfasts and an intuitive counselor who may have made the connection, it takes weeks to show them they will not die if they return to school.

Adults are frequent victims of this angst. When they are calm they can be given insight into this connection, enough perhaps to make them accept the need for change. The close connection of psyche and soma was suggested by a study a few years ago, which indicated that women had much greater anxiety a year after a bout of mononucleosis than they had had before their illness. Their nutrition may have been faulty before the sickness, and that could explain why they got sick. The sickness further depleted their ability to cope.

The therapy, of course, is to eliminate sugar-bearing foods or allergens, to nibble on foods that provide long-term energy (seeds, nuts, protein, complex carbohydrates), and to add B complex and vitamin C. (See Hypoglycemia.)

B_1, thiamin, is helpful for stress that could lead to anxiety. Choline helps. Many take inositol for anxiety. Calcium keeps me from noticing the world.

What a psychiatrist would label as an anxiety neurosis has one or all of the following symptoms: hypersensitive skin, hyperactivity, depression, apprehension, fatigue, headache, and insomnia. All of these can be relieved by Valium, but that just treats the symptoms. The symptoms are the body's response to biochemical changes. Find out why the chemicals are unbalanced.

APATHY □ A most obvious case of apathy was displayed to me some years ago when I walked into one of my examining rooms to find a six-week-old baby trying to focus on the ceiling tiles and waving his arms as if trying to get someone's attention, while his mother sat on a bench out of his sight staring into space.

No normal adult can *not* pay attention to a little baby who is trying to communicate. I wanted to scold the woman, but I realized she was sick. She had postpartum depression; eventually she recovered nicely. But what a good way to diagnose an adult who is depressed, sick, apathetic, withdrawn, or schizoid! Just get the adult and a one- to three-month-old baby together; if they do not start smiling, cooing, and giggling there is something wrong with them both.

Sometimes it is difficult to decide if depression follows apathy or whether apathy is already mild depression (q.v.). If the apathetic one is neglectful and unclean (dishes piled up, things not picked up, not bathing or brushing teeth, dirty nails, smelly, unshaven), a few shots of B_{12} (1000 mcg) are almost specific.

Lassitude ("I don't care") and reluctance to move are the first signs of scurvy, but they also suggest someone was indifferent (or apathetic?) about what was eaten. If little hemmorrhages show up at the hair follicles, that *is* scurvy and it requires immediate treatment! Low thyroid function will make anyone apathetic, but there would be other clues as well if that were the case. (See Anemia; Thyroid Problems.)

For some reason, magnesium, which sparks a large number of enzyme systems, is often low in the apathetic, indifferent ones. Manganese and zinc are also helpful. Protein may be low in the bloodstream after an infection or stress; a high-protein diet may help. Not just anemia, but iron deficiency, too, may cause apathy, because the cells are not being nourished properly.

One therapist suggests that "mental blunting" usually responds to shots of folic acid and B_{12}. These are the two B vitamins that are most effective as a first choice when someone becomes "withdrawn," which may be the first step before "indifference." It is difficult for a doctor to diagnose the condition. A flattened affect (expressionless face) is a sign of depression. A slowed pace and drooping shoulders may indicate to a spouse that something is happening. Admonitions, "Cheer up!" and "Have a happy day!" just make it worse. The trick is to read someone's body and detect the early signs before a full-blown depression is established.

With no good environmental reason to explain the apathy, one must assume that a chemical is not being produced in the brain. Enzymes make the chemicals, and the B vitamins act as coenzymes. Boredom leads to apathy; apathy leads to a poor appetite. Poor appetite leads to poor nourishment and inadequate vitamin and mineral intake, which leads us back to apathy and boredom. If one becomes apathetic, old friends tend to drift away. Good nutrition, therefore, leads to sociability.

ARTHRITIS □ Arthritis seems to manifest itself in unique ways depending on the individual with the sore joint. When I am stressed the last joint of the little finger of my left hand becomes sore and tender. Usually I've missed sleep or had too many things to do. I take some extra C, B complex, and extra dolomite, and in two days it's gone. Aspirin works also, but the pain keeps coming back every three to four hours until I do my vitamin and mineral routine.

I give a lot of vitamin B complex shots to the tired, the depressed, the touchy, the achy, and they tell me that their arthritis (or joint pain) also is less or is gone. Either I am making them feel better and they don't care about or notice the joints, or—and I would prefer this explanation—I am making their bodies healthy and they heal themselves.

I help one sixty-five-year-old woman who has had sore hand and hip joints for twenty years, probably a combination of rheumatoid and osteoarthritis. Every one to three weeks she comes in for a B-complex shot (B_1, B_2, B_3, B_6, pantothenic acid, B_{12}, and a little C). Over the years we have experimented, and if I add a little folic acid it works better. Sometimes she says, "Up the B_{12}," and I do, and she has a better week. If she is getting some flu bug, I will add some extra vitamin C. This is a muscle shot so it does hurt, but it is worth it. Her husband notices that she is more mobile and cheerful for several days after the shot. Vitamin C helps the body with pain control, presumably because it stimulates the manufacture of endorphins, the body's own narcotic. It also helps in the production of interferon, which fights infection; many arthritics are chronically infected with some germ or virus.

Hereditary factors make some people more susceptible. I know a woman who says, "All Norwegians have arthritis." Her extended family is loaded with it and she has various joint symptoms. In those with rheumatoid arthritis a majority (80 percent) have the histocompatibility antigen (HLA) marker DNA. This is a site on a chromosome that carries this troublesome antigen. But not all with rheumatoid arthritis show the antigen, and not everyone with the hereditary tendency will get the disease. Other factors, such as stress, allergies, vitamin deficiencies, and mineral imbalances, must be playing a role. Some painful joints will respond to cortisone drugs either taken orally or injected into the joint. If this hormone helps, it suggests, but does not prove, that the patient's adrenal glands are not producing properly and that improved nutrition could help.

Juvenile rheumatoid arthritis is a nasty form that can strike a young person down and wreck his or her whole life or at least alter it. It also has an antigen marker on an HLA chromosome in a way similar to rheumatoid arthritis. The standard plan is aspirin and physiotherapy, but along with this and before deformity sets in, megadoses to rebuild the adrenals and the immune system make sense. Emotional stress has often been the trigger to activate the disease in susceptible people. We know what stress does to the adrenals.

The obvious first thing to do when afflicted with a painful, stiff, or swollen joint is to see your doctor. X-rays and blood tests may be necessary to diagnose your case. Some arthritides are very destructive and need emergency care: pyarthrosis means pus in the joint, and the suddenness of onset and the severity of the pain are usually motivation enough to force the sufferer to get emergency care. These are the cases for which we try to save our antibiotics.

Once the wild infections and the injuries or twists that cause bleeding into the joints are dealt with, we are left with aches and pains, stiffness and resulting immobility, depression, and insomnia.

Rheumatoid arthritis typically begins gradually in the forty-five-year-old female. It runs a chronic course and more likely affects the knuckle joints. Blood tests should be able to confirm the diagnosis. The sedimentation rate is usually elevated.

Osteoarthritis also has a gradual onset but will affect both sexes and is more likely to show up after age sixty to seventy. It typically affects the last finger joints, the knees, and the hips.

If your doctor cannot figure out your case, you should consult a rheumatologist who is able at least to give you a name for your affliction and a treatment outline. These are chronic problems, so you must settle in with some doctor with whom you are comfortable; it's usually for the rest of your life.

I don't mean you'll be sick with arthritis for the rest of your life, but you'll need this pipeline to the latest research information. Your situation and body will change, and although you live in your body and are perceptive, you need the doctor to monitor your complaints and tests. The doctor usually starts with aspirin, the time-honored anti-inflammatory painkiller, and usually in big enough doses (20 grains every four hours) to bother your stomach.

The aspirin is valuable. If it relieves the symptoms to the point where you are mobile and pain-free, you can assume your condition is remediable if not reversible. It also allows an exercise and physiotherapy program to be effected. The worst side effect of arthritis is the muscle and bone wasting that follows the immobility due to pain and stiffness.

The next thing to do is to ask your doctor *not* to use cortisone except as the last thing on the list. Make him write it on the chart: "No cortisone." But find out if you have a condition that might respond to cortisone-like drugs. Polymyositis, allergic arthritis, and rheumatoid arthritis respond, sometimes dramatically, to cortisone, but the side effects are disturbing. If cortisone would help, one should try megadoses of vitamin C (5000 to 15,000 mg, enough to loosen the stools a bit); pantothenic acid (500 to 1000 mg), a cortisol precursor; B_6, 200 to 400 mg; vitamin E, 400 to 800 units; vitamin A, 25,000 units; zinc, 60 mg; and a no-sugar, no-white-flour diet. Adelle Davis pointed out that the pantothenic acid level in arthritics was 45 percent below that found in unafflicted individuals.

But along with that, or prior to trying to enhance the function of your own adrenals, you might try the four- or five-day distilled-water fast. It is amazing how many sufferers of reversible arthritis or arthralgia (joint pain) are eating some food that is giving them hives in the joints. Remember the allergist's touchstone: "Anything can do anything." One man's gas is another man's arthritis (or asthma or migraine or itch). If a food is doing it, one should know it in four to five days. Then foods are added back every day or two, and the reasonably aware sufferer is supposed to figure out his or her own poison. Elimination of milk and dairy products might take three weeks to benefit those suffering from allergy to cow's products. Corn, wheat, strawberries, eggs—anything can do it; it is usually the person's favorite food. A clue that may help the victim: if you had colic, ear infections, tonsillectomy, or bed-wetting as a child, dairy products may be the cause of your adult problems now, even though the "allergy" has moved to another organ. It is probably best to call this a food incompatibility since the mechanism has no relationship to the IgE-mediated eczema, asthma, and hay fever. The joint symptoms simulated the major arthritis classification sub-groups; some joint allergies act like rheumatoid arthritis, some like osteoarthritis, and some manifest themselves as classic spondylitis cases.

Dr. Norman Childers, a horticulturist, discovered a related type of sensitivity to solanine, a glycoalkaloid. This chemical, a toxin to some, will cause arthralgia in susceptible people eating tomatoes, peppers, potatoes, and eggplant. Tobacco has it also, but it does not bother all smokers. The symptoms of pain and stiffness usually are more common in the late summer in those eating these fresh vegetables in abundance. Once the pain is present it may take several weeks of avoiding foods in the nightshade family before the joints even begin to feel normal again.

Dr. William Kaufman discovered the safe and effective treatment of some forms of arthritis with megadoses of vitamin B_3, niacinamide. One builds up the dose to 2000 to 5000 mg a day in divided doses. In a month the patient may notice that he can turn his head farther—his joints have a wider range of movement. If not, let's move on to the next level of treatment—all with the blessing of your doctor, we assume.

Dr. John Ellis discovered that pain, stiffness, and swelling of the shoulders and fingers to the point of inability to use the hands were due to a type of neuritis in which the nerves would swell and impinge on the sheaths containing them, especially in the wrist where the median nerve passes through a narrow, bony, and ligamentous tunnel. The problem is called *carpal tunnel syndrome* (q.v.). The fingers ache like an arthritis, but it is basically due to encroachment on the nerves. Sometimes one of the small wrist bones becomes displaced and impinges upon the nerve. Surgery relieves the squeeze. Dr. Ellis discovered that these swollen nerves respond to pyridoxine, B_6, at about the 100- to 300-mg dose per day. Women on the Pill may be more likely to get this because the liver needs B_6 to metabolize the hormones. Associated symptoms are aches and pains in shoulders, arms, feet, and legs, especially at night. Walking and massaging helps some. The B_6 should be taken for about three or four weeks.

If all these are not quite the answer and you are back to the aspirin and thinking about getting your tonsils or gall bladder out or having your teeth extracted because you know some infection is responsible, a couple of other approaches might be rewarding first. (In general, if you have a chronic infection eating away at you, serious enough to cause arthritis, your erythrocyte sedimentation rate and your white blood count should reflect that infection.)

Some doctors are willing to order a hair test because it is becoming more reliable in confirming a clinical impression. Enough have been done now to reveal "trends" in certain disease states. Copper and iron may be high in the hair; some feel that these metals are stored in the synovial membranes (lining of the joints) where they cause damage. Arthritics in general are low in manganese and zinc, which have a reciprocal interaction with copper. It may be that copper goes to the inflamed tissues to help healing and is not balanced with the proper amount of zinc. Some feel that copper salicylate is helpful in inhibiting superoxide free radicals,* which tend to harm joint membranes. Aspirin and copper gluconate taken together may calm joints. Since manganese has an effect on connective tissue, zinc (30 to 90 mg per day for a month) and manganese (5 to 10 mg per day for a month) should be tried. Painful knee and hip joints in teenagers—especially those with pimply skin and white spots in the nails—should respond easily and quickly. Chronic refractory rheumatoid ar-

---

* Free radicals are molecules containing extra oxygen or electrical charges. Hydrogen peroxide (H_2O_2) and superoxide (O_2 plus one electron) are the main oxidizing molecules that can cause cellular damage. They are formed by the destructive action of pollutants, x-rays, and cosmic rays on unprotected tissues. They may play a role in inciting aging, allergies, and cancer. Superoxide dismutase, catalase, and glutathione peroxidase must be available to change these irritants into O_2 and water. (See Degenerative Diseases.) These protective enzymes require selenium and vitamins C, B_6, A, and E, but B complex and zinc are useful also.

thritis may respond to 150 mg per day of zinc. Although manganese is higher in the blood of arthritics than in normal people, for some reason a high intake of manganese is helpful. It is one of the first minerals lost when flour is milled. It is high in whole grains, seeds, legumes, and alfalfa—if the alfalfa was grown in manganese-rich soil. Similar foods also contain zinc.

Histidine, methionine, and cysteine, which are sulfur-containing amino acids, help to remove copper from the body—if that is the problem. Lovers of garlic (high in sulfur) may have less of the arthritis associated with high copper. Eggs would help, along with onions.

Calcium may be low in the blood of arthritics but high in their hair. High calcium, in comparison to magnesium, depresses the ability of magnesium to inhibit the action of hyaluronidase. This enzyme causes synovial-fluid breakdown and could lead to arthritis. (Vitamin C also works against hyaluronidase, hence its value in preserving the intracellular cement in cancer therapy.) Magnesium helps to solubilize the calcium. If the calcium-to-magnesium ratio is more than 20 percent higher than normal, magnesium should be added. Phosphates may help us—in bone meal, brewer's yeast, and lecithin.

Gold therapy may be the next thing to try if you and the doctor have gone down the checklist. It is especially good for rheumatoid arthritis; 75 percent of the patients improve. Newer forms of gold make the treatment safer now.

Other unexpected, beneficial side effects sometimes show up when we are paying attention to one symptom. I recall giving a forty-year-old woman vitamin B complex injections plus C along with a good diet and dolomite supplements. She took 2000 to 4000 mg of C at bedtime to help her absorb the calcium and magnesium. All these are the standard preoperative vitamins and minerals; she was due to have an obvious slipped disc repaired because of shooting pains in her leg. After four shots and two weeks of supplements, she no longer had the pain, and her somewhat reluctant doctor cancelled the surgery.

In the past few years I have treated many adults with chronic bronchitis, sinusitis, repeated upper respiratory infections, swollen glands, and skin infections. They seem to have impaired immune systems and cannot "learn" to fight off the usual bacteria lurking in and on these membranes, waiting for an opening. I stop the milk, the sugar, and the junk, increase their vitamin C, and when nothing much happens I give a few shots of a dead bacterial vaccine (M.V.R., Hollister-Stier, Spokane, Wash.). It is cheap and safe and gets rid of secondary bacterial infections sometimes with greater efficiency than an antibiotic.

I have used this vaccine in combination with the standard influenza A and B vaccine as an intradermal and hypodermic shot every one to three weeks in some arthritic patients, and have gotten what I thought was a great response. It somehow stimulated the latent immune system. It mobilized the defence. Just because we do not know why something works, we should not throw it out as a possible valid therapy. If coffee enemas work, use coffee enemas.

Natural treatment includes alfalfa, wheat grass, watercress, potatoes (unless they cause the problem), yams, celery, parsley, garlic, comfrey, endive, bananas, pineapples, sour cherries, and sour apples. Foods that produce an alkaline ash when working their way through the body seem useful. The alkaline influence helps to dissolve accumulations of deposits about the joints and in other tissues; thus a vegetable-juice fast would be important. Citrus may aggravate arthritis, however. An ancient remedy is worth trying; raw potato juice mixed half-and-half with water. Bromelain helps reduce the inflammation of rheumatoid arthritis. Cod-liver oil, 1 teaspoonful one hour before or three hours after breakfast or supper, helps some.

The parathyroid glands (just behind the thyroid) are responsible for the movement of calcium to and from the blood to the bones. If the calcium-to-phosphorus ratio is less than 2:1, no matter what the levels are, the parathyroid is stimulated; its hormone pulls calcium from the bones. This ratio is influenced by the diet, and we should try to take more calcium than phosphorus.

The ideal calcium-to-phosphorus ratio in the diet is between 1:1 and 2:1.

2:1 —dairy products and alfalfa sprouts
1:1 —fruits and vegetables
1:3 —grains
1:5 —nuts and seeds
1:8 —chicken, fish
1:12—red meat
1:22—organ meats. (See also page 421.)

Most refined foods are high in phosphates; soft drinks are very high. With diets high in phosphates, the calcium is pulled out of the bones and deposited about the joints. Restricting the calcium is inappropriate; it is the phosphates that should be curtailed.

(See Osteoporosis.)

ATAXIA □ If someone has been clumsy or poorly coordinated since birth, the assumption is usually made that it is due to some form of brain damage or cerebral palsy caused by a difficult delivery (premature, forceps, breech, lack of oxygen). A good neurologist can usually attest to the extent of the problem. (See Dizziness.)

But in the area that separates those with an easily diagnosed hurt to the nervous system from those who are well coordinated and adroit—the acrobat or juggler types—there is a great, gray mass of humanity where most of us find ourselves. We are probably all a little damaged cerebrally. I have a bad eye, do klutzy things, and notice that my left hand is about a quarter of a beat behind my right when I play the piano. People run into things, stub their toes, fall over, and it's not all low blood sugar or sadomasochism. Maybe you can blame your mother. If she did not get enough manganese in her diet when she was carrying you, the otoliths in your semi-circular canals, which play a role in balance, may not be formed properly. (It's probably too late for the manganese now.)

The B-complex vitamins are very helpful for those with poor coordination, because they act as coenzymes for the manufacture of brain chemicals. Some of the nerves have been damaged and are gone; but some must be just dormant there, ready to be activated. B_1 and B_{12} are the more important ones, but it is best to use the whole B complex. It would take a couple of weeks to sense a change. A study of clumsy children revealed that 5 mg of folic acid per week was helpful.

I have given B complex plus C shots to children for allergies or hyperactivity, and the parents would report in two or three weeks that not only were these conditions better, but that the child walked and ran more smoothly and seemed better coordinated. Usually these are subtle changes that only a mother can detect, but they are present nonetheless. As we age we expect to lose some positional awareness, but not everyone becomes maladroit. The condition suggests the nerves are not working optimally; nerve function needs oxygen, a constant supply of glucose, and vitamins and minerals.

If the problem comes and goes, that is, if there are good and bad days, the assumption can be made that a food (sugar or allergen) is causing a "tilt" somewhere in the nervous system. If the blood sugar falls, if the body goes into acidosis, or if there is an allergic swelling in some critical balance area of the brain, one would become temporarily uncoordinated.

Alcohol is the chief poison responsible for ataxia. I have heard of cases in which food fermented in the intestinal tract and the person became inebriated. They were called "drunk" by skeptics who were not willing to believe that a bunch of grapes could turn to wine in someone's duodenum. (See Dizziness.)

AUTOIMMUNE DISEASES □ A significant medical breakthrough in the last ten years has been the identification of a closely linked group of genes that provide the code for the structure of antigens on cell surfaces. The genes are also responsible for factors that regulate some immune responses. These factors are responsible for tissue rejection in organ transplantation: immune responses are manufactured by the organ recipient against the tissue antigens of the donor; the body manufactures antibodies against itself.

Human leukocyte antigen (HLA) can be measured; the test gives the doctor a clue about the disease in the patient under study and helps in the prognosis. A few of the diseases associated with this antigen are ankylosing spondylitis, gluten-sensitive enteropathy, insulin-dependent diabetes, systemic lupus erythematosis, and some forms of multiple sclerosis.

It is now believed that these diseases will appear in a susceptible person (one with HLA) if some stress or illness provides the trigger. For example, diabetes may show up in a youngster with the right HLA if he gets the mumps in the insulin-secreting cells of the pancreas.

Because of the antigen-antibody relationship in the onset of these diseases, cortisone-like drugs have been a godsend for the sufferers. The relationship also suggests that nutrition might have precluded the onset of the autoimmune disease, and that once established, the disease might be alleviated with super nutrition and supplementation.

B

BED CONFINEMENT □ The bedridden patient sets a mechanism in motion that may be more damaging than the original reason for getting into bed. Disuse atrophy of the antigravity muscles—calf, thigh, and back, mainly—begins within twenty-four hours of becoming horizontal; the longer the bed experience, the more atrophy results. This is why people are dizzy and weak after a long illness. No one made them do straight-leg-raising or calf- and back-strengthening exercises several times a day. When they stand, their leg muscles are not strong enough to hold them upright and to squeeze the deep veins to propel the blood upward to the heart where it can be pumped to the brain. They are so light-headed they fall back in bed again. Massaging the muscles is fine, but the bedridden patient must do the exercises himself; he has to use his *own* muscles to maintain the tone.

The bones decalcify rapidly with inactivity and especially during forced bed rest. The extra burden of calcium to the kidneys may not be soluble enough, and stones are common in bedridden people who are prone to them. Even those very healthy astronauts lost a lot of calcium during their time of weightlessness in space.

Surgeons are aware of the danger posed to the body by forced rest. They may correct the surgical condition, but in the process the patient gets a pulmonary embolus, because a clot formed in the slowly moving blood in the calf muscle, broke off, and lodged in the lung. Most surgeons try to ambulate patients as soon as they are conscious—sore incision, oxygen tube, I.V., reluctance, and all. To speed postoperative convalescence many surgeons inject 5 to 10 grams of ascorbic acid or sodium ascorbate directly into the ongoing intravenous line. The patient is awake in a minute or two and is usually able and willing to walk back to his room. The C metabolizes the remaining anesthetic and, of course, promotes the healing process.

Sick people need not take to their beds unless the fever or flu is so devastating that the victim is in danger of keeling over. The army (good old army) did some studies on hepatitis and mononucleosis. Soldiers with these ailments were assigned to the bed-rest group or the back-to-duty group. There was no difference in the outcome. The ones who had been up and about actually recovered more rapidly because they were in better condition.

Giving plenty of fluids to keep the patient hydrated and to keep the calcium soluble is smart. Bedridden and sick patients need protein (amino acids in the I.V. and little or no sugar), vitamin C, B complex, and some all-purpose minerals. Burns need zinc; stress needs B complex; C helps recovery and may combat infection.

BREAST CYSTS □ Breast cysts need a doctor's evaluation. It may be difficult to differentiate precancerous lumps from benign cysts that are aggravated by menstruation. Estradiol and estrone, female hormones from the ovaries, are breast irritants. The breast has estrogen receptor binding sites responsive to these irritating estrogens. One-third of breast cancer is related to excesses of these two hormones. But a well-nourished liver will convert them to estriol. This safe, nonirritating hormone uses these estrogen receptor sites and prevents the others from getting in.

Any woman with estrogen-excess problems should use the following diet and supplements, especially if she is taking birth control pills. Tyrosine is needed to help make thyroxin; it is abundant in potatoes, apples, sesame seeds, and mushrooms. Kelp (five to ten tablets) is helpful because of its iodine content. Folic acid, 1 to 2 mg per day, helps protect the body from estrogen excess. To help the liver convert estrogens to inactive compounds, choline (1 gram), inositol (500 mg), and vitamin B_6 (100 to 300 mg per day) are the woman's friends. B_6 helps to bring in progesterone, which reverses estrogen's effect. Estrogens prevent the most efficient use of oxygen, so vitamin E would improve that; the E (400 to 800 units per day) acts as an anticoagulant, useful since estrogens encourage thrombus formation. Zinc (30 mg) is necessary because it tends to replace copper in the body, and women with excessive estrogen or those on the Pill have increased levels of copper. Bioflavonoids (100 to 300 mg) will compete for the estrogen receptor sites and thus tend to reduce the impact of irritating hormones. Magnesium (500 mg) helps to shrink the benign cysts. It takes about two months on this program for the woman to perceive a decrease in the size and tenderness of the cysts.

In addition, all caffeine must be eliminated as well as foods containing methylxanthine. These chemicals, found in soft drinks, tea, coffee, and chocolate, stop the action of a catabolic enzyme, phosphodiesterase. This enzyme breaks down cyclic AMP, which has a growth-stimulating action. If unchecked, cyclic AMP will cause these sensitive tissues to proliferate—thus the fibrous tissue and cystic fluid. Nicotine is believed by some to aggravate breast cysts.

Allergies make all the above worse. Dr. Joseph B. Miller sees allergic connections with many of the above disturbing hormone-related problems. He uses a diluted solution of progesterone injected like an allergy shot calculated to relieve the discomfort of the swollen cysts.

To repeat, see your doctor if you discover any cyst or lump in your breast.

BREAST-FEEDING □ If you are pregnant and are not sure about nursing your child, at least go to the La Leche League in your town and pick up the enthusiasm of these women. The motivation seems to be more important than the equipment. Don't let your doctor, your in-laws, or your family talk you out of it. It is important to you as a person, as a woman, and as a mother.

Breast-fed babies get sick, but much less often than bottle babies, because early milk (colostrum) is full of white blood cells which seed an immune system throughout the throat and intestines. Their stools smell better, and they have a little edge over bottle babies in feeling secure and developing a good jaw. (Ask your dentist.)

Breast-feeding may tie you down somewhat, but the prospects for being allergy-free are so much greater in breast-fed babies that nursing is recommended as the only food source for the first year to eighteen months. Twenty-five to 50 percent of the iron in human milk is absorbed. But if pureed pears are given along with the breast milk, the absorption of iron is reduced by 80 percent. In the past the only reason to begin solids was to prevent the development of milk (cow's) anemia. Now we find that if solids are begun early, the allergic risk rises, and the iron is probably poorly absorbed until the baby is six months old anyway.

Infant-formula companies have tried to imitate breast milk but cannot quite do it. Some interesting facts:

Human milk has 278 mg of calcium per liter. If the mother increases her calcium intake, there will be no effect on the baby. If the mother increases her iron intake, no increase in her milk iron will occur. Zinc starts out at 3.7 mg per liter but is down to 1 mg at four months.

Hind milk (the last 2 ounces) has more fat; thus prolonged nursing usually helps the baby increase the time between feedings. Improving the diet will increase the fat. Adding more protein to a malnourished woman's diet will put more protein in her milk.

Human milk is high in cholesterol, but the baby's serum cholesterol is only 140 mg/100 ml of serum. Many breast-fed babies appear fat, but baby size is not equivalent to adult size.

If your milk supply seems inadequate, extra B vitamins could help. In cows, milk yield is reduced if copper is deficient in the diet (sulfur tends to antagonize copper). Milk production is reduced if molybdenum is too high in proportion to copper. Most of us get enough copper—maybe too much, due to acid rainfall and copper pipes.

If anyone asks you why your child is two years old and unbuttoning your blouse for lunch, you can say, "Dr. Smith said I had to." Or you can say simply, "I'm selfish; I don't want my child to cost so much—dentist, doctor, allergist." You also want your child to like you when he or she is fully grown. Nursing is a good way to promote this idea. As you nurse you say, "I love you; remember me when I'm ninety years old and need your help. I want you to be healthy when you're seventy so you can do it!"

The only real drag is the night feedings. I've tried everything, and there is no one all-purpose answer. (See my book *Foods for Healthy Kids.*)

BREATH AND BREATHING □ Shortness of breath suggests congested lungs, as in obesity, bronchitis, pneumonia, asthma, heart failure, tumor, a foreign object in the lungs. This needs medical attention.

Rapid breathing usually means the afflicted is demanding more oxygen than can be taken in by normal breathing. Anemia and anxiety sufferers show this. Ordinary walking will make a person who is out of shape breathe rapidly. Smokers often breathe more rapidly than nonsmokers. (See Thyroid Problems.)

The feeling of being unable to catch one's breath is often a sign of anxiety. Sighing respiration, often repeated, will exhale too much carbon dioxide and cause an alkalosis and sometimes fainting. If these anxiety attacks occur without an appropriate stimulus, the victim should examine her diet. (See Anxiety.)

Phlegm in the nose, throat, and windpipe usually is due to an inhalant (feathers, danders, wool, house dust) or ingested allergen (milk, wheat, eggs, corn). If the nose itches and invites rubbing and picking, inhalants are indicated. If the problem is mainly throat-clearing and zonking, it is due to food allergens, most often milk. A woman told me that she could not sleep because of her husband's snoring. She tried a variety of tricks—rolling him over, chin strap, sharp elbow in the ribs. There was little snoring if he stayed off milk; no milk, no cheese, and no ice cream really made him a quiet sleeper. B_{12} and B_6 help control snoring.

"Bad" breath is often a clue to the family: Dad is getting sick; Mom is about to have her period; Sis is about to have asthma; Uncle Ed has been drinking. A fruity, acetone breath may tell the family that Grandma's diabetes is out of control. Really "foul" breath, as if something has died, suggests that someone in the room stuck something up his nose last week and forgot about it. Other possibilities are an abscessed tooth, a rotten tonsil, or a lung infection, especially lung abscess. A few people have a real sewer pipe for a colon, and their bacteria manufacture some nasties that the liver cannot handle. (See Abdominal Discomfort.)

Chlorophyll (wheat grass, parsley), alfalfa, pancreatic granules, acidophilus might help change things. A food allergy can overstress the intestines; the unwelcome food just sits there because the body is rejecting it. Bacteria work on it and the fermented products are exhaled. If a four-day fast gets rid of a bad odor, it suggests this possibility.

Chewing cardamom or anise seeds freshens breath. Rosemary, myrrh, and goldenseal are helpful herbs. One teaspoonful of powdered charcoal in a glass of water first thing every morning will control bad breath.

BRUISING □ Bruising that results from minor injuries suggests a blood-clotting defect. If the platelet count is normal and no good reason accounts for the hemorrhages, then vitamin C in doses sufficient to cause some sloppiness of the stools should be tried. Bioflavonoids usually must be used with the C to help the capillaries hold the red cells inside the vessels.

BURNING FEET □ This sensation usually is due to a lack of or a special need for thiamin, vitamin B_1; 50 to 100 mg per day should eliminate the distress in about seven to ten days. Usually other B vitamins are deficient also, especially B_6.

I have heard that this condition may be seen with a pantothenic acid deficiency. If so, 100 to 200 mg a day would solve it.

BURNS □ Burns must be treated immediately with ice water. A towel repeatedly soaked in ice water should be kept on the burn for one to three hours. A burned hand or foot can be placed in ice water for hours—not minutes. This keeps a first-degree burn from becoming a second degree, and a second from turning into a third.

Minor burns can be treated with aloe vera, vitamin E oil, or raw onion slices or juice. The doctor is needed for more serious ones. Doctors all know that zinc supplements, used along with a high-protein diet, will help heal the skin faster; 30 to 60 mg would be about right.

Vitamin C helps for the effects of stress. Vitamin A helps the zinc help the skin.

BURSITIS □ Bursitis and tendinitis are the labels placed on many ill-defined conditions characterized by soft-tissue pain, usually about the shoulder. Bursae are thin, flat spaces lined with cells that permit muscles and tendons to glide across other tendons and bony prominences.

Friction, trauma, infection, and crystal deposits will inflame these areas. Miner's elbow, housemaid's knee, weaver's bottom, and soldier's heel are a few examples of this common condition.

Since not everyone gets the condition despite similar trauma, it suggests that sufferers have a genetic susceptibility, have had a previous injury, or are on a deficient diet.

If fluid is present, its removal may speed recovery. Some doctors will inject cortisone into the bursae. The fact that it helps suggests that a nutrition program to boost the output of the adrenals would be rewarding. (No sugar, no white flour; fresh fruit and vegetables are important.)

Pantothenic acid, 250 to 500 mg two to three times a day, would be a good place to start. Vitamin C, 1000 to 5000 mg; B_6, 100 mg; calcium, 1000 mg; and magnesium, 500 mg daily, should calm the soreness in just a week or two. (See Aches.)

C

CANCER □ The news is out, but I don't see too many people doing anything about it. The National Cancer Institute has announced that there is a link between diet and cancer. We need to eat less, adhere to a low-fat, high-fiber, low-alcohol diet. Fruits, vegetables, whole-grain bread, and cereals are to be emphasized.

We know of the cancer-causing effects of tobacco, x-rays, and ultraviolet light, but way back in 1977 the National Cancer Institute pointed out that "food" and alcohol contribute to cancer more than the other environmental villains.

Dr. Peter Greenwald, Director of the National Cancer Institute's chemoprevention project, announced that the NCI will spend millions of dollars on a project to check the nutrition connection. He said, "Laboratory studies suggest certain vitamins have an inhibitory effect on cancer." Well, finally.

The intake of fiber and roughage is aimed at cutting down on colon cancer, which is one of America's most common forms of malignancy.* Diet is believed to be largely responsible, and constipation is the problem. Under certain

* Cancer statistics as of 1982 based on data from the National Cancer Institute's Surveillance, Epidemiology and End Results Program:
    For the male, 34% of cancer deaths were caused by lung cancer, 12% were due to colon and rectal cancers, and prostate cancers accounted for 10%.
    For the female, breast cancer caused 19% of the cancer deaths,

conditions, substances in the bile can become carcinogenic; they exert this action on the colon when in prolonged contact with the colon wall. Dr. Dennis Burkitt discovered only a small amount of intestinal cancer in the African natives who were having two or three bowel movements a day. There is also a high correlation between breast and colon cancer and the long-term ingestion of large amounts of meat and dairy fats.

Who would think that something as good for us as food could turn around and do us in? But maybe it's Mother Nature's way of telling us that we haven't been eating the right food. It's too bad it has taken us so long to get the message. And of course the beef and dairy interests, the boxed cereal companies, and the sugar manufacturers are loath to believe this nasty connection. But half of all new cases of cancer are those of the gastrointestinal tract or the sex organs. Why is the U.S. so much worse on this score than most other countries?

In 1979, Dr. W. Richard Burack quite rightly tried to reassure doctors and lay people alike by pointing out that the apparent "epidemic" of cancer was due to a few population idiosyncracies. It was reported that in 1930 there were 118,000 deaths in this country from cancer, while in 1970 the figure had risen to 331,000. It would appear, on the face of it, that the cancer rate had about tripled. But in those forty years the population had risen from 117 million to 203 million; the population had aged, and the lifespan had increased about ten years. The proportion of our population over age sixty-five also had doubled. Thus, Dr. Burack concluded, cancer deaths have remained at the same figure of 130 per 100,000

---

lung cancer was 16% of the total, colon and rectal amounted to 15%, and uterine cancer stood at 5%.

In 1978 about 400,000 people died of cancer; it was the second leading cause of death—170 deaths per 100,000 population. Cancer accounted for 20% of the total deaths. (Heart disease accounted for 40% of the deaths in 1978.)

population since 1930. A big relief; we're not *all* going to die of cancer in twenty years.

The doctor did admit that cigarette smoking is wrecking our lungs, that alcohol consumption increases cancer susceptibility, that too many x-rays are being taken, that too much estrogen is being prescribed, and that excessive calories are being consumed. But as the medical director of a major chemical company he carefully pointed out the *nonrelation* of cancer deaths to the *twenty-eight-fold* increase in chemical production. With death rates staying the same and even going down (except for lung cancer) despite the increased use of chemicals, his conclusion was that chemicals have nothing to do with cancer.

You should know of more recent findings. The U.S. Department of Health, Education and Welfare said in 1980 that as many as 40 percent of all cancers may be caused in the workplace due to exposure to chemicals, asbestos, and pollutants. This goes counter to Dr. Burack's findings.

Well, the bell tolls for thee and me every time someone dies of cancer. I would like to believe that this disease is as unnatural as dental caries or an ear infection or a heart attack. The "average" death rate does not or should not mean the "normal" death rate. I do not happen to believe that God has a certain amount of cancer to pass out and He only gives it to those who can take it. There are reasons for cancer, and there are ways to protect ourselves and our loved ones.

We must go to our doctor and get a diagnosis and a treatment plan for any lump, growth, bleeding organ, weight loss, or changed bowel habit. Let the surgeon cut it out; let the diagnosis and prognosis be made. But let there be some choices.

You should be informed of the many paths to health, and then you should be the one to make the decision with your doctor's help.

Restriction of calories inhibits the production of skin and mammary tumors in mice. Correlations occur in human females. Estrogens act as cocarcinogens. The rate of manufacture is dependent on body weight. Heavy ladies are at considerable risk; it is a disease of more developed societies.

A high-fat diet increases tumor production in rats. A consistent relationship is seen in humans between fat intake and epithelial (skin, oral, genital) and endocrine tumors.

In 1975 a survey revealed an endometrial (uterine) cancer rate in American women of 34 per 100,000 per year. The lowest rates were found in Japanese and Nigerian women, 5 per 100,000. Fat consumption in the United States was 150 grams per person per day and in Japan and Nigeria but 40 grams. Women with intestinal cancer are typically tall and overweight. Diabetes increases the risk, as do hypertension and gallbladder disease. Those women who had polycystic ovaries had a higher incidence of this cancer, as did menopausal women who used estrogen replacement medicine. (The statistics make it sound as if every woman should have her uterus removed prophylactically.)

Several cancers are more likely to occur in animals with vitamin A deficiency. But a high intake of A does not always prevent a chemically induced tumor.

Arlin Brown, editor of the *Cancer Victory Bulletin,* says, "Nutrition is the most important factor in the cause, prevention and cure of cancer." Dr. Mark Hegsted of Harvard's School of Public Health says, "The major causes of death and disability in the U.S. are related to the diet we eat."

A few facts: Nitrates and nitrites in the food we eat turn to nitrosamines in the intestinal tract. The latter are carcinogenic. There is a high incidence of gastric cancer in the people living in the Andes; the nitrates in the water are probably related. Japan, Iceland, and Latin America have higher rates of stomach cancer, presumably because of the high concentration of nitrates in the soil. The gastric cancer rate has fallen in the U.S. and Canada, perhaps because of the ingestion of foods higher in vitamins C and E. Gastric cancer rates in Japan have begun to fall because the food service people are using fewer nitrites when fish are prepared. The Japanese are eating fewer pickled foods.

The more nitrogen fertilizer, the more nitrates in the vegetables. The manure piled up in the feed lots contributes to the nitrates in the water runoff. The higher the NO_4, the higher the cancer rates.

The statistics show that if diet were controlled, health habits improved, exposure to harmful substances minimized, and stress assuaged, three-quarters of the cancers could be eliminated. Elimination of smoking, obesity, and animal-fat ingestion are the primary targets of the Cancer Prevention Society as well as of the very conservative National Cancer Institute. Control of these factors could go a long way toward cutting down the death and disability associated with three-quarters of the common cancers. The remaining one-quarter of cancers involve the bladder, kidney, skin, and pancreas, as well as lymphomas and leukemias. These may be work-related and connected with chemical exposure. I assume Dr. Burack will have some cheerful answers when in twenty years it is found that his safe chemicals are responsible for some of these statistics. Remember how we fluoroscoped babies? Remember DES? What are we doing now that will embarrass us in about twenty years?

Rule: If man made it, it's probably dangerous.

EVERYONE SEEMS to be in agreement that the body harboring a cancer has a defect in some natural immunity. The cells growing out of control started because of an invasion of a virus, a germ, or a foreign chemical. This penetration occurred because the cell wall was deficient in some way. Cancer research has been turning to cell-wall biochemistry in an effort to learn what it takes to make the cells less penetrable. It is valuable also to improve the immune system of the whole body to minimize the spread. The immune system will not function well if the patient has had x-ray and chemotherapy.

A few things should be done by all of us as preventive measures:

- Have periodic checkups.
- Report lumps, bleeding, changes of bowel habits.
- Eat little beef; its fat content is up to 40 percent. The N-nitroso compounds found in human feces are mutogenic; that is, they can cause cancer. Eliminating fats cuts the levels of these compounds in half.

  Dr. Richard Passwater reports a relationship between cancer and a high intake of polyunsaturated fats. He urges that we keep the vegetable oils down to less than 5 percent of the total caloric intake; vitamin E is essential to prevent oxidation of these oils in the body.
- Eat enough bran and fiber to allow for at least two soft, easy-to-pass stools a day. One tablespoon of bran a day cuts mutogens by 50 percent. Vegetable eaters have fewer colon/rectum cancers.
- Eliminate all sugar from the diet. Stay slim.
- Avoid x-rays. Dental x-rays may be taken every year or two. Chest x-ray every one to two years. Don't get a G.I. series for every gas pain.
- Don't smoke. Smoking-related deaths claim 300,000 victims annually. Some adults quit after the official Surgeon General's report in 1964, but adolescents are making up for it—especially the girls.
- Exercise at least three times a week. Get off caffeine and chocolate.
- Keep a tranquil mind. Stress causes the pituitary to activate the adrenal glands, which then release large amounts of cortisol. Cortisol has an adverse effect on the immune system, especially T cells and the thymus.
- Diets high in fresh fruits and raw vegetables correlate well with low incidence of stomach cancer. Best: let-

tuce, tomatoes, cabbage, and fruits high in vitamin C. Higher rates of stomach cancer are associated with a diet of starchy foods, coffee, salted fish, and charcoal-broiled meat. The higher the amount of alcohol consumed daily, the higher the rate of pharyngeal and esophageal cancer.

Almonds are the best nuts. No milk. Organ meats are emphasized. Cold-pressed thymus gland and spleen tissue should help the anticancer immune system. Garlic does work. Calcium, magnesium, and zinc are worthwhile.

Here are a few things to be done in addition if you have diabetes or high blood pressure, if you smoke, drink daily, are overweight, eat sugar, are a woman on the Pill, work in or near chemicals, pollution, or smog, are irritable, have insomnia, cannot handle stress, do not exercise, have relatives with cancer, and don't do much about religion:

- Have periodic checkups; have your doctor look you in the eye and get you to change your lifestyle.
- Do the things listed above and take:
  Vitamin C, at least 1000 mg and on up to 10,000 per day, until your stools are a little loose; 2 grams of vitamin C a day cut the N-nitroso compounds in the stools by 50 percent (2 to 3 grams of vitamin C daily eliminates 60 percent of rectal polyps—considered precancerous). Dr. Linus Pauling and Dr. Ewen Cameron treated terminal cancer victims with 10 grams of vitamin C daily; the treated patients lived four times longer than those not treated, and a few had complete remissions.
  Vitamin A, 25,000 units daily.
  Vitamin E, 600 to 1000 units, blocks formation of nitrosamines.
  B complex, 50 to 100 mg of each—so your urine

stays yellow most of the time and you have dream recall.

Brewer's yeast, 2 to 3 tablespoons of the powder per day. Lecithin, 1 to 2 teaspoonfuls of the granules. Approach vegetarianism; add calcium and magnesium.

A few things to do if you have had a diagnosed cancer which has been removed:

- If possible, delay chemotherapy or x-ray irradiation until you have had a chance to build up your immunity.
- Do all of the above but try to exceed the 10 grams of vitamin C. Intravenous vitamin C can up the level dramatically; 50 to 100 grams intravenously two to three times a week may stop some tumors.* Pauling has found that the more severe the cancer, the lower the level of ascorbate in the patient's leucocytes.
- And add these:

    Selenium, 50 to 200 mcg per day. Selenium is part of an enzyme that protects cell walls against peroxides and toxic radicals in food and air. It may stimulate the immune system. Cancer rates are higher in areas where selenium is low in soil.

    Iodine (in kelp), 100 to 300 mcg per day.

    Vitamin A may do a better job on skin and epithelial tumors than on those arising from mesodermal tissues (sarcomas and lymphomas). Most tumors have receptors on their surface and if there are vitamin A receptors, the theory goes, the tumor would respond to big doses of A. Theoretically, vitamin A should work best on tumors of skin, head, neck, breasts, lung, gastrointestinal tract, and bladder. In a Norwegian

---

* Cathcart, "The Method of Determining Proper Doses of Vitamin C" and Klenner, "Significance of High Intake of Ascorbic Acid."

study of 8000 men, the incidence of lung cancer was 5 times greater in those on a low vitamin A intake.

Vitamin E helps the A work. And zinc is necessary to mobilize the A. A new form of vitamin A, 13-cis-retinoic acid, does not accumulate in the liver and hence seems to be less toxic than the natural oil-soluble A, so larger doses can be used. It has improved the immune competence of bronchial cancer patients in doses of 150,000 to 300,000 units daily.

Most natural cancer therapists use pancreatic enzymes three or four times a day. This helps the body digest food—especially protein—and good absorption improves the immune system. Cancer will not get a foothold if the immune system is adequate.

CARPAL TUNNEL SYNDROME □ This problem is now felt to be caused by a neuritis that can be reversed with the use of B_6, pyridoxine. The median nerve runs through the carpal tunnel in the middle of the palm side of the wrist; the nerve just fits between bones and ligaments. When inflamed, the nerve swells, and the swelling causes pain and aching in the fingers and hand. It is often worse at night. Massaging the fingers gives slight temporary relief. A surgeon will cut the ligaments, thus freeing the nerve from the pressure. The symptoms are gone, but the neuritis is still operative unless the patient gets B_6, 100 mg once or twice a day. Usually all is well in two to three weeks. It's worth trying before the surgery.

Pregnancy and hypothyroidism may trigger the neuritis that causes the symptoms.

CATARACTS □ Once a cataract has begun, its progress usually can be slowed, but I have never heard of a dissolution or removal except by surgery.

Vitamin E reduced cataract formation in the eye lenses of rats made diabetic. It took 35 times the amount of vitamin

E found in the normal diet. This suggests that vitamin E, 400 to 800 units; vitamin C, 1000 to 5000 mg; B complex, as listed on page 40; and zinc, 30 mg, would all be useful in preventing the cataracts so often found in diabetics.

Cystine and methionine have been used to slow the progress of cataracts. Controlling the blood glucose makes the most sense. Eye tissues are unable to handle the glucose, and sorbitol is formed. This substance is related to some cataracts. Bioflavonoids will control the production of sorbitol.

CELIAC DISEASE ☐ Celiac disease is also called nontropical sprue, idiopathic steatorrhea, gluten-induced enteropathy, and primary malabsorption. In certain people, gluten-containing cereal grains alter the mucosa of the small intestines. The lining cells die, the ingested food cannot be digested because the digestive enzymes cannot function, and absorption cannot occur through the damaged cells. Stools are frequent, glistening, large, foul-smelling, and they deplete the body of calories, vitamins, minerals, and protein. Cheilosis, numbness, and tingling indicate B-vitamin, folic acid, and iron losses. Tetany, fractures, and bone pain show that vitamin D and calcium are not being absorbed.

Stopping the gluten is the first step in treatment. Vitamin B injections would speed the recovery of the mucosa. Some victims of the trouble can even eat a little of the gluten-containing foods if they receive the shots in preparation for the gluten load. Oral vitamins may not be absorbed well enough to help the enzymes handle gluten. (See Abdominal Discomfort.)

CHEILOSIS ☐ These little cracks at the corners of the mouth usually are caused by the ingestion of some allergen—milk, chocolate, and citrus being the most common. Cracks or sores about the anal opening would help to confirm that a food is responsible. Talking and eating will cause the healing skin of the mouth to open again and again, so some lubricating oil (contents of a vitamin E or an A-and-D capsule) is called for to help keep the skin pliant. The condition can turn into impetigo, which would require an antibiotic ointment. (It is best to use an ointment whose base would not also be used internally, since it is easy to become sensitive to drugs that are used locally. (Neomycin and penicillin, for example, are common allergens.)

Vitamin B complex deficiency could be the cause of the cracks, although it would have to be a severe deficiency. Large doses of vitamin A will make the skin dry out (OK for oily, acne skin), and these cracks at the corner of the mouth or eye could be the first sign of vitamin A overdose. Cutting back seems like good advice.

CHEST PAIN □ Not every chest pain is a heart attack, and not every heart attack is associated with a chest pain. The most common pain is a muscle spasm between the ribs, which is usually more laterally placed (near the nipple) and feels as if the edge of the lung has caught on a rib. It hurts to breathe; sometimes it feels as if one has been shot or has broken a rib. If holding the hand tightly against the painful area and breathing against this splinting action relieves the pain, it is only a muscle spasm. This person needs calcium. A week of calcium supplements—best accompanied by magnesium—should put an end to this. It is called the rib syndrome and is associated with low calcium intake. Hypoglycemic attacks will allow it to show up, as will physical and emotional stress, since calcium levels rise and fall with blood sugar levels.

Shingles, a virus-induced neuritis, usually shows up first as a pain on one side of the chest; the pain follows the nerve parallel to a rib. Sore, red, small blisters appear a day or so later. The pain can last for years after the sores heal. Vitamin B_{12} shots, 1000 mcg intramuscularly, speed the healing. The sooner shots are started, the quicker and more complete the recovery. (Vitamin C helps fight all viruses also.) The disease often appears in a grandparent two weeks after a Christmas visit to the five-year-old who came down with chicken pox (same virus) the day the grandparent arrived. It can be severe and debilitating.

Various aches and pains in the chest wall, tight feelings, and vague uncomfortable sensations in the chest may also be relieved with B_{12} shots. Are they some harbinger of pernicious anemia? Chiropractors and kinesiologists can sometimes diagnose internal organ pathology by locating tight and tender muscles in the chest wall that are innervated by segmentally related nerves. For example, a tender, spastic teres muscle can mean a sluggish thyroid. The aches and pains associated with osteoporosis are supposed to be due to the collapsing vertebrae and the subsequent impingement of nerves. People with this problem often feel and move better after receiving calcium and magnesium intravenously; such a response would suggest that muscle spasm from low calcium is more responsible for the pain than narrowed spaces between the vertebrae. The tight muscles pinch the nerves and the irritated nerves cause a reflex muscle spasm as a "protective" mechanism. If this is the source of the pain, then the physiotherapist or the chiropractor can help; he should suggest at least some supplemental minerals.

Don't fool around with calcium for a heavy, crashing, substernal squeeze that may radiate down the left arm. That's heart attack symptomology, especially if accompanied by a rapid pulse and sweats. A doctor and an EKG are the minimal attention. The blood enzymes usually are elevated. If you recover, the Pritikin approach (no fat, no sugar) plus E, C, and magnesium may allow you to live a reasonably normal life.

CIRRHOSIS □ Cirrhosis of the liver does not necessarily mean the afflicted person has been drinking. Alcohol and its metabolite (acetaldehyde) or some immune response to alcohol is responsible for only one-third of the cases. Hepatitis, drug-induced liver damage, heart failure, damage from biliary tract obstruction, and metabolic errors account for the remainder.

This condition destroys liver cells, and they are replaced by scar tissue. Malaise, nausea, fatigue, are common symptoms. Some improvement should be possible at this stage if large doses of vitamins are given. No alcohol is permitted. Once jaundice, itchy skin, diarrhea, and dark urine have begun, the situation is usually considered hopeless; vitamins should be given by intravenous or intramuscular route (1 cc of a B complex plus C and folic acid every day or so).

The parotid salivary glands tend to enlarge in alcoholic cirrhosis, while the testicles shrink. The SGOT is greater than the SGPT (see Chapter 4); alcoholics with no obvious infection have an elevated percent of polymorphonuclear leukocytes.

Those with cirrhosis are prone to bleeding, fluid accumulation in the abdomen, disordered mental capacity, kidney failure, osteomalacia, and frequent infections.

Nutrition is the first line of control with cirrhosis.

CLAUDICATION □ Intermittent claudication is muscle pain in the legs or feet due to an inadequate blood supply to these muscles. It is aggravated by exercise. Pain due to atherosclerosis of the arteries supplying the legs can be so severe that it is present even if the person is at rest.

If the skin below the knee is cold and pale while the skin of the knee is warm, the artery supplying the lower leg is obviously narrowed. Palpation of the pulse in the foot may be difficult because so little blood is getting through.

Oscillometry and ultrasound testing of blood flow usually is done before angiography is attempted (injecting radiopaque dye into the femoral artery and taking x-rays).

In some people whose condition is not too far deteriorated, nutrition can reverse some of the damage. Vitamin E, 400 units and advancing to 1200 to 1600 units daily depending on the blood pressure, can relieve the pain in six weeks if it's going to work at all. No tobacco, no sugar, and no white flour is mandatory. Vitamin C, B complex, and a multiple mineral tablet help. Exercise—even just walking—is pushed to tolerance.

Some patients need arterial grafts, but a technique recently perfected by Charles Dotter allows for opening the lumen of the artery by passing a wire down into the obstructive area.

COLD HANDS AND FEET □ The circulation of warm blood through the capillaries of the skin is responsible for the warmth we associate with being alive. If anemia, bleeding, low thyroid, or chronic sickness is present, the body will conserve its heat by constricting the precapillary arterioles. Under these conditions the skin is usually cold and dry. I was taught in medical school that if the patient's hands are moist, he or she probably does not have low thyroid function; that usually creates cold, dry skin.

Cold, clammy hands usually are associated with anxiety. Just when you want to be cool, collected, and sophisticated, you feel the moisture dripping off your fingertips. Some people are built like that; on the other hand, it may be that they notice the world too easily. If one is ticklish and sensitive, it suggests that the nervous system is unable to screen out incoming stimuli. The B complex (50 mg of each), especially B_6 (try 100 to 300 mg a day until you have good dream recall), helps one notice the world less. Try 1000 mg of B_3. Calcium, 1000 mg, and magnesium, 500 mg, have a calming effect on the nervous system. These measures may help; you may still have problems, but you won't care so much.

Remember, low blood sugar can do all this. Food allergies also must be considered.

One trick to improve the circulation: walk in the bathtub in ankle-deep cold water for five minutes. Step out occasionally and then get back in.

COLITIS □ This is an inflamed colon. The most common form is that due to constipation alternating with diarrhea. It's called irritable bowel syndrome. It may have an emotional component, although the owner of the colon usually gets upset because of the uncomfortable messages he is getting from his nether regions. He thinks he may have just a little gas to pass, then discovers he has dumped a load. How embarrassing! The messages are not reliable. He may sit on the toilet for two days and after much capillary breaking and straining be rewarded with a worthless dollop. Then for two days he has five movements a day that would make a cow proud.

The most common source of this problem is dairy-product ingestion. Many people pass bowling balls a couple of days after eating even a small amount of milk or cheese. The bran or salad they took to soften the packed curd didn't blend enough with the dairy product to minimize its impact. Three weeks of a nondairy, no-white-flour, no-processed-sugar diet should end the ordeal. I've had patients who were about to have surgical exploration due to ingestion of dairy products; even one cubic inch of cheese would lock their bowels for a week.

The milk is surely to blame if one has a history of colic, vomiting, gas, ear infection, asthma, or rashes from infancy on. Rashes about the mouth and anal opening are the giveaway that food is responsible. A fast of four days may help to improve things enough to know that it is worth continuing. Wheat, corn, and eggs are the usual other irritants. (See Abdominal Discomfort; Allergies.) After a ninety-day fast from the food, it might be eaten once a week without all the trouble returning.

I have seen this constipation alternating with diarrhea in my infant patients when solid food was first begun. The milk would come through as a large, firm mass, then layered above that would be the digested remains of the oatmeal and applesauce.

A way to control the acute pain of a colitis attack is by fasting, which allows the bowel to rest. Sipping on juices would be safe; herb teas, such as goldenseal, slippery elm, licorice root, and capsicum, may be added. Camomile tea enemas will calm the colon.

Ulcerative colitis may start in childhood or adolescence and, like asthma, has genetic, emotional, and nutritional forces operating as causes. Because cortisone-like drugs have been able to control the cramps, weakness, and bleeding, it is assumed that an autoimmune or IgE-mediated process is operating. When medical management (diet and antibiotics) and cortisone enemata are no longer controlling the attacks, the surgeon steps in and removes the affected colon, since the risk of cancer is very great in neglected cases.

Dr. J. Siegel found a higher than expected incidence of hay fever, asthma, and eczema in a group of patients with inflammatory bowel disease. When the systemic allergy was controlled, the colon calmed down. It suggests a common etiology.

I have seen and treated *early* cases, diagnosed by competent gastroenterologists, where we were able to stop the progress of the disease. No sugar, no white flour, no dairy or corn products (allergic potential); plus as much vitamin C as would soften the stools; B complex (50 to 100 mg of each); calcium and magnesium; zinc, 30 to 60 mg; vitamin A, 10,000 to 25,000 units; vitamin E, 400 to 1200 units. After three to six months of a calm colon, the doses can be reduced until maintenance doses are established. I.V.s of calcium, magnesium, B complex, and C are given every other day while an attack is in progress; the B complex and C muscle shots are given on the other days, while the oral doses are taken daily. With all this the patient should require a little less medical management.

Crohn's disease (regional enteritis) is different but should be helped with the above routine. Cancer of the bowel usually reveals itself with a change of bowel habits without a change in eating habits. It is usually accompanied by blood, but don't wait. An exam with the sigmoidoscope reaches about 70 percent of colon cancers.

Because of the possible autoimmune or allergic nature of Crohn's disease and ulcerative colitis, and because cortisol can calm the symptoms, it is worth trying a program that would support the adrenals. Let the patient make enough of his own cortisol and he may not need outside help. Pantothenic acid, vitamin C, and B complex are called for. It has been found in ulcerative colitis that the intestinal mucosa is depleted of pantothenic acid. Coenzyme A is an enzyme needed for cellular function; pantothenic acid is a precursor of coenzyme A.

Don't give up.

CONCENTRATION □ Some people seem to be able to concentrate on a thought, a task, or a book and pay no attention to environmental emergencies (smoke, siren, phone ringing). I've seen it in my family. A "hyper" child, on the other hand, has a short attention span; he concentrates poorly, is easily distracted, and gets into trouble when he flits about the classroom.

Adults who were hyperactive as children usually carry their poor concentration with them throughout their lives, although the activity level may be reduced. They tend to avoid the activities that will embarrass them. For example, neurosurgery would be a poor career choice for such an individual; but maybe not pediatrics, where we jump from one patient to another in five- to fifteen-minute time slots.

Calcium, magnesium, and B_6 help most persons move away from the world a little, to be less dispersed mentally. B_1, B_3, and B_{12} will help concentration. Recent work indicates that lecithin becomes choline in the body, and that in the brain it forms acetylcholine, which is one of the brain chemicals that helps us think. L-glutamine has a similar effect; it makes glutamic acid in the brain, and this enhances acetylcholine production.

Of course, anemia, low thyroid, and hypoglycemia will prevent normal brain function. If a doctor has ever put you on Dexedrine or Ritalin for hyperactivity and if it had a calming effect, then you know that you did—and may still—have a biochemical peculiarity.

CONFUSION □ We're all a little confused. Life is tough enough, even when you have all your faculties. But some people are confused to the point of stupidity, and this is more probably due to a combination of genetics, pregnancy insults, and nutritional and stress factors.

If someone slowly slips into a confused state, with memory loss, disorientation, and confabulation, we ask about alcohol intake. If that is nonrevealing, a hair test is important to reveal possible heavy-metal poisoning (lead, aluminum, cadmium, mercury). Alzheimer's dementia is probably due to aluminum poisoning in some sensitive people. Calcium, magnesium, fiber, and garlic (capsules) will help pull aluminum out of the tissues so that it can be excreted. If the confusion is off-and-on, from one hour or one day to the next, it means that something in the diet is knocking the blood sugar down. (See Hypoglycemia.) Food allergies can wipe out memory.

A more recent cause of mental confusion is yeast overgrowth in the body in people who have had heavy doses of antibiotics, cortisone, birth control pills, or stress (q.v.). These patients, usually women, are fatigued and unable to remember what they did the previous day.

If confusion is associated with aging, hardening of the arteries, and high blood pressure, it is assumed that narrowing of the cerebral blood vessels is restricting the oxygen supply. A therapeutic test of inhaling oxygen should show if that is the cause. But so many of us over fifty and sixty years of age are eating so poorly, one must assume that nutrition can be blamed for part of this decreased mental functioning. The enzymes that manufacture the chemicals are vitamin and mineral dependent. Before these elderly, not-quite-with-it, ready-for-the-rest-home humans are written off as too far gone to help, we must try to supply what the brain needs. Magnesium, which sparks so many enzymes, should be at the 500-mg-per-day level. B_1 is best at 50 to 200 mg per day, and the rest of the B complex at 50 mg each; niacinamide at 1000 mg to 3000 mg a day (niacin works better, if the person can handle the flush it causes); vitamin C, 1000 to 10,000 mg; vitamin E, 400 to 1200 units. A good diet with nuts, seeds, raw vegetables, fruits, brewer's yeast—the usual—is also essential.

CONGESTIVE HEART FAILURE □ Congestive heart failure requires medical attention. The heart is stressed due to extra load (as with hypertension), excessive volume load (anemia), lack of adequate viable muscle (myocardial infarction), or valve defects that cause inadequate filling (congenital anomalies, mitral stenosis). The heart muscle hypertrophies, then dilates, then beats faster to compensate.

Most of the symptoms that accompany heart failure are due to the retention of sodium and water in the lungs, abdomen, and legs. Breathing difficulty or breathlessness suggests that fluid is backing up in the lungs because of the sluggish circulation. A more severe form is called orthopnia (breathlessness while lying down); some people have nocturnal attacks. This usually means the left ventricle has failed.

Ascites is the accumulation of fluid in the peritoneal cavity. Edema of the lower legs usually accompanies heart failure; it is worse after a day on one's feet and may be gone after a night's sleep.

Weakness, confusion, dizziness, nausea, constipation, stomachache (swollen liver), and nocturia all may appear with the failure.

An evaluation of the patient includes an x-ray of the chest for heart size and fluid in the lungs. An effort is made to determine and remove, if possible, the reason for the failure. Laboratory tests may show elevated BUN, SGOT, LDH, bilirubin. Protein is often elevated in the urine.

High-quality food plus sodium restriction are the dietary mainstays. Vitamins used for stress, especially the B complex, would be worthwhile.

CONSTIPATION □ This is the passage of firm stools. The frequency is usually decreased—perhaps once every three to five days—but this is not the criterion; the consistency makes the diagnosis. (See Abdominal Discomfort; Fiber.) If we could imitate our primitive cousins, we would have a mushy movement after every meal—well, at least two times a day. Easy-to-pass stools are associated with low frequency of appendicitis, hemorrhoids, colon cancer, and hiatus hernia.

You don't have to be a stool gazer to tell what's going on down there. You should be able to get a sensation that it is time, usually after a meal; this is called the gastrocolic reflex. You sit down on the toilet seat and with only a slight effort, you should be able to let it all go and get out of there in about five minutes or less. It should be brown, soft, sink minimally, and almost fall apart in the water. If it is a big struggle with much straining, your diet is wrong. (See Colitis.)

Milk and dairy products are the usual cause of constipation. They have no roughage and the curd turns into a hard rock which keeps that consistency until it is expelled. White flour, pasta, rice, and dough can all do the same because of their low roughage content. Just taking extra bran is not enough. The constipating foods must be discontinued.

Hypothyroidism is a common cause of constipation. Not enough fluid intake tends to constipate some people. Liver dysfunction and constant worrying will do it to others. Inositol, B complex, and potassium deficiencies will lead to firm stools.

Mineral oil as a laxative is terribly dangerous. It can be aspirated and it tends to prevent the fat-soluble vitamins from being absorbed. Cramping cathartics just give you Wednesday's bowel movement on Monday. It's treating a symptom and not the problem. Herbal laxatives are good, but roughage, bran, and fiber are the best. (Flax seeds, psyllium seeds, prunes, and figs help.)

Some will try increasing the vitamin C by 1000 mg a day until the stools are just a little soft. Exercise is a must, even if it is only walking two hours a day.

CONVULSIONS □ Convulsions are frightening episodes of unconsciousness usually associated with twitching or gross muscle shaking and falling. Obviously a doctor, usually a neurologist, is consulted to discover if a tumor, blood clot, or metabolic dysfunction is present. An electroencephalograph (EEG) is taken and occasionally a CAT scan. A high proportion of seizures is due to unknown causes; usually these have their onset in childhood or early adolescence. If they show up after age twenty, seizures are more likely to be due to injury or a tumor.

If all the tests are nonrevealing except that the EEG indicates "an irritable focus" over one area, and if the doctor has you try barbiturates, phenytoin (Dilantin), or valproic acid, you accept the prescription and fill it because the spells are nightmares to you. But your job is just starting. You have to live with your nervous system all the rest of your life; you must get it off "tilt." The doctor is treating the symptoms, the spells. He doesn't know exactly why you have the disease. It is called "idiopathic."

If one has the epileptic condition, one might expect seizures regularly and frequently. Some people go a week, others months, between spells. The tendency is there. Something triggers it, and that "irritable focus" sets off the next cell and the next until an obvious fit is produced. The drugs prevent the spread; you have to try to put out the original fire.

Our knowledge is imperfect, but maybe a short review of certain facts will help you choose a course of action. Eating, for some reason, makes a difference. The brain-wave test is different before a meal as compared with after. Dr. William Philpott has found that one-half of the epileptic population has abnormal carbohydrate metabolism, low B_6, low calcium, and low magnesium, which can allow a susceptible person to have seizures.

Lead poisoning could make one more susceptible. Low blood sugar in the person ready to convulse will trigger the attack. Most just faint.

The supportive nutrition program might just allow an epileptic to get off the medicine sooner than the standard four years of being seizure-free. One should insist on a good laboratory screen test of the blood and a hair analysis with special interest in the heavy metals and levels of manganese, magnesium, and calcium.

The nutritional approach would be the standard no-sugar, no-junk diet, with six nibbled meals a day. Calcium, 1000 mg; magnesium, 500 mg; B complex, as listed on page 40; extra B_6 (especially if dream recall is poor) 500 to 1500 mg per day; folic acid, 1 to 5 mg a day; biotin, 200 to 400 mcg a day; manganese, 5 to 15 mg per day (one-third of those with seizures are low in manganese); zinc, 30 mg per day. Taurine is supposed to help. Glutamic acid can help. Folic acid and B_{12} should be in the supplements.

The seizure-prone person should notice a calmness, an evenness, in three to four weeks. Another EEG might be appropriate. If there are no breakthrough seizures in six months, a reduction in the medication might be considered. There must be no sudden withdrawal from an antiepileptic drug.

CORONARY ARTERY DISEASE: Fats, Triglycerides and Cholesterol □ Every two to three weeks an expert announces that he or she has an answer to degenerative diseases in general and to vascular breakdown specifically: stop the lard and the butter because those fats hit your aorta like a hockey puck. It seems logical that high levels of fat in the diet would lead to high levels of fat in the bloodstream, and that this would be associated with atherosclerosis (thickened blood vessel walls infiltrated with cholesterol, fat, and early calcium deposits) and narrowed blood vessels. The 40 percent fat in the typical American diet seems to be the chief contributor. Even thirty years ago, autopsies done on American soldiers killed in action revealed that 70 percent of these twenty- to twenty-two-year-olds had coronary atherosclerosis and that 25 percent had more than 50 percent narrowing of one coronary artery. So it's not that more of us are living longer and getting the degenerative vascular diseases; someone or something is *doing* it to us.

The ingestion of saturated (hard) fats is very effective in raising the serum cholesterol level. Lowering the cholesterol level by eating polyunsaturated fats is difficult. A high cholesterol level in the bloodstream (greater than 250 mg per 100 ml) is associated with increased risk of a vascular disease (angina, heart attack, thrombosis, embolus). But, of course, many people have fatal heart attacks with very low cholesterol levels (150 to 190 mg per 100 ml). On the other hand, the low incidence of vascular troubles of the high-fat-consuming Masai (milk and blood) and the Eskimos (blubber and seal oil) is legendary.

The American Heart Association announced eleven years ago that cholesterol in eggs was the cause of high cholesterol in our blood and that we had to cut back to three eggs a week. A number of egg-loving researchers worked feverishly to vindicate hen fruit. (Would God wreck a chicken?) Much to the embarrassment of all those who had proscribed the egg, it was learned that 50 to 75 percent of everyone's cholesterol is manufactured *inside* the body; most people can eat twenty eggs a day and their cholesterol level will stay the same. The lecithin in the egg probably contributes to the emulsification and speedy digestion of this excellent food (every other protein is compared with the high quality of egg white). We all need cholesterol. If one does not eat enough, the liver will make it. The body uses it as a major constituent of cell membranes; 50 percent of the myelin sheaths of nerves is cholesterol. It is essential to the manufacture of hormones, and at least one-third of the production of cholesterol is used to form bile acids needed for fat absorption. Finally, the amount of cholesterol in the diet is not the significant factor in the development of atherosclerosis.

Cholesterol, then, is a risk factor but not *the* risk factor. The cholesterol content in the American diet is much the same as it was in 1909—500 mg per person daily. It seems prudent to keep cholesterol at or below a level of 200 to 210 mg per 100 ml of blood.

WHAT HAPPENS to the fat we eat? Ingested fat is emulsified and hydrolyzed by bile and lipase into fatty acids, monoglycerides and cholesterol. Inside the cells of the intestines they are recombined into small fat droplets, called chylomicrons. Triglycerides make up 95 percent of these droplets. Inside the cells of the arterial walls the chylomicrons are broken down again into fatty acids, glycerol and cholesterol. If not used as fuel, the fatty acids are stored around the body as fat. The cholesterol remnants are taken up by the liver. If the food supply of cholesterol is ample, the liver reduces its production. Triglycerides are also formed from sugar and alcohol.

The liver uses triglyceride, cholesterol, phospholipids, and protein to make a very-low-density lipoprotein (VLDL). This is hydrolyzed when it reaches the bloodstream (as above); the fatty acids and glycerol thus produced serve as sources of energy for the various body tissues. Further processing turns VLDL into intermediate and low-density lipoprotein (LDL). This latter is taken up by the cells. But since the cells cannot degrade cholesterol, it needs a carrier to return it to the liver. The liver produces high-density lipoprotein (HDL), which travels out to the cells and returns the cholesterol back to the liver for reuse. Thus high amounts of VLDL or LDL encourage atheromatous deposits; high levels of HDL tend to reduce that risk.

About 10 percent of the population have abnormalities of these lipid transport systems; most are genetic conditions.

Some are due to pre-existing disease. Many are aggravated by obesity and faulty diets.

The following is a brief summary of the five types of hyperlipoproteinemia, including their lipid patterns and suggested treatment. If you have one of these conditions, you need an internist to guide you through the diagnosis and treatment. It requires a lifetime of follow-up.

Type I has an easily identified layer of fat particles (chylomicrons) floating on top of the plasma. We all have these triglycerides if we have recently eaten a fatty meal, but if they appear after an overnight fast (blood drawn before breakfast), it places the patient into this type. The cholesterol is usually normal or high, the triglycerides are greatly elevated (greater than 1000 mg/100 ml), and the high-density lipoprotein is usually absent. It is often a genetic problem (lipoprotein lipase deficience), so it may appear in childhood. Patients with this often have xanthomas (yellow fat tumors) and enlargement of the liver and spleen. The condition is associated with diabetic acidosis and hypothyroidism. The treatment is a boring low-fat diet. It is interesting that a high level of these chylomicrons does not in itself produce a higher risk of cardiovascular disease, but the abdominal pain and pancreatitis of Type I can be reduced by keeping the triglycerides below 800 mg/100 mg of serum. Dietary fat ingestion is kept below 30 grams a day (1 ounce).

Type IIa is fairly common. It is characterized by a high LDL and a high cholesterol level. It is genetic and is often associated with early cardiovascular disease. *Type IIb* patients have high VLDL, LDL, cholesterol, and triglycerides. They may be associated with hypothyroidism, a kidney disease (nephrosis), and obstructive liver disease. They are treated with thyroid hormone, niacin, and cholestyramine (which sequesters bile acid in the intestines so fats are not absorbed). A low-saturated-fat and low-cholesterol diet is standard (under 300 mg per day). The IIb patients improve with a low-carbohydrate diet and the maintenance of ideal body weight.

Type III is rare. It shows a high level of intermediate lipoproteins, cholesterol, and triglycerides. It is important to recognize Type III early, as it leads to cardiovascular disease. It is genetic. Dietary carbohydrates and fat should be severely limited. Thyroid hormone might help. Niacin has proven valuable; niacinamide, the other form of vitamin B$_3$, does not seem to be effective. Clofibrate works as niacin does: reducing the liver synthesis of VLDL.

PERCENTAGE OF CALORIES FROM FAT IN VARIOUS FOODS
(SATURATED AND UNSATURATED TOGETHER)

50 to 90% fat:

Cream cheese, avocado, rib eye beef, weiners, olives, sausage, pork luncheon meats, cheese and cheese spreads, tongue, eggs, ground beef (regular), salmon and tuna (canned in oil), pork (loin and butt), ice cream, granola, chicken (roasted with skin), beef (porterhouse, T-bone), pecans, walnuts, macadamia nuts, filberts, Brazil nuts, almonds.

40 to 50% fat:

Pork and lamb (shoulder), salmon (red sockeye, canned), whole milk, potato chips, cashew nuts, peanuts, pumpkin and sunflower seed kernels.

30 to 40% fat:

Tuna in oil (drained), low-fat yogurt, creamed cottage cheese, lean beef, turkey (flesh and skin, dark meat), leg of lamb, low-fat milk, perch, sturgeon, swordfish, coconut (90% saturated).

20 to 30% fat:

Chicken (white meat), turkey (white), clams, mussels, oysters, herring, bass, salmon (pink), liver (pork, chicken, lamb, beef).

10 to 20% fat:

Tuna (water pack), haddock, cod, flounder, sole, halibut, perch, pike, sea bass, snapper, crab, lobster, porridge, bread, skim-milk cheese, brown rice, blackberries, strawberries, and most peas, beans, and lentils.

Less than 10% fat:

Most breakfast cereals, uncreamed cottage cheese, chestnuts, skim milk, buttermilk, fruits, white rice, whole-wheat flour, soybeans, garbanzo beans.

Type IV is fairly common. The VLDL is increased along with triglycerides. The cholesterol levels may be normal or elevated. A reasonable level of triglycerides (less than 200 mg/100 ml of serum) should be the minimum goal, as this type leads to cardiovascular disease also. If obese, the patient must lose to ideal weight. Alcohol is taboo, no sugar is to be eaten, and of course a low-fat diet is important. Estrogen therapy and oral contraceptives will aggravate this type.

Type V is a mixture of types I and IV and is treated accordingly.

Although the general level of fat ingested is an important consideration (best under 20 to 30% of total calories), new research indicates that the fats derived from fish oils, called omega-3 fatty acids, are more protective than those derived from vegetables, called omega-6 fatty acids. Fish membranes remain fluid in very cold water because they contain these omega-3 fatty acids. Both omega-3 and omega-6 fatty acids are essential (EFA) because the body cannot manufacture them. Linoleic acid, an omega-6 fatty acid, must be consumed at about the 1–2% level of total calories to prevent a deficiency. It is the source of arachidonic acid which is needed to make some prostaglandins.

Omega-6 fatty acids constitute 50 to 70% of safflower, corn, cottonseed and sunflower oils. The more helpful omega-3 fatty acids are in linseed, salmon, cod liver oils and mackerel; they contain about 8 to 12% of the beneficial eicosapentaenoic acid.

Cow's milk, lard, chicken fat and beef are all low in omega-3 and omega-6 fatty acids and high in saturated fats. Coconut oil is 88% saturated fatty acids.

WHEN VASCULAR PROBLEMS occur, diet control is always attempted first and is successful in the majority of cases. These rare cases of genetic hypercholesterolemia and hypertriglyceridemia need diet control and often drugs for management. One must remember that low thyroid function (q.v.), alcoholism, nephrosis, or use of oral contraceptives will alter the laboratory results. A thin person with elevated lipids usually has the familial form. Exercise will increase the HDL level, as will a little alcohol. Obesity, smoking, and sugar ingestion lower this protective HDL.

You have a few clues about your chances of avoiding cardiovascular disease if you know the following: your family history of sickness, your weight, your sugar and alcohol intake, your smoking history, your fat intake, and your exercise level. Your doctor can and should tell you your blood pressure, and you can insist on seeing your blood-screening results. To be accurate, the blood lipids should be tested at least twelve hours after the last meal; if tests are abnormal, they should be repeated twice before acceptance of the diagnosis.

If your cholesterol level is above 225–250 mg per 100 ml, or if the triglyceride level is above 150–200 per 100 ml, some intervention is prudent, since higher levels are associated with vascular disease. About half the patients doctors see have elevation of blood lipids. But only about 10 percent of the population is afflicted with the genetic, more serious hyperlipidemias.

Do we have to worry if we are not in this group of hyperlipoproteinemics? We do, but not as much. But read on and see if you might qualify.

The following are the risk factors most experts agree should be monitored:

1. Elevated cholesterol and triglyceride levels in serum

2. Blood pressure elevation

3. Obesity

4. Smoking

5. Lack of physical exercise

6. Elevated blood uric acid levels

7. Diabetes

Observers of vascular disease feel that fat in the diet cuts down the blood flow, causing red blood cells to become "sticky," that is, they clump together, further reducing the supply of oxygen to the tissues. This poor nourishment of the blood vessels causes weakness which then allows the cholesterol and fats to invade the damaged cells, thus narrowing the vessels further. Excess sugar intake is also associated with adhesiveness of blood platelets. Platelet clumping is the first step to clots and thrombosis.

These two conditions, often working together, are responsible for the vascular problems that take so many of us too early. One is the atheromatous plaques which are formed by the influx of lipids and lipoproteins—usually the low-density ones—into the arterial walls. Platelets are the other factor. These form thrombi, the final insult, plugging up the vessels and producing heart attacks, strokes and pulmonary emboli.

A logical program would be to test the lipid levels of young people only if there is a family trait of blood fat transport abnormalities and cardiovascular disorders. Lifestyle may contribute more to vascular disease than do the lipid levels. Obesity, imbalanced diet, poor intake of nourishing foods, alcoholism, diabetes, liver and thyroid disease, and use of oral contraceptives all seem to be more related to high risk of vascular disease than the blood lipids alone. The risks from smoking, high blood pressure, and lack of exercise should be stressed more than getting a checkup and a blood test.

What the researchers are finding (and what most of us are seeing by looking around) is that huge amounts of fatty acids are being stored as triglycerides on a lot of bodies. Serum cholesterol and triglyceride concentrations are best correlated with obesity. If a person is fat, he or she is more likely to have blood lipid elevations.

Heredity factors and excess insulin secretion help to explain some of this. If quick sugars, like sucrose and dextrose, are consumed in higher-than-needed amounts, the sugar is stored as glycogen (in liver or muscle) or is converted to fatty acids and then stored as fat, with the help of insulin. Researchers are now speculating that the rapid increases of cardiovascular deaths may be a result of the increased sugar in our diet rather than the increase of fat. In England the rate of death from coronary disease rose tenfold from 1926 to 1939. This increase is correlated with increased ingestion of sugars rather than fat.

The American Heart Association (1978) recommends that we reduce our cholesterol intake to less than 300 mg per day and the fat level to less than 30 percent of the total calorie intake of the patient with elevated cholesterol. In the entire policy statement only one phrase suggests that refined sugar plays a role: "Acquired hypertriglyceridemia may be related to alcohol or excessive calories and carbohydrates." Where have these leaders in vascular research been? Sugar (white, brown, corn syrup, maple syrup, molasses, and honey) turns into fat. My mother knew that. I knew it before I went to medical school.

Fats, sugar, and salt are too high in the American diet. A few years ago a study in New York revealed that 45 percent of the ten- to fourteen-year-old students had a cholesterol level of over 180 mg per 100 ml—too high for that age group.

Those who have a genetic need to watch their cholesterol level must achieve a diet low in saturated fats. Beef is especially sneaky, because the fat is all through the interstices of the lean part of the meat. Some fat can be trimmed from pork; plenty is still left in the pink meat. The fat in hot dogs, 18 percent in 1899, was almost double that in 1968. We have been told that many products labeled "vegetable oils" will "reduce cholesterol levels" and are safe. This assertion is false. Some vegetable oils are highly saturated and would be dangerous or at least inappropriate. Some nondairy creamers use coconut oil, which is highly saturated. Palm oil is saturated; so are the fats listed as "hardened" or "hydrogenated." These oils and processes are used only to prolong the shelf life of foods.

Milk may not be the villain it was once thought to be. When attempts were made to increase the cholesterol level in the blood by using two quarts of whole milk per day, cholesterol levels stayed the same. A "milk factor" may be at work inhibiting the enzyme that synthesizes cholesterol in the liver. Yogurt was more effective in raising blood cholesterol levels, but whole or skimmed milk helped reduce the levels. Butter, taken alone without the milk, did raise the cholesterol levels. Hard cheese raises the cholesterol, but cottage cheese and sour cream don't. The cholesterol-lowering property of milk may be in the fat-globule membranes; butter doesn't have this.

(Maybe something other than butter could be used to make the bread slide down more easily. It is said that the use of butter on bread began in medieval times. Guards on the castle wall were suspicious that the stewards bringing their food might be dropping the bread in the courtyard, wiping it off, and returning it to the tray. But if the bread were spread with butter, then bits of dirt, straw, and manure would reveal whether the bread had come straight from the oven or not.)

Not all milk is good for us. Dr. Kurt A. Oster, emeritus chief of cardiology at Park City Hospital, Bridgeport, Connecticut, believes that homogenization of milk releases a chemical, xanthine oxidase, that may initiate the original lesion in the blood vessel wall. His worldwide observations indicate that in places where milk is consumed raw or only boiled, the cardiovascular disease rate is low. In countries where the milk is pasteurized and homogenized, the vascular disease rates shoot up. Finns have a high rate, presumably from a high intake of homogenized milk. Folic acid, 20 to 80 mg per day, plus vitamin C in large doses, are xanthine oxidase inhibitors.

Do we need any fats at all? Fatty acids are used as an energy source, as a carrier of fat-soluble vitamins, and as an aid to digestion. Because cholesterol and fat are found in breast milk, it is assumed that it is necessary for the growing brain. Once the brain and body have grown, a little bit of fat, especially linoleic acid, is needed for the integrity of the skin. The Scots have one of the highest death rates from coronary occlusion in all of Europe (the rate for Finns is higher). Recent research in Edinburgh and in Finland revealed that the diets of those suffering from vascular troubles were very low in essential fatty acids (EFAs), which include linoleic acid and arachidonic acid. These EFAs must be obtained from a dietary source because the body cannot make them. These fats are precursors to prostaglandins and are able to inhibit platelet aggregation. The Scots and Finns have a diet high in saturated fat and low in polyunsaturated fats (where EFAs are). Cholesterol levels were not different in the group that suffered the coronaries.

Dr. Pritikin would have us believe that to avoid vascular trouble—and to treat it—we must cut out fats and oils, saturated and unsaturated. Nuts and seeds are taboo, except chestnuts, which have no oils. He gets remarkable results, but many people have had difficulty sticking to the diet because it is so boring and so difficult to get used to. He does stop refined sugar, white flour, and other junk. Might he be less rigid with the fats since he is getting good results from the discontinuation of sugar? In any case, one way or another, we have to get linoleic acid; it *is* essential.

Are polyunsaturated oils—those rich in unsaturated chemical bonds—a suitable substitute? Have all the corn, safflower, peanut, and cottonseed oils been a real help? Can we substitute these for the hard (saturated) fats and so banish worry about our vascular system? Dr. Pritikin says *all* the fats are bad for us. He keeps his patients under 10 percent fats and oils (the average American diet is at 40 percent or more fats and oils). If we were to replace the saturated with polyunsaturated at the same percent of total calories, some problems might follow. Vitamin E is always needed to prevent oxidation of the unsaturated bonds. Premature aging may result if these fats are damaged. Oxidation of the excess unsaturated fatty acids may produce free radicals, which can damage cells. The old-age pigment, lipofuscin, may be the result of this damage. Gallstones have been known to increase in those consuming more unsaturated fatty acids (cholesterol concentrated in bile). (See Degenerative Diseases.)

If unsaturated oils are used in cooking, heat plus oxygen produces toxic substances which could be carcinogenic. If there were some way we could know how our hearts and minds will be at age ninety, then we would know what to do now. I'm sure you know people who eat a steak every night after a couple of highballs and live to be eighty-five years old. However, alcohol consumed with a fatty meal produces a rise in lipemia greater than that produced by either one taken alone.

Are the doctors who recommended diet control for "at-risk" patients satisfied that this is the end-all of cardiovascular disease? A few years ago a survey revealed that those scientists interested in arteriosclerosis problems in twenty countries around the world felt there was a connection between vascular problems and diet and that some recommendations should be made about reducing animal fats and refined sugar. After the McGovern Committee suggested in 1979 that we cut down on dairy and animal fats, reduce the intake of sugars and salt, and increase the intake of fruits, vegetables, and whole grains, the dairy interests complained, the beef industry objected, and the sugar trust said their product was pure. The American Medical Association, in an effort to bring order out of the conflicting opinions, made a policy statement: "No one has proved that diet has anything to do with disease," (what about caries, obesity, cirrhosis, hemorrhoids, some cancers, diabetes?), "and furthermore, if Americans changed their diets, it would seriously disrupt our economy." Some doctors, like Gilbert A. Leveille, professor of food science and human nutrition at Michigan State University, feel the whole population should not be subjected to a diet that may benefit so few. He feels that Americans do not suffer from diseases because of what they eat.

But consider these disturbing facts: heart attacks are increasing in China despite low-risk factors; in many countries the heart attack rates vary by as much as 400 percent despite similar dietary fat intakes; the heart attack rate in Finland is 13 times higher than in Japan, but the hypertension rate is only 2 times higher. The heart attack rate in Greece is one-tenth that in the United States. Some feel the consumption of olive oil (2 percent of all calories consumed) is protective; it has monounsaturated oleic acid. Greek men have low serum cholesterol associated with these high levels of oleic in their body fat. Whom do we believe? Everyone is right, but not completely. Maybe some other factors—just as well documented—should be recognized by doctors in the U.S.

For instance, heart disease death rates, although accounting for more than half of all deaths, have been falling in the last fifteen years. Age-adjusted heart disease mortality declined by 20 percent in the United States between 1968 and 1976. But the average American was eating twice as much beef and the sugar intake was still rising. Americans were eating fewer eggs, but as we have seen, that fact really has nothing to do with heart attacks. They did eat 40 percent less saturated fat and 55 percent more polyunsaturated fat than in 1950. In 1955 more than 50 percent of males smoked; in 1975 about 40 percent did. There was an increase in sales of bikes, tennis rackets, and sports equipment in general. Coronary-care units probably contributed by preventing a significant number of deaths.

Dr. Emil Ginter believes that the improvement in cardiovascular statistics is due partly to a shift in dietary habits but is better correlated with the increased consumption of vitamin C by Americans. Now we have to find out if the survivors are the ones swallowing ascorbic acid. A dose of 1000 mg a day seems to be the minimum that will help increase the liver production of P-450, an enzyme that speeds the conversion of cholesterol to bile. Vitamin C helps increase the amount of HDL cholesterol, the safer form. Vitamin C also lowers overall cholesterol levels about 12 percent in one year of use. When iron (in the absorbable ferrous form) is taken with fatty acids, a peroxide is formed together with the unabsorbable ferric form. Vitamin C reduces this. Vitamin C also helps the body make chondroitin sulfate A, the "mortar" in healthy arterial walls. (Cholesterol attaches only to damaged cells.)

Other lipid investigators believe that someone must be swallowing all those vitamin E capsules and that the increased use of d-alpha-tocopherol explains the increased survival rates. Vitamin E has the following benefits: it dissolves clots in veins, prevents clot formation and pulmonary embolism, decreases the need for oxygen, works as a vasodilator and opens up collateral circulation, and restores normal capillary permeability. Vitamin E also relaxes and diminishes scar tissue, preventing scar tissue contraction. It also improves the athletic performance of humans, dogs, and horses. Dr. Evan Shute has been working with vitamin E for about fifty years and believes that there were 10,000 fewer heart attacks in 1980 because 40 million people are taking big doses of vitamin E. A dose of 300 units used to work in 80 percent of patients, but now, with smog damage a factor, he feels that patients must use 1600 units. Oxygen, enzyme action, and oxidizing chemicals in smog are the converters of unsaturated fats into peroxides. These peroxides damage cells. Vitamin E prevents this oxidation. The more unsaturated fatty acids are consumed, the more E is required.

Lecithin is a phospholipid that helps to emulsify fat. It is digested and absorbed like a food, but the constituents (especially choline) re-form and help the transportation, metabolism, and excretion of cholesterol. Twenty to 30 grams of lecithin per day, along with restricted sugar and fat, often will lower cholesterol and increase the HDL (7 to 10 capsules is equivalent to 1 tablespoon of lecithin granules, and 2 tablespoons equals about 30 grams. Because lecithin has a large amount of phosphorus, calcium and magnesium should be taken along with it.

Alfalfa has been helpful in lowering the cholesterol levels and dissolving arteriosclerotic plaques in some monkeys fed a diet high on cholesterol and fat. High-fiber diets also are linked to a low incidence of heart and artery disease. Pectin, high fiber, and bran in the intestinal tract have a cholesterol-lowering effect. Oats seem to be helpful.

Homocysteine is a toxic amino acid whose presence encourages the atherosclerotic process. It is rendered harmless with vitamin B_6—which may explain why women on the Pill have increased vascular problems, since the Pill requires B_6 for its metabolism. Maybe the primitive people who eat lots of high-fat and high-protein foods do not have atherosclerosis because they don't cook their meat as we do and hence have more B_6 to handle the homocysteine.

Epidemiological studies indicate that those living in hard water (calcium) areas have fewer heart attacks. One function of calcium is to combine with the fat and cholesterol in the intestinal tract and prevent their absorption. Calcium deposits may form in the blood vessel walls, but only if these walls are damaged.

The fact that arterial muscles are more spastic in low magnesium solution may explain the sudden-death syndrome that sometimes follows a recovery from heart attack. Some of these people can be identified prior to their fatal illness by a hair analysis showing low magnesium. The average daily intake of magnesium in the United States has decreased by about 20 percent in the last seventy years.

Hair samples of arteriosclerotic patients are often low in zinc and chromium. (See Hair Analysis in Chapter 4.) Zinc helps tissues heal, and chromium is known to help regulate glucose metabolism. Those fed a high-chromium diet have fewer plaques in the aorta. Little chromium is found in the vessel walls of Americans compared with those of Africans or Asians. Silicon is normally abundant in arterial walls; a good source of silicon is fiber.

Manganese is needed by the body in lipid metabolism. Lipids are low in selenium; 100 mcg of selenium each day is about right.

Inositol in doses of 250 to 600 mg per day helps the body regulate lipids.

Niacin will help to reduce cholesterol. The dose should be increased slowly until 3000 to 6000 mg per day are being consumed. It produces a disturbing flush.

Garlic and onions in good-size daily amounts have a favorable effect on the blood vessels.

Vegetarians have a particularly low incidence of coronary disease. In those over sixty-five, the mortality rate was 30 percent less than the rate of the meat eaters.

To better your chances of avoiding coronary heart disease (especially if you have high blood lipids and your family has a history of vascular disease), you may want to follow the following suggestions with your doctor's help:

1. Stop sugar; cut out salt.

2. Reduce saturated fat, margarine, butter, beef, pork.

3. Stop smoking.

4. Exercise three to four times a week strenuously enough to get your heart rate up to 130 beats per minute, and maintain that rate for fifteen minutes.

5. Eat three to four meals a day. Use the four-day rotation plan, that is, eat the same food only every four or five days. (See Allergies.)

6. Increase bran, fiber, roughage, until you have at least one soft bowel movement a day.

7. Take vitamin C, 1000 to 10,000 mg per day, depending on bowels, allergies, and infections.

8. Vitamin E, 400 units, is standard. If high blood pressure is present, vitamin E may aggravate it, so build up slowly. If angina, varicosities, hemorrhoids, or circulation problems are already present, try to get to 1200 to 1600 units.

9. Take lecithin, 10 to 30 grams per day.

10. Do not drink homogenized milk. Use skimmed with a drop of cream or 1 percent milk. If you have gas or allergy problems, get calcium from oyster shells or calcium gluconate (1000 mg). Magnesium, 500 mg, should accompany the calcium. Best taken at bedtime with 1000 mg of C.

11. Add zinc in 30-mg doses, more if you have prostate trouble. Also include chromium, 1 mg; manganese, 5 mg; and selenium, 100 mcg. Brewer's yeast is also good.

12. B complex, with 50 to 100 mg of each of the Bs, is a must. The B_6 may have to be increased until dream recall is adequate. Most B-complex capsules have inositol in them. Niacin works to reduce lipids, but the flush is uncomfortable; build up slowly. B_6 helps many enzymes involved with metabolism.

13. Try to be more of a vegetarian unless you are a Masai or an Eskimo. If you love eggs, and if your cholesterol is OK, eat them only every four days—not because of the lipids, but because of any possible allergy problem.

14. Unsaturated fatty acids which contain essential fatty acids may help. Linoleic acid combines with zinc to make alpha E 2 prostaglandin, which helps open up blood vessels. With little of these acids and zinc in the diet, prostaglandin F 2 will be the predominant product form. It tends to cause vasoconstriction.

Omega-3 and omega-6 fatty acids will reduce cholesterol and low density lipoprotein in the plasma. But only the omega-3 fatty acids from fish oils have a triglyceride reducing action. Ingesting 4 to 8 grams per day (about 1 to 2% of the

daily caloric intake) of these omega-3 fatty acids will probably reduce plasma lipid levels and platelet adhesiveness.
One should not just add this eicosapentaenoic acid to the
diet; fats in general should be reduced. Using cod liver oil
may add too much of the vitamins A and D.

CYSTIC FIBROSIS □ In this condition, believed to
be inherited, the mucus-secreting glands of the body produce a thick material which prevents proper function of the
lungs (bronchitis) and pancreas (malabsorption) and excess
salt concentration in sweat.

Most patients have succumbed to respiratory complications by age twenty to twenty-five. Now Dr. Joel Wallach has
indicated that it may be a selenium deficiency acting with or
without genetic factors. The basic defect is an inability to
protect membranes from oxidation injury. Dr. Wallach noticed that a similar illness in animals is corrected with selenium. Selenium and vitamin E protect tissues from oxidation; there is a higher incidence of cystic fibrosis in areas of
the United States where selenium is known to be low.

If the diagnosis is made early, the following might control the illness before scar tissue has formed: selenium, 20 to
300 mcg; E, 100 to 800 units; zinc, 25 to 50 mg; copper 1 to 2
mg; B complex; vitamin C. These should be used along with
the standard vitamin A, D, and essential fatty acids. But some
long-chained polyunsaturated fatty acids interfere with selenium absorption.

It is hoped this information will be helpful for any parents who know that cystic fibrosis is in the family tree somewhere, and whose child is developing some suspicious
symptoms.

D

DEGENERATIVE DISEASES □ As we age, we all
have to expect a few aches and pains, a slight elevation of

blood pressure, some sleepless nights, memory loss, gray hair, flabby skin. But, we say, God give us the strength to go on as long as we are useful and then go suddenly. For some of us, it's a process of wearing out slowly all over. Others are so unfortunate as to acquire some nasty, devastating failure in one organ while the other organs are still functioning fairly well.

Stress, allergies, pollution, sugar, and mean people all wear us down. If we notice a weakness in our early years, something can be done to shore up that area so the expected degeneration will be evenly distributed in each organ. If your body is in great shape but your brain is just a few feeble synapses, what's the point? If you had known you were going to live this long, wouldn't you have taken better care of yourself?

An interesting theory of disease has been offered by the nutritionist Jeffrey Bland. He believes that disease involves the inefficient transfer of energy. The degeneration of tissues is associated with lipid peroxide formation. This peroxidation forms pigments which choke off cellular function. One of these pigments, lipofuscin, becomes especially noted in the heart.

Drugs will induce peroxidation, which causes cross linkage of DNA strands in the nucleus of cells (cancer connection?). Cell membranes are affected, especially the red blood cells. When oxygen combines with the carbon molecules in cells, energy transfer is reduced. Some cells die. Degeneration sets in.

The liver is essential in detoxifying the body. Vitamins C and B increase cytochrome reductase, which aids the liver in detoxifying enzymes.

Vitamin E increases the P-450, another key enzyme that helps prevent peroxidation.

Selenium is an antioxidant; it reduces the peroxidation. Sulfur helps too.

Polyunsaturated fats are more easily attacked by oxygen;

these peroxides are known stimulators of carcinogens. A high-sucrose diet increases the peroxide damage to the liver.

Deficiencies of iron, zinc, and copper cut down the P-450 function. Another enzyme, superoxide dismutase, is protective. Glutathione peroxidase contains selenium and controls peroxidation. Cancer is more common in selenium deficient animals.

Pick out a few areas where you are weak and concentrate on those. I'm a skin and mucous-membrane person, so I take plenty of A, C, and zinc along with the Bs. Remember, once you slip, it's hard to feed yourself well enough to get back to normal functioning again. If you feed yourself right in the first place, perhaps you won't slip. Or maybe not until you're ninety-five.

According to Dr. William Philpott, the following should be taken as a defense against degenerative disease:

Vitamin C, 1000 mg
Vitamin B_6, pyridoxal-5-P04, 50 mg three times a day
Vitamin B_2, 100 mg
Calcium, 1000 mg
Magnesium, 500 mg
Zinc, 30 mg
Folic acid, 30 mg
Vitamin E, 400 units

DEPRESSION □ Someone estimated that about 40 million people in the United States and Canada have a significant few days of depression every month. Two-thirds of them are women whose menstrual cycle is the triggering factor. In some of the depressed, a trauma (death, divorce, financial reverses, unemployment) is quite obviously the inciting event. But in most of the withdrawn, quiet, weepy ones there was no cause, or the stated reason is too feeble to explain the depth of the response. ("I flunked my driving test." "The cake fell." "My mother-in-law is coming for a few days.")

After a death or loss, it takes time to work out one's grief. It takes about six months; we deny, we feel angry and guilty, and then acceptance comes and we say "I'm OK now." We usually eat less when saddened, and this stress tends to put us in a deficiency situation. Vitamins and minerals are necessary to help the brain enzymes produce enough brain chemicals to keep us sane and cheerful.

A depressed person should be recognized when still in the period of apathy (q.v.); it is always easier to treat depression in the early stages. With some people it is quite obviously due to diet: sugar, food additives, processed foods, allergens. Moods may swing as fast as it takes to eat a doughnut followed by coffee and sugar. Many have a craving for some food they must eat daily. (See Allergies; Hypoglycemia.) The speedier the ups and downs, the likelier it is that food is causing the depression. The depressed person, however, has no insight into the inappropriateness of his response. Some loved one may have to forcibly change the person's diet.

Medication prescribed by the doctor (for example, Elavil) may be lifesaving, since suicide can happen to the least likely person. But the fact that the medication is at all helpful means that some brain chemical is not being produced in sufficient amounts.

Norepinephrine and acetylcholine are chemicals made by enzymes that don't function without certain vitamins and minerals. The whole B complex usually is used to help those enzymes; vitamin shots may be necessary to initiate the improvement, because intestinal absorption may be faulty. B_1 (thiamine), 200 to 1000 mg daily, helps also to fight the fatigue that accompanies depression. B_6 (pyridoxine), 300 to 500 mg daily, is an old friend and is especially beneficial if the menses make the depression worse. B_3 (niacinamide), 100 to 5000 mg daily mixed with enough niacin to create a flush (100 to 1000 mg daily), helps cerebral metabolism and promotes cheerfulness. Pantothenic acid (a cortisol precursor) at 1000-mg doses is important because many forms of depression stress the adrenals. PABA, choline, and biotin have helped. Vitamin C helps all systems, and at least for a while, a dose big enough to loosen the stools would turn the emotions around (10 to 15 grams per day). Magnesium (as oxide, 300 mg three times a day) is a spark that often gets many of these enzymes going; sometimes it works all by itself (it acts like lithium). Vitamin A helps some people (10,000 to 30,000 units a day). When control is achieved, the prescription drug can be reduced slowly and then the vitamins can be cut back to a maintenance dose. Usually something good happens in about two weeks, but a month is the minimum trial before beginning to look elsewhere. I have had patients who were taking all the "right" nutrients and nothing happened until they got the nutrients either intravenously or intramuscularly. (Low thyroid, yeast, and heavy-metal poisoning would slow the response.) Perhaps the easiest type of depression to treat is the postpartum blues: B_{12} and folic acid seem to be ideal. Some give anywhere from 1000 to 10,000 mcg of B_{12} in a muscle shot daily along with 1 to 20 mg per day of folic acid. I usually mix B_{12} (1000 mcg) in a syringe with folic acid (5 mg) and inject it daily or have a spouse do it. Most women are improved in three days. Some need a maintenance booster every week or so. (I wonder if these people are destined to develop pernicious anemia at age fifty? Is depression an early sign of pernicious anemia?)

These things are not given in a vacuum. Some people need psychotherapy as well as a loving touch. But no psychotherapy works if only the lower "gorilla" brain is all that is available. Therapists must feed their clients some nuts, seeds, or cheese at the beginning of the treatment hour.

Most psychiatrists believe that depression can manifest itself with these clues: The infant, if depressed, cries with colic and bangs his head. The six- to eighteen-month-old is apathetic and withdrawn, while the two- to six-year-old acts out his depression by temper outbursts, running away, or by being accident-prone; they call themselves bad. The adolescent uses denial, but the depressive equivalents appear as boredom, restlessness, inability to concentrate, losing interest easily, and jumping to new occupations. Fatigue is common. Hypochondriasis. Delinquent behavior. Sexual promiscuity. Shoplifting. Depression is at the root. It is the person's reaction to loss. But we have also seen all those symptoms and signs in the hypoglycemic, in the hypothyroid, and in those with food allergies.

A low-protein diet following stress will lead to depression. Some people are depressed if they have been overloaded with iron; but an iron deficiency also will lead to apathy and depression, as can zinc and manganese deficiencies. These minerals are needed to help make many enzymes function.

I am disturbed when I see people receiving lithium for a depression that is clearly diet related. Lithium is indicated for the manic-depressive type—the person who is up for six months and down for six months. It is very useful. Many have found that if lithium works, magnesium often does too. It is cheap and safer. Bipolar, or manic, depression has a genetic factor operating. If lithium is helping, those who are taking it should know that the blood test to monitor the level is best taken ten to twelve hours after the last dose. Another consideration: the kidney mechanism that is involved with sodium reabsorption also handles lithium; if a lithium patient suddenly decreases his sodium intake, he might have a rise in lithium levels. By eating a great deal of salt, on the other hand, he may knock the lithium down, and the depression could be renewed.

If the depression is unipolar (no highs) and if the same condition is found in close relatives, Elavil is one of the best medications. It doesn't work as well with a depressed person who has many relatives with alcoholism and antisocial behavior. (I would assume the latter case is due to hypoglycemia, and the best prescription would be to restrict sugar and take large doses of B complex.)

DIABETES □ Diabetes is really many diseases involving the body's sugar metabolism. It is considered a hereditary illness and may appear in a child after a virus infection (for example, when the mumps virus destroys the islet cells in the pancreas where insulin is made). About 20 percent of siblings of children with overt diabetes have the tendency to the disease or already have it. Testing the urine of a brother or sister of a diabetic child is best done after a meal or during an infection. Dr. Alva Strickland found a higher percentage of red hair and freckles in diabetic children than in control subjects.

Pregnancy may precipitate diabetes in a susceptible person. Eighty percent of adult-onset diabetics are overweight when the disease is diagnosed. Obesity and excessive consumption of calories tend to create a resistance to insulin. Hamsters genetically predisposed to diabetes will not develop the disease if their diet is limited as compared to those that are allowed to eat as much as they want. In a study, the latter all developed diabetes. It suggests that the more we eat, the more the pancreas puts out insulin, and the more insulin, the lower the blood sugar falls and the hungrier we get.

Insulin helps the body to store calories as fat. When the blood sugar of a diabetic falls, the person gets hungry and eats again, often a quick carbohydrate. Up shoots the blood sugar to a level high enough (above 160 mg percent) to allow diagnosis. Many diabetics have a normal amount of insulin; the problem is that the insulin is not controlling the blood sugar level as it should.

When obesity is combined with high blood sugar, there is a relative deficit in number of insulin receptors. (These are cellular structures to which the insulin molecule must attach before it initiates its unique function of converting glucose to glycogen or fat for storage.) When calorie intake is reduced, less insulin is produced, less insulin reaches body cells, and they respond by producing more insulin receptor sites. The insulin produced is more efficient and blood sugar is kept at normal levels. A *lean* person who develops diabetes will more likely have to take insulin for control.

Most maturity-onset diabetic cases were obese when they were diagnosed. This suggests that the high amounts of insulin secreted due to the carbohydrate ingestion somehow blocked the receptor sites on cells when the diabetes became manifest. Most obese diabetics have elevated amounts of insulin.

Dr. James Anderson, associated with the University of Kentucky Medical Center, Diabetes Department, has done research and written books about the subject. He feels that diabetics in our country are consuming too much fat and not enough fiber-rich complex carbohydrates. These foods have the property of releasing their energy over several hours, in contrast to the thirty minutes it takes for sucrose and quick sugars to hit the bloodstream. The high-fat diet that is the habit of most people in our country creates an insulin insensitivity.

He points out that the incidence of vascular disease, heart attacks, and gangrene in the diabetics of Japan and India is much less than in those of England and the United States, because peoples of the former two countries eat a much higher amount of vegetables, grains, and fiber-containing fruits and a much lower amount of meat and fat. As a consequence, he feels, the insulin needs of people in England and the United States are higher.

Seventy-five percent of the deaths of diabetics in our country are due to heart attacks. Carbohydrate restriction means the proscription of sugar but not of carbohydrate foods: whole grains, potatoes, beans, peas, and other vegetables that give up their calories over a long period of time after ingestion. These complex, long-acting vegetables and fruits must be urged on the diabetic along with foods with a high fiber content; then the diabetic will begin to notice less need for insulin, and control of blood sugar fluctuations will be easier.

In South Africa forty years ago only 5 percent of routine hospitalized patients had diabetes. Now 45 percent have the problem. Is this what modernization does? Here is another fact: every year a number of former desert dwellers who have moved to Israel become diabetic. All have a similar genetic makeup. The longer their exposure to sugar, it seems, the greater the likelihood of their getting this carbohydrate malfunction.

Diet controls 90 percent of maturity-onset diabetes. The diagnosis is usually made by the glucose-tolerance test, in which 100 grams of sugar are swallowed. The fasting sugar should be no greater than 110, the one-hour level below 160, two-hour below 120, and the three-hour down again to 110. The test would best be extended to five or six hours to see what the level goes down to. Some hypoglycemics are at 300 at one hour and down to 40 at the fourth hour. Those who are above these arbitrary levels and show no symptoms are called chemical diabetics. If obese, they will easily slip into diabetes. For them diet control is almost an emergency. (See Obesity.)

Dr. William Philpott believes that 50 percent of diabetics do not have the classic aninsulinemic diabetes; that they are suffering from carbohydrate mismanagement and would better qualify for the food-allergy category (q.v.). He insists that "diabetics" should fast and then be tested with one food per day, with simultaneous checking of the blood sugar. "The hyperglycemia is an acute allergically evoked carbohydrate disorder and a miniature diabetes mellitus attack." Symptoms usually accompany the blood sugar fluctuations.

Diabetes is a stress, and stressed people need increased vitamins and minerals. Of course, cutting out sugar and junk food is essential. These people need to find out to what foods they are sensitive and to take large amounts of supplements:

B_6, 100 to 500 mg; B_3, 100 to 500 mg; C, 1000 to 5000 mg— more if infections are a problem. Vitamin C is low in the blood platelets of diabetics. The B complex helps reduce nerve damage (50 to 100 mg of each per day at least). Vitamin E, starting at 100 units and building to 400 or 800, cuts down on artery complications (thromboses) and helps the body store sugar as glycogen. Brewer's yeast, 3 tablespoons a day, supplies some chromium. This B complex and chromium has been shown to be a glucose-tolerance factor; the combination allows the body to get by with less insulin. Zinc is needed for insulin activity and fat-tissue function. Calcium depresses the activity and absorption of zinc; the hair test in diabetics often shows a high calcium-to-zinc ratio. Manganese is often low in diabetics and is needed for glucose utilization; it also helps produce insulin. Vitamin A helps. Excess magnesium in proportion to calcium will suppress insulin activity.

The incidence of unstable or insulin-dependent diabetes includes most juvenile-onset cases and those 10 percent of adult-onset cases who *really* tried to diet and were unsuccessful in controlling the symptoms. Compliance means changing the whole lifestyle, getting on a no-sugar diet, stopping foods to which they are allergic, counting calories and achieving ideal weight, taking B-complex shots, and exercising. If there is still no control, these people will require insulin shots. Poor control with the shots, despite measuring food and calibrating the dose depending on the blood sugar, may be due to the appearance of a foreign-substance response (antigen-antibody reaction) to the animal insulin. This often produces the fragile/labile diabetic who has wide swings of blood sugar. Glucagon from the pancreas and pituitary growth hormones are factors producing instability in control. Insulin by shot never works as well as the patient's own, so every effort should be made to increase the natural insulin. Insulin-induced coma may lead to brain damage.

Having diabetes might just force the patient to take better care of himself. Anastasia Chehak, R.D., a licensed diabetic educator and nutritionist, has found that the key to successful diabetic management is for the patient to put himself under the care of someone who believes in continuing education and constant review of essential information. Motivation, cooperation, monitoring of blood sugar, attention to food intake, exercise, and stress control are all part of the continuing care that has to be part of the diabetic's life.

It is important for the patient to know that new advances are constantly being made in the field. Management is not just a matter of getting an insulin shot every day. Diabetics should be connected with someone involved with the American Association of Diabetic Educators. Turn a deaf ear to anyone who says sugar and white flour are OK.

DIARRHEA □ Most of us get diarrhea every once in a while; usually we call it the flu. When it comes in the middle of a speech, a class, a wedding, it is called stress.

In most cases, one or two runny days means the one- or two-day flu; weakness, cramps, sweats, and pallor are other signs. Taking a lot of water to prevent dehydration is good. Apple juice might restore some lost minerals. Bananas are usually safe, but the more you eat, the more cramps you'll have. So stick to fluids and keep up the vitamin C—unless you think a big dose is aggravating the diarrhea.

If someone has the "intestinal flu" and it lasts more than a week, it is not flu; it is something else. (See Abdominal Discomfort; Colitis.) A specific diagnosis of salmonella or shigella (bacteria infection) must be made. Salmonella diarrhea is supposed to smell like rotten eggs; it just may be the bacteria releasing hydrogen sulfide. If no diagnosis can be made and it is not giardiasis (caused by a parasite), it is called chronic nonspecific diarrhea. By now, it may have slipped into a malabsorption problem because the intestinal lining has been eroded and everything that goes down acts like a dose of salts.

Food allergies can develop suddenly after the stress of a

virus disease. A water fast of four days would reveal the source of the trouble; a new food is added daily until the looseness returns. Having thus identified the offender, avoiding it for ninety days may allow the intestine to forget that it is supposed to shoot it out the other end.

If the problem is chronic nonspecific diarrhea, however, it will not respond to time. Drugs help, but they just treat the symptoms. The treatment is whatever works, so experiment is called for. Acidophilus capsules might change the intestinal flora into something more friendly. Essential fatty acids might do the trick: safflower or cod-liver oil—perhaps a teaspoon twice a day for a few days. Some swear by garlic capsules two to three times a day. In some people a zinc deficiency is associated with diarrhea and a rash (acrodermatitis); 30 mg of zinc two to three times a day might put an end to the diarrhea.

Folic acid deficiency is common in our country because we are not eating the leafy vegetables. A low level is related to diarrhea, and of course, the diarrhea would contribute in turn to a folic acid deficiency. A borderline deficient person may compensate until he gets the flu; the diarrhea will not clear until he gets a shot of folate. Folic acid helps restore bowel enzymes.

After starvation and diarrhea, a temporary atrophy occurs in the lining cells of the intestines, where many digestive enzymes are located. Slow introduction of foods is called for so as not to tax the minimal production of digestive juices. Sprue is a form of malabsorption that leads to delayed absorption of protein, B_{12}, vitamins D and K, folic acid, minerals, and water. Vitamin shots are often necessary. (See Abdominal Discomfort.)

One must be healthy to be healthy.

Naturopaths recommend the following: for acute diarrhea one should stick to juices—blackberry, sauerkraut, and tomato. One part cabbage juice to three parts carrot juice should help replace the fluid loss and provide the body with the lost minerals (especially potassium); drink 4 to 6 ounces every two hours.

Other favorites: teas of slippery elm, gentian, okra, amaranth, or cinnamon. Toasted rye flour is supposed to plug one up.

When improvement is obvious, cooked vegetables, millet, whole-grain rice, and sour milks may be added.

A preventive method that can preclude travelers' diarrhea: two tablets of betaine hydrochloride after each meal. Hydrochloric acid is supposed to kill the bacteria in the stomach. Raw garlic has an antiseptic effect.

DIET □ The optimum diet to maintain perfect health is probably a myth. We are all so different, due to genetic, pregnancy, and environmental factors, that we must individualize nutrients just to get near something suitable and perhaps sustaining. The recommended daily allowances (RDAs) the government has suggested as a guideline apparently are only for survival.

Many of us have genetic needs or dependencies, not just minor deficiencies. Years of experimenting and stumbling about have revealed that many people require large doses of certain vitamins and minerals in order to control some rather nasty problems. If the government says we only need 2.5 mg of B_6 (pyridoxine), but a pregnant woman finds that she needs 50 to 100 mg of it to control her nausea and vomiting, is she cheating to take that amount? Does her nausea and vomiting have to mean that she is rejecting the baby and is bad and must see a psychiatrist?

Don't believe what you hear. Do you always believe the government? Did they measure you when they decided you should only need 5000 units of A? If I have less than 25,000 units I get phlegm and hyperkeratosis. If I were still living in Scotland and eating haggis, oatmeal, and applesauce, I might be OK. If you were still living in Africa, Greece, Hungary, Germany, or wherever your ancestors came from, you might be genetically more suited to the natural foods grown there.

We all have certain basic needs to maintain life. A gram or so of protein per kilogram of body weight is usually enough for us grown-ups.* Now you must decide if you should be vegetarian, carnivorous, or omnivorous. The illness history of your relatives may help you decide. If your family is full of obesity and diabetes, has high cholesterol and triglyceride levels, is prone to atherosclerosis and malignancy, then you should seriously consider becoming a strict (vegan) vegetarian. But remember, you will often be short of B_1, B_2, lysine, methionine, iron, calcium, and vitamin D. Some vegans find it difficult to get adequate balanced protein because they don't know about complementarity, how to combine seeds, nuts, and grains to get all the amino acids. The B_{12} can be made up for with soy sauce, tempeh, certain seeds, beans and nuts, and certain root nodules (for the bacteria thereon). A supplement combining the nutrients that are low in the diet would make it better. Vegans may find that they need to salt their food (sodium chloride) because they are getting a high amount of potassium with little sodium. If much phytate is consumed (grains) in unleavened bread, a zinc deficiency could occur, because phytate combines with and carries out the zinc. A short, pale, pimply vegetarian has probably not gotten enough iron and zinc. (Using yeast in cooking destroys the phytate.) Soy proteins may cut absorption also.

You would be happy to know, however, that it is difficult to be a vegetarian and also be obese; one usually cannot get enough of the low-density carbohydrates into the stomach to gain weight.

Those who eat a lot of animal meat are running a risk, especially in the blood pressure, cholesterol, and cancer departments. Because meat is so full of phosphorus, meat eaters are in danger of having low body calcium; high phosphorus tends to interfere with calcium absorption. Omnivorous

---

* For example: 1 egg contains 6 g protein; 1 oz milk contains 1 g protein; 1 oz meat contains 6 g protein (approximately); one 1-inch cheese cube contains 4 g protein (approximately).

women lose 35 percent of their bone calcium mass from age fifty to ninety. Milk-and-egg-eating vegetarian women lose but 18 percent. They both should be using calcium and vitamin D supplements from age twenty-five on. (See Osteoporosis.)

B_6 is needed to synthesize protein, so a supplement (100 mg) should be used daily if the protein in the diet is high. A protein deficiency could lead to low albumin, edema, and obesity. Magnesium is needed if dietary protein is high. A high-protein diet may make the body lose copper. Meat and milk users should *not* use table salt, because the sodium in meat and dairy products is fairly high.

Meat eaters should take extra calcium. They should try to eat only 2 or 3 ounces at a time of the leanest piece available, and avoid beef. Beef/pork fat is hidden all through the meat. The rind on pork can be trimmed away. (It seems outrageous that so much time and money is spent feeding steers and hogs when we could have or should have been eating the feed itself—corn and soybeans—at a fraction of the cost.)

You take your choice. After our younger years, most of us find that animal meat sits heavily upon us; this is probably a function of reduced hydrochloric acid. The gas and bloat you get after a big meat dinner is probably God saying, "You're eating too much."

Unless you are one of those who feel good when they eat meat, you will probably do well to eat it less frequently. At the very least, restrict the beef, try to rotate the types of meat, and somehow get calcium (1000 mg) and magnesium (500 mg) ingested daily.

(See Allergies; Hypoglycemia.)

ALLERGISTS have found that rotating the diet will prevent the development of many food sensitivities. No food or food group should be eaten daily, if possible; drink milk and eat dairy products only once every four days. Foods eaten daily or frequently will stress the body's capacity to metabolize them and reactions will develop. Many find excess gas, fatigue, diarrhea, aches, headaches, irritability—anything—may appear.

In general, humans should eat a low-calorie mixed diet, with samplings of all the edible foods available. Don't have high-fat or sugary foods in the house. Replace them with high-fiber raw foods.

Take the supplements suggested for your age or your disease or condition and try the following diet. It is safe and good for you.

Breakfast: One orange or piece of fruit (better than juice).
One bowl of oatmeal (rotate with egg, fish, chicken piece, liver, or other whole-grain cereal).
Glass of milk (2%) or high-calcium-type tea.

Snack: Handful of nuts (rotate with other nuts and seeds).

Lunch: Mixed green salad, raw vegetables, or cole slaw.
Bowl of beans or sandwich (rotate with chicken, turkey, cottage cheese, lean meat, or old-fashioned peanut butter).

Snack: Whole-grain bun or granola.
Can of vegetable juice or (better) raw vegetables.

Dinner: Soup (not canned); salad.
Protein (rotate soy, legumes, lean meat, fish).
Steamed vegetable; baked potato or brown rice.
Tea.

Snack: Low-fat cheese or nuts and piece of fruit.

Sleep well; awaken refreshed.

DIPLOPIA □ Double vision, or diplopia, may be present at birth. Surgery is the usual therapy for this. If it appears later in life, it may be due to alcoholism (q.v.), a blow on the head, botulism (poisoned food), low blood sugar, or multiple sclerosis (q.v.).

A doctor's diagnosis should be sought. If a reason cannot be found, you may have to do some detective work yourself. If it suggests the likelihood of neuritis, try the huge oral and intramuscular doses of B complex (100 mg of each of the Bs four times a day for three weeks).

(See Neuritis.)

DIVERTICULOSIS □ Diverticulosis is considered a disease of developed countries, in which little dietary fiber is consumed. Fifty percent of adults in Western civilization have this problem by age eighty. It is assumed that pressures inside the colon produce a little balloon of mucosa through the muscular wall. If the stools are full of fiber, bulk, and water, they easily are evacuated. If dry and hard, the muscular walls of the colon hypertrophy and pressure increases in the lumen, pushing out these small pockets.

The symptoms may be nonspecific: cramping, changes of bowel habits, sensation of incomplete evacuation, and vague tenderness. (See Abdominal Discomfort.) The doctor orders a barium enema x-ray and finds the diverticulae.

They can get worse or infected (diverticulitis) and be as serious as appendicitis. Some bleed. All this from eating constipating foods! Milk is the worst offender. (See Fiber.) Lettuce leaves won't help. No white flour; no sugar.

DIZZINESS □ Dizziness is the subjective feeling of unsteadiness, weakness, and turning. In vertigo, the victim has the sensation that the surroundings are whirling about him. Some serious problems must be ruled out first: alcoholism, hypertension, hypothyroidism, endocrine conditions, and infections.

Usually hearing loss and ringing in the ears accompany

the intense, disconcerting, and overwhelming sense of dizziness—sometimes called Ménière's syndrome (q.v.). (See
Labyrinthitis.) The fact that the symptoms come and go suggests that the blood sugar is fluctuating, that a hive is involving the inner ear, or that a blood vessel is bounding next to a
swollen, sick nerve. Some researchers have found high insulin levels and low blood sugar levels. The afflicted one
should try to write down what he or she ate for the few hours
before the attack.

Magnesium is important (500 mg per day is about right).
B_1 (thiamin) helps the nerves; B_6, B_{12}, and pantothenic acid
help, implying that an allergic process is involved. The cilia
may be lost from the semicircular canals, which help control
balance; vitamin B should help. Manganese might just help
uncoordinated movements. (See Ataxia).

For light-headedness, consider the possibility of anemia,
which would call for iron, B_{12}, and folic acid. Get an examination and a blood test.

DREAMS □ We can find out a lot about our deep
selves by having our dreams analyzed. (I stopped dreaming
about lions after my father died.)

Dream recall and memory problems usually respond to
pyridoxine (B_6). I find that about 20 percent of the population
cannot remember their dreams, and a smaller percent think
they do not dream at all. Women have more trouble recalling
dreams because of their extra need for B_6 to metabolize the
female hormones; those on the Pill need extra B_6.

A dose of 50 mg of B_6 on Monday morning should be
enough to tell you on Tuesday that you did dream the night
before. Some need 100 mg per day. Too much B_6 too close to
bedtime will sometimes "produce" too many dreams and
wakefulness.

Dr. Carl Pfeiffer has found that if B_6 doesn't do it for
memory, then manganese, 5 to 15 mg a day, should be the
next choice. Some people lose their memory because of a
yeast infestation (q.v.).

Memory is important in learning and especially reading skills, and I have helped many children (and some adults) in this regard with large doses of B_6.

"Bad" dreams, scary dreams, night terrors, usually are associated with the adrenalin release that occurs in many people who eat some sugary food or an allergen at bedtime. The blood sugar rises and insulin pours out, reducing the blood sugar rapidly; this releases the adrenalin. The adrenalin gives the scary connotation to whatever dream is in progress. The sleeper may awaken with big pupils, rapid heart, and profuse perspiration. This is an adrenalin attack—it doesn't *have* to be an anxiety attack (q.v.).

E

EARACHE ▫ We associate earache with childhood, but whenever there is a way of communication open between the pharynx and the middle ear, there will be infection—usually painful—behind the eardrum. It develops somewhat the way sinusitis does. An infection gets in, the opening seals over (Eustachian-tube lining swells from infection or allergy), pus forms, eardrum bulges, victim screams. Antibiotics are the standard treatment.

In children there is a high correlation of allergies (milk especially) and the incidence of middle-ear infections. From the first attack we recommend the discontinuation of cow's milk—even in the nursing mother's diet. After a few attacks, however, fluid behind the eardrum may be trapped, requiring drainage, suction, and the insertion of a little tube into the eardrum to aerate the middle ear. The tubes are left in place until the child is about seven years old, after which the anatomy of the area has changed enough that the risk of infection is less.

The nutritional routine for the infant, child, or adult, is to stop the suspect food (milk, sugar), increase the dose of vitamin C until the stools are a little loose (500 to 5000 mg is the average), and increase the vitamin A to 10,000 to 25,000 units a day. When a cold strikes, many have found that increasing the C by 5 to 10 times and doubling the A for a few days will slow the cold down and abort the ear infection. But don't fool around: an earache needs an ear look and usually an antibiotic. A good clue: if the stuff coming from the victim's nose is green or yellow, it suggests a germ and an antibiotic would be appropriate. If the mucus is clear or milky, it may be only a retracted ear drum, and we might try prayer along with the C and A for a day.

The presence of a cold suggests a nutritional slip. Those little viruses are just waiting for a chink to open up in the immunological armor. Then they leap in. The virus lowers resistance so the bacteria can follow.

Dr. Jack D. Clemis, former president of the American Society of Otolaryngologic Allergy, said at an American Medical Association meeting three years ago: "There is mounting clinical evidence that allergy plays a dominant role in disorders of the Eustachian tube, middle ear, and mastoid." If the diet change (you really have to stop eating whatever it is you love to eat every day) and the extra vitamins C and A are not helpful, then some testing for inhalants seems appropriate. Allergies to house dust, wool, or animal dander usually reveal themselves by the sneeze, itchy nose, and watery eyes that occur with close association.

If the sinusitis, bronchitis, or ear infection always follows a cold, and if the cold mucus turns to thick yellow or green pus before the ear attack, many patients will find that a series of shots of dead bacteria (their own or a stock solution) will provide the necessary immunity buildup so the next cold will stay a cold or just dry up without the secondary bacterial infection. (See Respiratory Symptoms.)

EDEMA □ Water accumulating in the tissues is usually a sign of sluggish circulation, which explains why swollen ankles accompany heart failure. The heart is too weak to pump out all the blood, so extra blood backs up; the lungs fill (shortness of breath), the liver becomes swollen, and the ankles fill up. What's called for here, obviously, is to see the doctor and get the heart failure corrected.

Puffy lids, dry skin, constipation, slow pulse, and sluggish thinking would suggest low thyroid function (q.v.). Hypoalbuminemia will allow fluid to leak into tissues.

Women commonly notice that the rings they wear fit tightly two days before their periods begin; the headache, the touchiness, and the period follow, in that order. Most find that just 50 mg of B6 daily is enough, but it must be begun a week or two ahead of time. Pregnancy edema (and nausea and vomiting) needs 150 mg of B6 daily, an occasional vitamin shot, and a diet reevaluation. Salt (sodium) usually is restricted, as it adds to the burden. But some puffiness is normal. Diuretics are considered dangerous in pregnancy edema and should be the last medicine to be used if nutrition is not working. Potassium orally will help balance the sodium. Magnesium has proven helpful in nonspecific puffiness.

Bioflavonoids have been helpful in reducing capillary-wall permeability, thereby decreasing capillary leaks and resultant edema.

If serious disease can be ruled out, exercise and deep breathing may help. The up and down motion of the diaphragm to its maximum excursions helps move lymph fluid away from the tissues.

EMBOLISM □ An embolism is a blood clot that has lodged in an artery, producing a lack of blood to the tissues served by that artery. The common situation is for a clot to break off from a leg vein, travel up through the right side of the heart, and lodge in a pulmonary artery. It is a not-uncommon postoperative event. Pregnancy, injuries to the pelvis and lower extremities, burns, heart failure, or any condition that would require prolonged bed rest may be the cause.

Occasionally pulmonary embolism leads to pulmonary infarction—hemorrhage, collapse, and destruction of lung tissue. The small emboli usually resolve and leave little scar tissue. Shortness of breath is common. A feeling of "impending doom" is often reported if the embolus is large. Chest discomfort, not unlike that of myocardial infarction, is reported. Rapid heartbeat is usually found. The white count rises. Pulmonary function tests are abnormal. An angiogram might be worthwhile.

Because the vascular system is involved here—a clot breaks off of a thrombus, becomes an embolus, and lodges in an artery—vitamin E is of great value. Some authorities will move the units up to 1200 to 2000 daily while monitoring the blood pressure.

EMPHYSEMA □ Emphysema means overinflated. The lung damage occurs in the tiny air sacs in the tissues that meet the capillaries and send out oxygen and pick up carbon dioxide. The walls of the sacs break down and the air spaces enlarge, destroying the elastic tissue and the capillaries simultaneously. Air exchange is reduced.

Shortness of breath (dyspnea) is the most common symptom, but it develops only after the disease is well established. Almost all the victims are cigarette smokers. Many feel that the dyspnea is due to their age or to cigarettes per se ("I'll be OK because I can quit smoking any time I want"). These are the people who stand on the down escalator.

The chronic bronchitis that is usually associated adds to the shortness of breath. In the late stages, the patient is ill, thin, and dyspneic on slight exertion. Wheezing becomes pronounced as the bronchial tubes become filled with mucus. It may be twenty years from onset to the first appearance of symptoms. At the end stage the victim needs oxygen just to be able to turn in bed.

I have treated a few men with advanced emphysema. Vitamin B complex plus C injections were helpful in making them more comfortable. It is amazing how difficult it is to get these obviously crippled people to quit the cigarettes.

Vitamin E will help some; build up to 800 to 1600 units a day.

ENDOMETRIOSIS □ Endometrosis is the growth of endometrial (uterine lining) tissue on other areas of the pelvis outside of the uterus. The peritoneal tissues try to encase and subdue these "foreign" endometrial cells with fibrous scar tissue. The symptoms mimic many other gynecological disorders, since the tissue responds to ovarian hormones; there is proliferation and bleeding. Symptoms will quiet down between menstrual periods and during pregnancy.

Pain occurs at the time of menses in most patients with endometriosis. Dull pain low in the abdomen and the low back is characteristic. Sterility occurs in 50 percent of patients. Many have pain on intercourse.

Direct observation of the lesions with the laparoscope makes the diagnosis.

Many with this condition have a thyroid problem. A morning temperature consistently below 97.6° (orally or axillary) would suggest the need for thyroid gland supplements. Vitamin E, 400 to 800 units, may calm the problem.

EXERCISE □ Those who exercise strenuously do not need a lot of extra protein, as once was thought. Some long-distance runners prepare themselves better for a run by using up the glycogen in their muscles and then eating starchy foods—bread, corn, pasta, potatoes, some beans—to fill up the muscles with glycogen. This seems to help them run the twenty-six miles of a marathon, but it doesn't work for everyone.

Exercise is a stress, so the B vitamins are indicated. In one study, those doing contact sports and taking vitamin C and citrus bioflavonoids had fewer injuries than those without these supplements. Runners in particular become zinc deficient; 30 to 60 mg of zinc is about right as a supplement on running days. Vitamin E levels drop in those doing heavy exercise; 400 units every four to six hours might keep the body running efficiently, since it helps to oxygenate the tissues.

Joggers need some monitoring by their doctor to see if the cardiovascular system is working optimally and is able to handle the increased heart rate. Tolerable vascular stress two or three times a week is believed to increase the collateral circulation around any narrowed vessels. Pounding on the hard pavement can break the red cells in the foot capillaries, causing blood to appear in the urine. Choose the best time and place to avoid air pollution while jogging.

Aerobic exercise is that which is done in the presence of adequate oxygen. In the anaerobic form oxygen is deficient and toxic metabolites accumulate; lactic acid is one. This causes the pain and stiffness the day after overuse of the muscles. It can be harmful to heart muscle.

Mitochondria are enzyme-filled structures in each cell that produce energy from dextrose, fatty acids, or amino acids. Water, urea, and carbon dioxide are formed. A gradual increase in exercise each day or every other day will increase the efficiency of the mitochondrial enzymes. Fat and carbohydrate are burned more completely. If one is sedentary, the mitochondria shut down. There are fewer enzymes to burn the fat; lard accumulates.

The mitochondria need vitamins and minerals to act as coenzymes to function properly. The B complex, vitamin E, manganese, zinc, iron, and chromium seem to be the principal ones involved in energy production.

To get oneself in the aerobic training area, the twenty- to thirty-year-old would need to have a pulse rate up to 160 to 175 beats per minute for twelve or so minutes three times a week; this is the way to attain ideal fitness. But the sixty-year-old would only need to push up to about 120 or so beats per minute. One should be breathing deeply but not gasping for air. Working out with someone helps to keep motivation high, but a fitness-oriented doctor or trainer should monitor the buildup. Swimming, dancing, yoga, jumping rope, or anything that will sustain this pulse rate is suitable.

Eating a piece of pie (500 calories) and then trying to walk it off in an hour will give a net gain.

Exercise		Uses up (per minute)
Walking	at 4 mph	7 calories
Jogging	at 5 mph	12 calories
Cycling	at 12 mph	10 calories
Swimming	leisurely	6–8 calories
Skipping rope	vigorously; landing on both feet	13–14 calories
Rowing, outdoor	at 6.5 mph	14–15 calories

An exercise fitness program will increase the levels of high-density lipoproteins (the safer kind), elevate the mood, and reduce the perception of stress. It is known to increase the secretion of endorphins, our own private painkiller. Exercise improves job performance and is associated with better health indices and greater longevity.

Exercise is called the eighth nutrient group—right along with water, oxygen, protein, fats, carbohydrates, vitamins, and minerals.

Do something—turn to the section on Obesity.

EYES □ Most of us are aware that nutrition can affect the eyes—for example, that vitamin A deficiency can lead to night blindness, or at least make it hard to see things in the dusky light. If you do have this trouble, try a few thousand units more than the RDA of 5000 units. If night blindness is associated with a "nutmeg-grater" feeling on the skin surface of the upper outer arms and thighs, vitamin A is surely deficient. Try 25,000 units a day for a month; it should help both eyes and skin. Red and crusty eyelid edges also respond to vitamin A.

If the white conjunctivae have dilated (or at least obvious) capillaries over the surface, B_2 should clear it up (25 to 50 mg a day). Blepharitis, or scaling of the eyebrow skin, is related to seborrhea; try zinc (30 to 60 mg), B_2 (25 to 50 mg), B_6 (50 to 200 mg), all daily, as well as essential fatty acids (q.v.).

Yellow plaques in the lids usually are due to pathological hypercholesterolemia. Get the blood test and do something about your diet. (See Coronary Artery Disease.) Cholesterol often gets deposited in an arc in the iris. If the arc is gray, it indicates aging or premature arteriosclerosis.

Nearsighted people may be low in chromium; a study indicated that nearsighted people consumed 3 times as much starch and sugar as the farsighted (chromium is missing from processed food). But a deficiency of vitamin D also may cause a progression of myopia. Cod-liver oil (A and D) sounds like a good thing for the eyes. Zinc is found in high amounts in the eye; it is necessary for the metabolism of the A.

Contact-lens wearers often complain of burning and drying sensations; these usually indicate a need for the B complex, especially B_1 and B_2 (riboflavin). Most wearers will benefit from taking 25 to 50 mg of all the Bs daily. If vitamin A is deficient there may be a drying of the eyeball surface; contact-lens wearers should take 10,000 units of A if this occurs. Smoking interferes with the oxygen and carbon dioxide exchange on the surface of the cornea; lens wearers therefore should not smoke. Vitamin C deficiency (and decreased bioflavonoids) will show up as engorged little blood vessels about the edges of the eyeballs.

The movements of the eyeballs are influenced by vitamin B_1. Deficiency of thiamin (B_1) due to alcoholism and a very inadequate diet will often cause double vision and crossed eyes. (But multiple sclerosis and botulism also may be heralded by double vision.)

━━━━━━━━━━ **F** ━━━━━━━━━━

FASTING □ Fasting is a valuable method for differentiating reactive hypoglycemia from a nasty insulin-secreting tumor of the pancreas that requires surgical removal. The patient drinks only water (distilled is best) and the blood glucose level is monitored as it slowly falls, usually without any symptoms. In the normal person or in those with reactive hypoglycemia, the glucose level slowly sinks from 80 to 90 mg percent down to 50 to 60 mg percent in 72 hours.

The blood insulin falls slowly, since no glucose has been ingested to stimulate the pancreas to secrete the insulin. If insulin appears in the blood inappropriately, it suggests further investigation.

The four-day water fast is useful also in discovering food allergies. The first three days are tough because of withdrawal symptoms (headaches, irritability, restlessness). Withdrawal symptoms indicate an addiction to something eaten frequently, usually the person's favorite food. On the fourth day, when all the food (and allergens) have gone through, the faster feels weak but happy, relieved, light, "open," and cheerful. Then a new food is eaten daily until the symptoms recur.

This test is more accurate than skin tests for food allergies. (See Allergies.)

Fasting as part of a weight-loss program is rarely helpful and, indeed, could be dangerous, because only 35 percent of the weight loss comes from fat stores; the rest is from lean muscle tissue.

Many people really feel refreshed after a fast. They explain the lift as a "cleansing," or that the body organs had a chance to "rest." The improvement they notice is probably due to the absence of reaction to chemicals created when allergens were consumed.

FATIGUE □   So many of us are fatigued that it might almost seem to be the normal human condition—except for the few among us who bounce out of bed, exercise, work, sing, love, play, and get by on seven hours sleep, all without using uppers. Are they cheating? Do they take quick naps that refresh them without the rest of the world knowing? (My own trick is a six-hour day: eat, work for four hours, nap for ninety minutes, and then up and eat again.) Genetics must have something to do with it, because many of these alert, tireless folk are eating junk, booze, and *no* extra vitamins!

Anemia is the first thing that comes to the doctor's mind when fatigue is the chief complaint. Needing laboratory confirmation, the doctor has a blood test taken. If the hemoglobin, hematocrit, and number of red blood cells are normal, he will get the white blood count, sedimentation rate, and a urinalysis. These should tell him if there is some infection or a growth that might be sapping the patient's strength. The doctor must search for low thyroid function, diabetes, cancer, or emotional problems. Depressed, apathetic people usually are fatigued, but often it's hard to know if the depression causes the fatigue or the fatigue causes the depression.

Suppose the doctor is very thorough but finds no good medical reason for your bone-weary fatigue. Do you just take to your bed and have someone wait on you until you die of weariness? Sounds asinine. You thank the doctor for the psychiatric referral, but promise you will do a few other things first.

Get your laboratory readouts and see if your results are in the upper, middle or lower third of the normal range of what the laboratory says is OK. You may be at the lower end of iron and thyroid levels for *your* body. Try some ferrous gluconate for a month along with vitamin C. Use kelp tablets, five a day for a month (can encourage a sluggish thyroid gland) after taking your morning temperature (see Thyroid

Problems). Manganese is needed to help thyroid function (5 to 10 mg per day for a month).

Magnesium is low in the diet of many of us; 500 mg a day relieves the touchiness and irritability that lead to fatigue; the world moves back a pace or two. Magnesium is good, too, for morning fatigue. The most common cause of A.M. fatigue is the food eaten at bedtime, a sugar or allergen that causes the blood sugar to sink below a working level. These people have trouble facing the day.

Zinc sparks a lot of energy-related enzymes and would be especially valuable for the adolescent who is pimply, tired, and has white spots in the nails, or for the tired older man who finds his sexual powers slipping and his urinary stream narrowing. Vitamin C helps the whole body and helps the minerals gain access into the body; 2 to 3 grams a day for a month should tell you if it's worthwhile. Pantothenic acid helps if allergy is prominent.

When all the tests are normal, fatigue usually responds to B complex in doses of 50 mg each two or three times a day. The urine should appear bright yellow and dream recall should improve. Biotin will help. PABA has been used at the 1000- to 4000-mg doses. L-glutamine and B_{15} (pangamic acid) also have helped some of the fatigued. (Pangamic acid is usually in the 50-mg size; three to six a day should help in three to four weeks.) Vitamin E is successful if the fatigue is due to circulation or oxygenation deficiencies (400 to 800 units a day). Potassium deficiency often is associated with fatigue, especially in the allergic, those who oversalt their food, and those on diuretics.

If one is drowsy but cannot sleep, B_6 may help, but too much (200 to 400 mg) might make for restless sleep due to vivid dreams.

B_{12}, 1000 mcg, combined with 5 to 10 mg of folic acid as an intramuscular injection will often lift the spirits of the depressed and banish fatigue. If the shot helps the next day, even for thirty minutes, it suggests that one is on the right track; now talk your doctor into doing it more consistently.

If fatigue is an off-and-on thing, it should be easy to figure out that some food is responsible. Energy requires sugar—not the quick stuff, but an even supply that will nourish the brain and body more evenly. (See Allergies; Hypoglycemia.)

Exercise is an important part of the treatment of fatigue; it oxygenates tissues.

FEMALE HORMONES □ Many of the problems of women respond to nutritional supports. It suggests that someone (men? the world?) is stressing them or that they have a vitamin dependency. Stress certainly makes the body use more of the B complex; B_6, in particular, is the female's friend. Female hormones, estrogen especially, increase the metabolism of tryptophan, which demands B_6 (pyridoxine). If they are low in B_6, women may get depressed, irritable, surly, and the response of a nonempathetic husband or boy friend will make the problem worse. Use of the contraceptive pill exaggerates the tendency. However, 50 mg of B_6 two or three times a day usually takes care of the problem within one cycle. Pregnant and premenstrual women with swollen tissues can be relieved with B_6; taking 50 mg orally (or a few shots) usually helps in a few days. (See Edema.) Neuritis, aches in arms, hands, fingers, leg cramps, loss of feeling in hands and feet, all respond to B_6. Prematurely born infants are often low in B_6, which suggests one possible cause for the early delivery. Acne that flares at menstrual times is usually improved with 50 to 100 mg of B_6. Many studies indicate that the "modern" diet does not supply even the 2 to 3 mg recommended—a piddling amount.

Estrogens raise the serum copper with a resultant loss of zinc; 30 mg should be good along with B_6 to neutralize the estrogen reactions. Women on the Pill who are drinking water from copper pipes may be depressed because of a B_6 deficiency and the loss of zinc. A high amount of copper in the hair analysis may mean a high amount of estrogenic substances. This copper is needed by the liver in a metalloenzyme to convert estradiole and estriole to estrone (the safer noncarcinogenic form). The hair loss that may occur in women on the Pill may be due to a high amount of copper in the body.

Sex hormones shift folic acid enzymes away from female tissues; thus folic acid is recommended for women. One to 5 mg of folic acid a day has been known to eliminate cervical (uterine opening) dysplasia, a precancerous condition. Oral contraceptives raise serum fats, but vitamins and minerals reduce the levels. Vitamin E can alter lipids in the blood, and lipids are involved with breast cancer.

Iodine and thyroid dysfunctions are related to some female problems: vaginal infection (trichomonas, or yeast), Bartholin gland cysts, and breast pain. Pregnancy induces a goiter in women who were subclinically deficient in iodine before conceiving.

(See Blood tests for hormones, Chapter 4.)

FERTILITY □ If you want to help newlyweds, throw brown, not polished, rice at them. They both need all the B complex they can get down to make up for the junk they might have eaten during their adolescence and courtship.

If the couple has established that they are ready to start a family, but nothing happens, an investigation by a gynecologist should be launched. The future father must be checked out also; it's not always a female problem. If his live sperm count is not up to standard, he would require a good diet and all the nutrients that help the female (see below). Vitamin A and zinc are necessary for adequate sperm production. After about a month things should improve. If semen is too viscid, vitamin C will help.

If her tubing is patent, her ovaries put out eggs, her thyroid is functioning, and the doctor says, "You're OK," she should try the following at least:

Vitamin C, 1000 mg as a minimum
B complex, 50 to 100 mg of each of the Bs
A weekly shot of B_{12}, 1000 mcg (intramuscular) for three weeks
Folic acid, 1 mg
Vitamin E, 400 units
Vitamin A, 10,000 to 25,000 units daily for a month
Zinc, 30 to 60 mg
Licorice-root tea

Fertility is affected by smoking. One study revealed that female smokers had a 40 percent higher infertility rate than nonsmokers; about a third of male smokers had reduced motility of their sperm. Alcohol affects sperm and potency; alcoholics are more likely to have reduced counts. Drugs affect conception and genital function; a methadone user told me it took about twelve hours for him to have an orgasm.

Anything that can affect the body cells will affect the cells that make up the next generation. Remember, those babies have to grow up and take care of us.

FIBER □ The more we deviate from the way Mother Nature set us up to live on this earth, the sicker we become. It is too bad that it takes decades for an unnatural diet to cause the diseases of civilization. If we ate a slice of white bread and had an attack of appendicitis inside the hour, we would be able to see the connection. The time from the dietary indiscretion to the actual pathology is so long that the relationship is difficult to perceive. But the evidence seems incontrovertible now. We have a Stone-Age intestinal tract, and we *must* eat Stone-Age food: roughage.

Appendicitis appeared in England in the early nineteenth century and became more common after 1900. In 1925 an English doctor described two cases of then-rare coronary artery occlusion. Diverticular disease has been diagnosed with some frequency only since 1930. Gallbladder disease, varicosities, hemorrhoids, pulmonary emboli, hiatus hernia, and cancer of the colon and rectum are rare in those living on a high-residue diet (for example, a primitive African tribal diet). These diseases of civilization were rare before the turn of the century and have become common since the extensive ingestion of milled and bleached flour and refined sugars. Because it took a few decades from the removal of the fiber to the compilation of the statistics that indicated the relationship, we are reluctant to believe the connection because it doesn't happen to everyone. We are loathe to change now because we love that soft, billowy bread and the sweet taste of lemon meringue pie. We are hooked.

Dr. Dennis Burkitt clearly pointed out the connection and has indicated another epidemiological pearl: appendicitis "becomes common in a community several decades before a major rise in frequency of any of the other noninfective bowel diseases." Diverticular disease, tumors of the colon and rectum, and ulcerative colitis have appeared with some frequency in the past fifty years, long after appendicitis surfaced in 1900. These are not genetic conditions; they are environmental. Burkitt blames the roller mills set up in the 1870s for the processing of grain. Fiber made up about 0.35 percent of last century's bread; now it is a feeble 0.15 percent, and less bread is being eaten. Cereal fiber intake also has fallen. Sugar consumption is up. Fruit and vegetable fiber has less impact on the bowel function than does grain fiber. Mother Nature assumed that man would be eating the foods growing on the planet, so she gave us a long (20- to 40-foot) intestinal tract, just right for the foods we are supposed to eat. We are now eating foods designed for a 10-foot-long gut. We need the fiber as a carrying mechanism to expose the proteins, starches, minerals, and vitamins to the absorptive areas. We also need this mucoid vehicle to carry some of the noxious wastes out the other end—and fast. The high fiber content holds moisture and transit time is rapid. African natives' stools may weigh 300 to 500 grams, compared to the Western bit of inferior, dried-up 100 grams. The transit time for these native stools is usually less than twenty-four hours; "civilized" people carry their sludge around for three days, and it is hardly worth dumping when the time comes. Many natives feel that if they do not have a good stool after each meal something is wrong.

If stools take a long time in transit, bile salts are changed to cholic acid, a carcinogen. The long contact of this chemical with the bowel mucosa in a susceptible person could lead to the development of cancer. The Finns eat 80 percent more fiber than do the Danes; both eat about the same amount of fat. Cancer of the colon is 4 times more frequent in Danes.

Straining at stool seems to lead to varicosities, hemorrhoids, and hiatus hernia. Intake of fiber-rich foods and cellulose may protect against hypercholesterolemia. Doctors who treat rural African natives have never seen gallbladder disease or stones. Three-quarters of Swedish women over age seventy have gallstones.

Because these conditions, like tooth decay, are so common in Western men and women, the doctors feel they are part of life; we're expected to get one or all of them as we age. How, then, can we bring people to understand that our Western diet is abnormal and that it leads directly to these preventable conditions? There is plenty of evidence. For example, in a study using diabetic adults, 70 percent of them were able to stop their insulin when they were fed a high-carbohydrate diet and 15 grams of fiber.

Crude fiber is what is left over after plant foods are boiled in acid and then in alkali. But dietary fiber is the plant residue that gets to the colon: pectin, hemicellulose, cellulose, and lignin. Changes in fiber alter not only the bulk consistency and transit time but also the chemistry of the stool contents and the rate of absorption of the calories. Fiber decreases the absorption of water, bile acids, and cholesterol from the intestines into the body. In a twenty-year study, the men who consumed 9 grams of fiber daily had a lower rate of coronary heart disease than the men who ate 6.7 grams daily. The sheer bulk of fiber makes the eater feel full sooner; therefore there is less chance of obesity. Fibrous foods take longer to chew and swallow. The high-fiber diet helped patients who wanted to lose weight. Just by substituting bread with high fiber for that made with bleached white flour, they could lose weight without hunger. Some of their calories went out with the bulkier stools.

Since none of the cereals contains pectin and few fruits and vegetables contain lignin, one must consume a variety of whole grains, fruits, and vegetables to get all the fiber. Each part plays a role. Lignin can bind with bile acids and get them out through the stools. This helps to eliminate some of the formed cholesterol. Subjects consuming from 12 to 16 grams of pectin daily for several weeks had a reduction of serum cholesterol of 8 to 30 percent. Rolled oats, barley, pectin, and alfalfa have this ability to lower the cholesterol by binding with and carrying it out. Bran has no effect on serum cholesterol. Pectin can help stabilize the blood sugar, since it tends to slow the rate of glucose absorption. The fiber content of the American diet is now down to 3+ grams a day compared to 7 grams one hundred years ago. We need to up our intake so our bowels can make our bodies better. A 1977 study clearly showed the improvement that 6 to 7 grams of dietary fiber could bring to patients suffering from diverticular disease. All improved.

Despite all this, the Institute of Food Technologists is dragging its feet; maybe they are used to their bowel habits. They say, "Use of dietary fiber should be looked on with reservations. The feeling of urgency about use of fiber in the nutrition should not cause the public to change." They may never have had the feeling of urgency. Most people in our country have never had a normal bowel movement.

We should swallow about 1½ ounces of bran per day. Most start out at 1 or 2 teaspoons of miller's bran a day and build it up depending on the size and form and frequency of the resulting bowel movements. Lettuce and other salad in-

FIBER CONTENT OF FOODS

Very little or none: white bread, white crackers, white rice, white pasta, fruit juices.

Low fiber (up to 1 gram per 100 grams of food): Whole-wheat bread, brown rice, shredded wheat, oatmeal, asparagus, cabbage, carrots, celery, corn, lettuce, spinach, tomatoes, applesauce, bananas, grapefruit, pineapple, prunes, raisins.

Moderate fiber (up to 2 grams per 100 grams of food): 40% bran flakes, raisin bran, legumes, broccoli, cauliflower, parsnips, pumpkin, rutabaga, apples, most berries.

High fiber (2 to 4 grams per 100 grams of food): All-bran, wheat germ, artichoke, fresh blackberries, dried figs, dried dates.

gredients are less than 1 percent fiber; whole-grain breads and cereals are the best. Seeds are high in fiber; most berries have little seeds that give texture. Nuts and vegetables will help.

These same foods have phytic acid and oxalic acid, which could combine with the calcium, magnesium, iron, zinc, and chromium in a good diet; supplements, therefore, might best be taken at different times than the cereals. However, if yeast is used to bake the bread, phytase is released, which destroys the phytic acid, and so mineral absorption is not affected.

Spastic and irritable colon may be helped with bran, as it normalizes the stools; loose ones are more formed and hard ones are softened.

Usually if patients merely avoid processed foods, white flour, and refined sugar they will get enough fiber to imitate the primitive caveman diet. One to 4 teaspoons of bran (miller's) a day in soup or on cereal should be about right. Rice bran, bran cereal, buckwheat, are all high in bran.

If a doctor wants to treat your diverticulosis (or bowel dysfunction) with the soft and bland outmoded diet, he is treating it with the cause.

FRACTURES ◻ If you are hit by a car, you are entitled to a few fractures. Not everything is caused by faulty nutrition. (Exception: the driver may have had the wrong drink before driving.)

Immobilization to alleviate the pain and allow the healing process to proceed also tends to let calcium run out of the body. Atrophy is not uncommon in bones and muscles that are not being used. A walking cast, exercise, and electrical stimulation are all accepted therapies to promote healing. Nutrition is involved because any injury is a stress and stress depletes the body of C, B complex, calcium, and zinc. These should be increased for the broken body.

Calcium added to the diet of someone who is confined to bed and already losing calcium might be too much for the kidneys to handle and stones might form in those predisposed. Using 500 mg of magnesium, 100 mg of B_6, and 400 units of vitamin D along with the 1000 mg of calcium should nourish the bone and prevent calcium stones in the urine.

Most fractures occur in elderly women who have not kept up on their calcium intake. Many have spontaneous fractures because their bones are so demineralized. A step off the curb can do it. Many of the elderly do not walk because they are so sore and tired, and being sedentary, they lose calcium more rapidly. (See Osteoporosis.)

FUNGUS ◻ We are all covered with germs, viruses, fungi, and yeasts. An invasion of any of these sufficient to cause a recognizable illness is supposed to mean that our usually efficient immune system was not fed properly or was so busy with another stress that it could not handle a sneak attack. Doctors are seeing more fungal and yeast infections (q.v.) because of the widespread use of antibiotics.

The children who get ringworm of the occipital (back) part of the scalp are more likely to be the ones who sit in the front row of the theater (because they are nearsighted?—zinc deficient?) watching the screen with their heads resting on the back of the seat.

Ringworm of the skin is rather easy to treat, but the hair regrowth (in children) and nails in adults does take a while. A dermatologist should consider the possibility that nutrition was partially to blame for fungal invasion, and along with the appropriate medication he should (with warnings about possible side effects) remind the patient to use vitamin A, 25,000 to 75,000 units a day; zinc, 60 to 90 mg a day for three to four weeks and then a lower dose; and iodine, five to ten kelp tablets a day (iodine usually comes as 0.15 mg per tablet, so 0.75 to 1.5 mg is about right).

If you have ever had a fungus, you might assume your body is weak in this department and might continue these nutriments in lower maintenance amounts forever.

G

GALLSTONES □ The proportion of the population who have gallstones is rising. Autopsy examinations reveal that over 60 to 70 percent of the elderly have stones. Most have no symptoms. In medical school, we were told that pain in the upper right quadrant of the abdomen in a woman who was fair, fat, and forty meant gallbladder disease. Now it is encountered in twenty- to thirty-year-olds. The diet change to sugars and fats is largely responsible.

Bile is composed of bile salts, lecithin, and cholesterol. If the cholesterol concentration exceeds the emulsifying ability of the lecithin, the cholesterol starts to precipitate out. The stones are not opaque to x-rays unless calcium gets combined in the stones, allowing them to be seen in the films. If they are small, they pass through into the intestines and out. If large, they stay in the bile duct. If the stone is the same diameter as the lumen of the bile duct, it may start to pass but get stuck, causing a sharp, stabbing sensation.

Women, because of their estrogen production and especially if they are on the Pill, are more likely to have gallstones. These people use up more vitamin E, which is a key factor in fat metabolism. Gallstone incidence may be up because of the increased use of polyunsaturated fats, which require vitamin E to prevent peroxidation. Exercise and weight reduction will reduce the chance of stones. Heredity is a factor; if your mother had them, you may be susceptible.

The prevention diet consists of fruits, vegetables, fiber (pectin is especially important), a minimum of beef and animal meat, no sugar, few saturated or unsaturated fats. (See Coronary Artery Disease.) Vitamin C helps turn cholesterol into bile acids. Lecithin, biotin, inositol, help emulsify the fats. Olive or corn oil (2 tablespoons a day on a salad) is supposed to help. Vitamin B$_6$, 100 to 200 mg daily, is good.

If you need surgery, your abdominal pain and your surgeon will tell you. If you are all doubled up now reading this, it is a little late for nutrition.

GANGRENE □ Tissues that are deprived of oxygen, as in frostbite, crushing injuries, or occluded arteries, will die. Diabetics in particular are prone to poor circulation, occlusive vascular disease, and gangrene of the toes.

Vitamin E can act as a preventive because of its effect on the blood vessels. It improves the circulation by reducing the adhesiveness of platelets, dilating the capillaries, and increasing the oxygen-carrying capacity of the red cells. It will not bring dead tissue to life, but a cold, pulseless foot might have its circulation improved enough to save it from amputation. Vitamin E usually is used at the 400-unit-per-day dose; the threat of losing an extremity would suggest big doses. If there is elevated blood pressure, increases must be built up carefully: 800 units of E for two or three days, then 1600 units for two or three days, then keep the daily level at 2000 to 3000 units until the circulation is improved; then slowly lower the dose. It does seem preferable to amputation.

GLAUCOMA □ We are led to believe that it's normal for pressure to build up in the eyeball as we age. But some elderly people just don't get glaucoma. Heredity must have some connection, but the key seems to be nutrition. How else to explain why some of us will get it and others are never bothered? Stress is a triggering factor. Caffeine can make glaucoma worse.

Dr. Ben Lane has found that glaucoma patients are more likely to be low in vitamin C intake; they were taking only 60 mg daily (the RDA). The mineral chromium also was at a low level in many of those with high intraocular pressure.

This pressure is the most common cause of blindness in adults. All eye doctors check the pressure when doing the yearly checkup for new glasses. If pressure is up and drops are prescribed, use them. But up your vitamin C intake, and ask the doctor to have your hair minerals tested. You might teach him or her something about nutritional support.

Vitamins A (25,000 units) and E (400 to 800 units) help. Calcium should be at the 1000-mg level daily.

GOITER □ The swollen lower throat once was common enough in some areas of the world as to be considered normal. Then someone discovered that an iodine deficiency explained it. Use of iodized salt in these deficient areas has made goiters a rarity.

The thyroid gland has all the ingredients needed to make thyroid hormone *except* iodine. The thyroid-stimulating hormone from the pituitary continues to urge the thyroid gland to produce its hormone, but the gland responds only to the extent of swelling up with cysts full of unfinished hormone. Meanwhile, there is insufficient thyroid hormone in the circulation to tell the pituitary and the hypothalamus to stop their stimulating activities.

Kelp is the common, inexpensive form of iodine (each tablet usually has 0.15 mg). It does not have sufficient trace amounts of other minerals that we all should be getting.

Taking thyroid hormone also should dampen the manufacture of thyroid-stimulating hormone from the pituitary. See your doctor. (See also Thyroid Problems.)

GOUT ☐ Raised uric acid levels in the blood may signal a future painful gout attack. The joint most commonly involved is the one where the big toe joins the foot, but it often appears too in the ankles and knees.

Urate crystals form in the white cells in the painful, swollen joint. Colchicine and indomethacin are the standard treatment. Probenecid helps reduce the high serum urate levels. Allopurinol prevents synthesis of uric acid from purines.

Diet is partially to blame, along with a hereditary tendency. The blood levels of a number of chemicals were tested after some normal volunteers ate an American diet— about 30 to 40 percent sugar. The cholesterol, triglyceride, and uric acid levels rose in all, suggesting that gout is not just a disease of the affluent meat eater. It is everyone's disease. Dr. John Baum has explained that uric acid levels rise with alcohol intake. Caffeine—present in coffee, tea, and many cola drinks—is a trimethylxanthine and will not convert to uric acid. But sugar in after-dinner coffee and liqueurs is a culprit. Extra fluid intake keeps uric acid in solution.

Uric acid levels rise when we are faced with stress, but they fall during hard work. Because coffee drinkers are often coffee addicts, and because the coffee makes the blood sugar bounce around, it probably should be restricted in the gouty. Following the ideas suggested under "Hypoglycemia" should help.

GROWTH ☐ Once you are a full-grown adult (the established age is twenty-five), you are fixed for life—or until you start to shrink after age fifty, when the vertebral discs start flattening out. If you are really short (under 5 feet 2 inches), if all your relatives are 5 feet 3 inches to 5 feet 11 inches tall, and if an endocrinologist has said there was nothing wrong with you in that line, you may have suffered from some nutritional deficiency. If you now have a child who is on the bottom percentile in growth, nutrition can help; the possibility of an emotional or heart or kidney problem must be ruled out, however. Take a morning temperature to check thyroid function (see Thyroid Problems).

Vegetarians who eat a great deal of unleavened bread may not get all the zinc they need for proper growth; the phytates bind zinc and it is largely unabsorbed. White spots on the nails would be a clue.

For a slowly growing baby, 4 mg of zinc per 1000 ml of formula will overcome the problem. Anemia creates ano-rexia, apathy, depression, and failure to thrive. In this case, a nutritional problem can become an emotional one. Iron would help prevent alterations of the intestinal lining, which develop in anemic people.

The B vitamins are all worthwhile, but folic acid in par-ticular affects the intestinal lining cells and thus absorption (folic 1 mg per day). Daily doses of vitamin C, ranging from 500 to 10,000 mg, always help. Manganese usually is defi-cient in our foods and does affect growth (5 to 10 mg per day). Iodine (0.15 to 0.75 mg a day) helps the thyroid to make thyroid hormone.

If you are short, you may still be suffering from the above nutrient deficiencies. Your family may have a dependency on one or more of the suggested nutrients.

═══════════════ **H** ═══════════════

HAIR □ The luster and manageability of hair give some testimony to the general body nutrition. The hair is protein, so a diet that is low in protein, especially in the sulfur-containing amino acids (cystine, methionine), pre-vents the hair from looking healthy.

Zinc in combination with vitamin A has much to do with

the skin enzymes that lay down protein (see Acne). Low zinc levels in the body can lead to hair loss or brittle hair that lacks pigment. Some people have had luck reversing early gray hair with PABA, pantothenic acid, and folic acid. The formula even works on some mice. Dark hair is associated with a high zinc-to-copper ratio. Gray hair usually has a lower zinc-to-copper ratio. (White sheep have little copper in their wool; black sheep have a high concentration of copper. Work that into a dinner-table conversation.)

Lack of a beard might be due to a very low zinc level. Depigmentation of the hair in children is associated with severe malnutrition; alopecia is more likely to occur in severely malnourished adults. However, Carlton Fredericks points out that the prisoners of war who suffered monumental malnourishment seldom lost their hair. Evidently all the body's enzyme systems shut down when protein is severely restricted. Low thyroid function will change the character of the hair (see Thyroid Problems).

The B complex helps every cell, but 500 mg to 1000 mg of niacinamide is especially helpful in making hair "manageable" and improving its luster. Vitamin E stimulates hair growth and color. Lack of sheen and luster as well as any dandruff problem should improve with vitamin A, 25,000 units daily. It will take a few months to see the difference.

Split ends, dry hair, and dandruff improve with vegetable oil. If the hair is oily, removal of animal fats from the diet would make sense. Both dry and oily hair should be better with B complex (B_6 is good for seborrhea), E, C, kelp, bone meal, and cod-liver oil. These nutrients help everything.

Shampoos, rinses, soaps, and sprays are not as important as what happens inside the growing hair follicle at the root where the hair shaft is being formed. Nutrition counts. After three months, ask your hairdresser or barber if he or she can tell what supplements you've been on. Jojoba oil on the scalp may stop dandruff.

(See Alopecia.)

HALITOSIS □ Vitamins B$_3$ and B$_6$ help some halitosis sufferers, presumably by aiding digestion. (See Breath and Breathing.)

HEADACHES □ I'm a headache person. Years ago I read somewhere in psychiatric literature that headaches are a sign that the victim is turning aggression inward upon himself. If he would be more open, verbally or physically, he could minimize the pain. But his parents taught him never to show his emotions; that was a definite no-no. So his normal feelings of anger had no outlet and he somatosized the energy. Instead of headaches, someone else might have an ulcer, or hypertension, or asthma; an inadequate conscience would permit animal behavior.

Although I was outgoing and friendly, it is true that I rarely released angry feelings. When I did, I ended up with a headache. Maybe I was punishing myself for the *expression* of the hostile feelings. Guilt did it.

My years in practice of being helpful, cheerful, sympathetic, and available gave me headaches on Mondays and Thursdays, the high-stress days. I couldn't get mad at a baby for having croup at 1 A.M., and I couldn't take it out on my wife and children, since they had nothing to do with the great inconvenience of illness in my patients. Was I tired and overworked? A lot of sleep only made it worse.

Then my dentist told me I was having too many cavities. I stopped eating the half-pound of cookies I'd been nibbling on every day—and the headaches disappeared. The stress of fifty phone calls on Monday and my partner being away on Thursday still was operative, so I began to pay attention to the nutritional factors of illness. I discovered that the body can cope with a lot of stress if the diet allows the brain, liver, adrenals, and pancreas to function optimally. (I stopped getting cavities too.)

The headache mechanism is thought to be a generalized swelling of the brain or of the blood vessels, sufficient to stimulate the nerve fibers in the meninges, the membranes covering the brain. The brain must be served with oxygen and glucose to support its high-energy metabolism (it is the busiest organ of the body). If the supply of fuel is diminished, the vessels dilate to allow more blood to enter as a compensation. If the blood sugar suddenly drops from 100 to 50 mg/100 ml of serum, the available fuel is cut in half, and before sugar can arrive from storage in the liver, the victim of the hypoglycemic attack might get a headache, or pass out, or feel shaky and hungry.

The dilated blood vessels cause the throbbing, pounding, full feeling in the head synchronous with the heartbeat. This sensation is called a vascular headache. A migraine is a vascular headache with a strong genetic component. It is more usually seen in females, although cyclic vomiting, a migraine equivalent, is more typical in boy relatives of women with migraine.

Doctors tend to feel that if a disease is familial, the patient is stuck; they write out a prescription for something (Cafergot) and tell the patient, "See you once a year." But if someone has the gene, shouldn't the disease manifest itself every day? Why would a woman go along fine for weeks, and then, just when the boss comes to dinner, her head falls off? Something or someone caused a sufficient stress to make those susceptible blood vessels go into spasm and overdilate. Levels of circulating basophils and lymphocytes are reduced in migraine patients, suggesting a defect in cell-mediated immunity.

Two things can be done: reduce the stresses, and nourish the vascular system so it will not be so responsive to the stressors. We all have stress, but in some the nervous system seems to allow the perception of stress to get through the filtering devices too easily. The cortex assumes something awful is about to happen and alerts the hypothalamus, which sends the message to the pituitary, which sends it on to the adrenals by neural and humoral pathways. The cortex may be extrasensitive genetically due to inadequate production of specific brain chemicals or some poison that may be lowering the threshold of response.

I have treated patients with appropriate nutrients that should have helped them attain adequate function, yet the headaches continued until they quit their awful jobs. Most of us, however, seem to be able to handle all of life's cruel jokes so long as we stay away from sugar and foods to which we are sensitive and take some B complex along with calcium and magnesium.

A good checkup is mandatory to rule out a tumor or blood clot causing increased intracranial pressure. Blood pressure elevation may cause headaches. Aluminum and lead poisoning could make the brain swell enough to produce pressure. Hypoglycemia will make the blood sugar rise and fall and trigger the pain.

Food sensitivities are becoming more recognized as an important factor (see, for example, a 1980 article in *The Lancet,* which reported that two-thirds of severe migraine patients are allergic to certain foods); usually it is the food the patient loves and is, of course, addicted to. If the doctor asks, "Are you allergic to food?" the patient will often give a negative answer because he does not know that there is a connection between the corn he had on Sunday and the headache he had when talking to the boss at 11 A.M. on Monday.

Skin tests are unreliable in tracking down allergies, and the expensive RAST is not always diagnostic. Sublingual testing, as described by Dr. Doris Rapp, can identify the offender. But perhaps the best way to figure out your body's unique response to foods is to use the four-day water fast. (See Allergies; Fast.)

It is rare, however, to be sensitive to only one food or food group. If every food to which one is sensitive were eliminated from the diet, many people could only drink water. Many have found that their food allergies are less devastating, or at least the symptoms can be minimized, if they eat each food no more frequently than every four days. The body usually can handle this amount of "allergic load."

Dr. Joseph Miller has found that food-allergy injection therapy is highly effective and dependable in quickly providing protection; it allows the patient to continue eating many of the allergenic foods with little or no headache. Sodium cromoglysate (inhaled powder), used as a preventive in asthma, will protect victims of food sensitivities if taken orally on a daily basis. The cost is prohibitive, however. Some will take five capsules just before a big special meal.

I have relieved a number of patients from their incapacitating headaches by the use of intramuscular shots of the B complex (B_1, B_2, B_3, B_6, B_{12}, and pantothenic acid) given every two to ten days. Patients usually inject themselves. These evidently improve the allergy control system, help the intestinal enzymes break down the foods into nonsensitizing simple amino acids, carbohydrates, and fats, and help the adrenals put out physiological amounts of cortisol to suppress the allergic reaction.

Cluster headaches are considered a migraine variant but usually occur suddenly in men between twenty and forty years of age. They awaken between 2 and 6 A.M. with an intense boring pain, usually around one eye. Some consider it to be the worst pain known to man. It is accompanied by redness and watering of the eye and stuffiness of the nostril on the side of the pain. The pain may radiate all over the face and jaw and into the neck. After several devastating nights the attacks stop and may not return for weeks, months, or years.

Alcohol, nitrites, and histamine are known to trigger attacks. Falling blood sugar at 2 A.M. due to the ingestion of allergens or sweets at bedtime could allow this miserable pounding to begin. Seeds, nuts, and protein at bedtime along with calcium (1000 mg) and magnesium (500 mg) might prevent the blood sugar drop.

Dr. William Philpott has been able to control the wild fluctuation of blood sugar that follows the ingestion of an allergen by having the patient take 1000 mg of C, 1000 mg of calcium, and 300 mg of B$_6$ about thirty minutes before the food challenge. The bad reaction (headache, irritability, or whatever) just doesn't happen.

Birth control pills and estrogen taken by postmenopausal women will give headaches to headache-prone persons. A high sodium intake also is associated with headaches. Headache sufferers should put the following foods off limits.

Headache-producing foods: Alcohol (especially red wines and champagne), chocolate, chutneys, cheese (except cottage), fatty foods, fried foods, fish (pickled or fried in batter), bay, chili, cinnamon, citrus, pineapples, bacon, ham, hot dogs, salami, liver pate, pickles, goose, duck, asparagus, eggplant, onions. Cut down on coffee. Look out for monosodium glutamate.

HEARING IMPAIRMENT □ Hearing impairment in adults is most likely caused by nerve damage (virus, excessive exposure to high-decibel noise, and aging). Children become hard of hearing because of middle-ear infections and the resultant secretory middle-ear problem (see Earache). Since some primitive tribesmen have perfect hearing at an advanced age, we assume chronic noise exposure is the culprit in causing the loss of hearing in modern civilization.

An examination by an otolaryngologist should reveal if a neurosensory or conductive (fluid in middle ear) condition is responsible. Repeated ear infections and fluid accumulation should be treated, but allergies are the most common reason for the tendency. Milk is number one, but any food can do it. Increasing the C, B complex, A, and zinc should help control allergies and reduce the infection rate.

Nerve deafness is worth treating with C and B complex, but there is no guarantee of control. I once gave a man a B complex shot (0.7 cc) for fatigue. He called the next day to say that the ringing in his ears that he'd had for ten years was gone. Ringing may be a harbinger of deafness; it is usually the first clue of an auditory neuritis.

HEARTBURN □ The medical term *symptomatic gastroesophageal reflux* refers to the burning sensation at the lower front of the chest (near the heart) following meals.

Around the lower end of the esophagus there is a ring-like pressure zone that is supposed to keep the stomach contents, acid and pepsin, from regurgitating into the esophagus. Some foods (oil of peppermint, garlic, onion) have a relaxing affect on this muscular sphincter. Fat also relaxes the muscle and may explain why indigestion so often follows a fatty meal. Coffee produces a direct effect on the esophagus, not a reflex relaxation of the muscle. Alcohol relaxes the muscle tension of the sphincter and decreases peristaltic force. (This is why drunks who are fat have trouble holding their dinner in place when untying their shoelaces.) A cigarette after a meal also will relax the muscle gate and allow acid to bubble up.

Obesity can produce heartburn just from pressure, as happens also during pregnancy.

Small frequent feedings are best for heartburn. Protein will increase the muscle tension and help contain the food in the stomach. The fat content should be as low as possible. Calcium and magnesium as antacids might be suitable at the end of the meal. Dolomite or a calcium/magnesium tablet would be a good way to get the day's mineral requirements in.

Low amounts of hydrochloric acid produced by the stomach will often produce the same symptoms as excess acidity. In this case, it is sour food that is bubbling up. Antacids would be wrong for this condition. Hydrochloric acid tablets would help to keep that sphincter closed.

HEART RATE □ A doctor's examination, usually accompanied by an x-ray and electrocardiogram, should reveal the cause of heart rate irregularities. Heart failure must be corrected.

If the examination reveals no gross or obvious problem, nutrition could be a therapy. A rapid heartbeat may appear after ingestion of sugar or a food to which one is sensitive. In fact, food allergies often are diagnosed by the Dr. Coca pulse test: when the blood sugar rises and then falls rapidly due to an overproduction of insulin, adrenalin is excreted into the bloodstream and, of course, stimulates the heart to race along. The pulse usually rises about twenty to thirty minutes after the food is swallowed. From a resting pulse of 60, some will have a rise to 90 beats per minute just from holding the food in their mouth or having an extract of it dropped under their tongue. Some exquisitely sensitive people will have a *slowing* of the heart rate when exposed to their allergens.

A rapid, fluttering heart may not be getting sufficient oxygen to beat neatly and forcefully. Vitamin E, 400 to 800 units daily (increase slowly), should help.

Premature ventricular contractions, or ventricular tachycardia, are frequently controlled with the proper amount of magnesium. Some hair analysts cite low levels of magnesium in the hair of persons with cardiovascular disease leading to heart attacks. These patients would be more likely to have ventricular fibrillation as a complication of the coronary occlusion.

Drs. Emanuel Cheraskin and W. M. Ringsdorf have found an association with cardiovascular health and the height of one of the waves in the ECG (P_1). They found that a lower P_1 wave is associated with a higher intake of vitamin C.

HEAT □ Adaptation to heat is difficult. You're still hot even when you take everything off. Drinking a lot of fluid will help, because sweating and vaporization of the sweat cools off the body. If you pass a dilute urine four to five times a day, you know your body is not dehydrated.

Salt tablets are now felt to be less important for the laborer or exerciser, because an ordinary diet has plenty of salt. A strict (vegan) vegetarian might have to take extra sodium chloride (table salt) in order to balance his relatively greater intake of potassium.

Prickly heat, usually seen during times of heat and humidity, is due to inflammation of the sweat glands. Vitamin C handles this easily (1000 mg two to three times daily). Heat is a stress, so the B complex is also helpful.

HEMORRHOIDS □ Why do we joke about these? The victims don't often find them funny, although they usually have brought them on themselves by eating the low-roughage diet now commonly in use in our civilized society.

Among other possible causes, liver disease and venous congestion will encourage growth of hemorrhoids. Also, women in pregnancy and childbirth have more trouble because of the increased pressure on the pelvic and anal veins. But plenty of people have pressures in their veins and never get these dilated and painful veins around the anal sphincter.

Vitamin E has been used internally and externally and can even shrink some of these veins if the diet is changed also. B_6 (50 to 100 mg daily) is important. Surgery may still be necessary, but one would heal more quickly if supplements were taken.

Sitz baths will calm the pain. Cold witch hazel lotion is soothing too.

(See Constipation; Fiber.)

HERPES I (CANKER SORES) □ These pesky sores are due to the herpes simplex virus. The virus lives inside the nerve endings near the lips and gums. When a stress strikes (sunshine, citrus, chocolate, walnuts, fever, menstruation), the virus migrates to the local mucous membrane and multiplies. Because it is a virus, vitamin C should be able to stop it, but huge doses are needed—20,000 to 50,000 mg per day. Some victims have experienced worsening of the sores due to vitamin C. Apparently, however, this is due not to the C but to the corn from which the C was manufactured. Some corn remnants are left in the powder and these people are allergic to corn. If that connection seems unlikely, perhaps the high acidity of ascorbic acid is doing it; try sodium ascorbate or calcium ascorbate.

The virus thrives on the amino acid arginine (found in walnuts and chocolate). It does poorly on lysine, however, and this amino acid, taken daily in pill form at 500 mg to 1000 mg per day, generally suppresses the symptoms. Ascorbate in solution, locally applied, will help also. Opening up a vitamin E capsule and rubbing the contents onto the developing sore usually can stop the pain and the progress.

Skin and mucous membranes are healthy if they get an optimum amount of zinc and vitamin A; 50 to 100 mg of elemental zinc daily would meet the need. Dr. Robert Cathcart suggests increasing the dose until some stomach distress appears, then backing off. Too much zinc over a prolonged period will cause a copper deficiency and anemia. Lactobacillus capsules, three times a day, are helpful.

Some therapists have found niacinamide (500 to 1000 mg) beneficial; others use pantothenic acid (250 to 500 mg three times a day) at the first sign of the tingling. Low thyroid function may allow development of the sores. Treating the patient as if he had pernicious anemia in some cases has helped (muscle injection of B_{12} and folic acid). But the most effective method is to raise the general level of health of the whole body; this reduces the susceptibility to the stress of the causative factors.

Herbs that help control recurrences are indigo weed, Oregon grape, and goldenseal.

HERPES II (GENITAL HERPES) □ This virus produces blisters on the genitalia that erode in twenty-four to forty-eight hours to become painful ulcers. These open sores take about two weeks to heal. Recurrences are common, but are usually less frequent with aging. (The herpes I virus is responsible for about 15 percent of these genital lesions.) If herpes II virus is present in the genital tract of a woman at childbirth, her baby may develop a devastating type of encephalitis; caesarean section is the usual recommendation. The same virus is thought to be related to a cancer of the cervix. Ten percent of women with no symptoms and no visible evidence of lesions are found to be shedding the virus from their cervical areas.

The virus is ubiquitous. Most fifty-year-old people show antibodies to the virus, a sign of past infection. But these antibodies are not strong enough to prevent recurrences.

The virus duplicates in nerve ganglia near the site of these recurrent sores. The infectious virus will migrate via the nerve fibers to the skin and produce the blisters.

Since impaired immune response, sickness, stress, menses, exposure to cold, and fatigue will allow the virus to get re-established, all these problems should be controlled with diet and nutrition as much as possible. Sex may only be the trigger. Those with cell-mediated immunity defects may have the persistent, chronic type.

Satisfactory treatment has not been found. Antiviral drugs show some promise. As the lesions characteristically fade and recur, any treatment given coincidentally with a remission is given the credit.

Vitamin C, 10,000 to 20,000 mg taken orally, will heal the lesions faster than the drugs, but it must be taken at the first twinges. Lysine, 500 mg twice a day, helps the oral type; 500 mg a day might work prophylactically to lessen the recurrence rate. Lactobacillus capsules three times a day are helpful for some. Vitamin E oil topically promotes healing and cuts the pain temporarily. Zinc, 30 to 60 mg daily, improves the healing ability of the skin. They should all be tried, and maybe at the same time.

All this is a strong argument for sexually active men to always use a condom and for women to use the diaphragm. Never have sex if open lesions are obvious. (Is it polite to ask?) Avoid stress.

HIVES □ Itchy blotches on the skin are not always due to chocolate or strawberry ingestion, although that is a start in the detective work of finding the cause. Drugs and chemicals are probably the most common causes (see salicylate list under "Hyperactivity"). Saccharin and sulfa drugs are common hive makers. Benzoates, universally used as preservatives, will cause hives. Yellow dye #5, a tartrazine, will frequently set the skin going (in Tang and candy corn, for example).

Hives can be triggered by sunlight, cold, dust, molds, and even the yeast Candida (see Yeast Infections). Exertion, sweating, and stress will bring them out in some.

Hives can be fatal if the larynx is involved, so the condition must be taken seriously. It is assumed that the response is due to histamine released from the mast or basophil cells. Antihistamines should suppress it. But in some people, the IgE antigen-antibody response is not demonstrated, so injection desensitization will not help as it would in pollen hay fever.

Calcium will counteract the histamine release, so it is valuable if everything else has been done without success to find and eliminate the offender. Since cortisone-like drugs will suppress hives, the nutrients that encourage their maximal function should be used (C, pantothenic acid, B_6, calcium, zinc, and A).

I have stopped hives with 1 gram of calcium (gluconate) plus C (5 grams) intravenously. Very gratifying to the patient and to me.

HYPERACTIVITY □ Adults can have this problem. You may know or be married to someone with the symptoms: the short attention span, distractibility, tendency to fly from one activity to another, never satisfied, fun to know but hell to live with. They can easily get a bad self-image; they are sensitive, goosey people.

Part of the problem is genetic and part of it is biochemical. These people are very prone to develop symptoms of allergy or diseases of a "psychosomatic" nature, usually because they have hypoglycemia; sugar ingestion upsets them. Their restlessness, foot swinging, or rocking may indicate a calcium and magnesium deficiency. Indeed, many crave milk, which may suggest a calcium lack.

B₆ (100 to 400 mg a day) helps the brain make some of the chemicals they need; the dosage should be increased until they have good dream recall. Manganese is low in some and also relates to poor dream recall.

Food allergies make many people hyperactive. A fast may be the only way to tell. If four days of fasting make the afflicted person be calm and unflappable, then the problem is a food allergy.

Dr. Ben Feingold found that salicylates caused hyperactivity in susceptible people. It is difficult but worthwhile to try a no-salicylate, no-additive diet for three weeks. Many find that if they make their own adrenals healthy with vitamins and minerals, the additives will not bother them.

Salicylates are found in: Alka-Seltzer, Anacin, aspirin, Bromo-Seltzer, Bufferin, Coricidin, Empirin, Midol, Pepto-Bismol, candies, cosmetics, gum, lozenges, mouthwash, oil of wintergreen, toothpaste, almonds, apples, apricots, cherries, grapes, nectarines, oranges, peaches, prunes, raspberries, strawberries, wines.

HYPERINSULINISM ☐ This excess secretion of insulin in response to slight rises of the blood sugar is very similar to hypoglycemia (q.v.). I would assume that if someone notices the symptoms of low blood sugar all the time, not just in isolated episodes, then he would be classified as having too much insulin.

It is now felt that there is more to "low blood sugar" than low blood sugar. The insulin that is released to handle the high blood sugar has an independent effect on the brain. The blood sugar fluctuations do not always reflect the brain sugar fluctuations. Indeed, in some patients during the glucose-tolerance test a brain-wave test may show abnormalities consistent with inadequate cerebral nourishment while the levels of blood glucose are still within normal limits. An insulin level taken simultaneously may reveal a greater-than-average level. The patient usually becomes depressed, hostile, or unconscious.

When there is a lack of laboratory correlation, the severity of the nervous system symptoms suggests the diagnosis of hyperinsulinism. Unfortunately, however, doctors tend to believe the values on the lab slip rather than the patient sobbing on the floor.

Usually the four-day fast calms the pancreas to the point where less insulin is needed. Then the victim may try to sneak in small amounts of foods that have been infrequently eaten in the past (to avoid the common food allergies).

This would be a stress situation, so the B complex should be taken (100 mg of each), plus C and a generous amount of calcium and magnesium. Serum calcium rises and falls with the secretion of insulin; the more the insulin, the lower the calcium. This calcium washout often makes the patient tense and touchy—more than would be due to hypoglycemia alone.

HYPERKERATOSIS □ This condition is diagnosed by feel. The skin over the back of the upper arms and the front side of the thighs feels like a nutmeg grater. Rough, bumpy skin, and to a certain extent the thick fish skin that some people exhibit, can be smoothed out with vitamin A; 10,000 units a day might be a small dose for some. Usually no more than 40,000 to 50,000 units is needed. My maintenance dose is 25,000 units. Vitamin A toxicity is possible, but usually is associated with larger doses than this. Headache would suggest discontinuing the A.

Those with rough skin, with colds that do not respond to vitamin C, and with a history of warts are probably vitamin A dependent and would need 2 to 10 times the recommended daily allowance of 5000 units. Those with hyperkeratosis and acne and warts should really be helped with the high doses of A.

Vitamin E makes the A work more efficiently, and zinc helps the skin also. If a close look at the skin reveals little hemorrhages at the point where the hairs leave the skin, and if the hairs are growing in a corkscrew shape, these are signs of scurvy; weight loss, overwhelming fatigue, and listlessness would complete the picture.

HYPERPARATHYROIDISM □ Hyperparathyroidism is caused by the increased secretion of the parathyroid glands, four tiny nodules of tissue found just behind the thyroid gland in the neck. An increased amount of calcium shows in the blood test.

A tumor can cause the trouble, but the gland will secrete extra hormones as well if the calcium level falls. This can occur if a high phosphate level appears. (See Osteoporosis.)

The symptoms may be nonexistent or vague and mild. Apathy, anxiety, depression, confusion, muscle pain and weakness, hypertension, nausea, vomiting, constipation, kidney stones, and arthritis are but a few. X-rays show demineralization of bone.

If a parathyroid tumor is present, it must be removed, but breast and lung cancer also will cause a rise in calcium and must be ruled out. Excessive milk and antacid ingestion will raise the calcium in the blood, as will estrogens and an excess of vitamins D and A.

HYPERTENSION (HIGH BLOOD PRESSURE) □ From 1971 to 1975 a National Health and Nutrition Examination Survey was conducted in the United States. It uncovered some disturbing aspects of this healthy, "best-fed" nation in the world.

About 20 percent of adults from age twenty-five to seventy-four (sample was about 10,000 people) have high blood pressure (that is, either systolic blood pressure of at least 160 mm mercury, or diastolic blood pressure of at least 95 mm mercury, or both).

Hypertension is about twice as prevalent among black as among white adults.

Hypertension is more prevalent among adults living in the South. Another survey showed that 8 percent of 10,000 high-school seniors in Savannah, Georgia, had hypertension.

The educational level and the size of the family income are inversely related to the prevalence of high blood pressure. The higher the income and the more units of education completed, the lower the percentage of those with high blood pressure.

Weight showed a positive correlation with blood pressure readings. The greater the weight, the more likely that pressure would be up. The really upsetting finding was that about one-half of the adults with definite high blood pressure had never been told by a doctor that they had it.

Ninety to 95 percent of those with hypertension have "essential" hypertension, that is, there is no obvious anatomical or physiological reason for the problem. It might be correctable if due to coarctation of the aorta, a kidney anomaly, or a hormone-secreting tumor.

Many adolescents have borderline, or labile, hypertension. Here the blood pressure is normal some days and elevated at other times (90 mm of mercury would be the dividing line for the diastolic pressure in the adolescent). This condition is often the harbinger of the persistent essential high blood pressure (see Adolescence, Chapter 5). Apparently some of us get ulcers; some, migraine; some, asthma; and some, high blood pressure. There is no doubt that the tendency to the condition runs in families. Studies of twins indicate this. Adopted children do not acquire the blood pressures of the natural children in the same household.

Blood pressure is a function of the cardiac output (the vascular volume) multiplied by the vascular constriction (re-

sistance of the peripheral blood vessels). Increased vasoconstriction results from increased activity of the sympathetic
nervous system. Rather than just blocking the response of the
beta-adrenergic receptors, we ought to be turning off the
sympathetic nervous system. Stress would obviously play a
role here, so the perception of stress might best be damp-
ened.

The brain (perception of stress) affects the hypothalamus, which stimulates the vasomotor center in the top section of the spinal cord (medulla). These messages are relayed
to the sympathetic nerve ganglia along the spinal column.
Nerve impulses travel to the adrenergic nerve terminals that
stimulate the adrenergic receptor sites, and the muscles in
the arterial walls contract. Blood pressure rises.

The kidneys exert an important controlling function on
the blood pressure. An enzyme, renin, is released from the
kidneys if the blood pressure drops, sodium levels fall, potassium rises, or if there is neurogenic stimulation. Renin acti-
vates two other chemicals: angiotensin I and angiotensin II;
this latter one has a vasoconstrictive action on the blood vessels. The blood pressure rises. Angiotensin II also stimulates
the secretion of aldosterone (from the adrenal cortex); its
action helps to retain sodium in the body and to allow potassium to be excreted. Fluid volume rises and blood pressure
increases. This vasoconstriction and increased volume are
the triggers to shut off the renin.

Malignant hypertension is often seen in younger patients
with high levels of renin. They are more likely to suffer
strokes and cardiovascular damage. Renin doesn't shut off
when the blood pressure rises. Propranolol is almost specific
for those with hypertension associated with high renin
levels.

Patients with low renin levels and high blood pressure
are more likely to respond to diuretics. A twenty-four-hour
urine sodium measurement before treatment seems wise.
These patients should respond more readily to the low-so-

dium, high-potassium diet than the patients with high renin levels.

Increased intake of sodium and water without increased loss would lead to increased blood volume, or total body fluid. If, in the presence of increased volume, the peripheral vascular resistance did not decrease, the net effect would be an elevated blood pressure.

Thiazides (diuretics) are first used to lower blood pressure. Their main action is to cause a decrease in salt and water content of the body. They may also relax arterial wall muscles. The side effect is low potassium, but this can be corrected with oral potassium supplements and a low-sodium diet. The sodium intake is supposed to be cut to about 1 gram a day. This is difficult except for vegetarians and highly motivated people.

Methyldopa is often used next if the diuretics are not sufficient to lower the blood pressure. It acts by interfering with the production of catecholamines (like adrenalin), which have a hypertensive action.

Propranolol blocks responses of the beta-adrenergic receptors, which are responsible for bronchiolar smooth-muscle relaxation, rapid heart rate, and renin release from the kidney.

These drugs and others used are well intentioned, since high blood pressure must be reduced. But beyond that it would be worthwhile for everyone who has any elevation, no matter how slight, to try a few home remedies also.

Salt (sodium-containing plain table salt) must be avoided. It should not be used in cooking or left in a saltcellar on the table. Those people who salt everything before they taste the food have to change their habits. Morton's "Lite Salt", kelp powder, mixed herbs, and all spices make a satisfactory seasoning because they have relatively more potassium than sodium. I have found that the majority of salt sprinklers are "looking" for flavor enhancement because they are low in calcium, magnesium, zinc, or B-complex vitamins. Within a week of these supplements, most of them stop salting their food.

week of these supplements, most of them stop salting their food.

A study conducted recently at the University of Oregon Health Sciences Center revealed that hypertension might result sooner from a calcium deficiency than from a sodium excess. I would like to believe that low calcium could produce a muscle spasm in the arterial wall muscles.

In many studies of patients with hypertension there runs a pattern: those who were ingesting more potassium than sodium were more likely to have normal blood pressure, and those who had elevated blood pressure were more likely to be taking in more sodium than potassium. The average American diet contains 6 to 20 grams of sodium a day; we need only 1 to 2 grams.

In a study of Mormons, who used no caffeine, alcohol, or nicotine, the blood pressures were all normal, but the group that were vegetarians had an even lower level of blood pressure. Vegan vegetarians have the lowest blood pressures of all; it's OK unless it makes one weak. They get a high amount of potassium in their diet. Lactovegetarians get a fair amount of sodium from the dairy products. Certain cheeses (Roquefort, camembert, gorgonzola, processed cheeses, cheese spreads) are high in sodium and therefore should be avoided by hypertensives. Carnivores get a lot of sodium, and then, when they salt their steaks, have french fries, canned peas, and a cheese dressing on their salad, they are asking for it. But not every salt lover is hypertensive, nor does salt-love correlate with sodium levels in the blood; high amounts of sodium in the urine correlate better with high blood pressure. As a corollary, high amounts of potassium, compared to sodium, in the urine were more likely associated with normal blood pressure.

A high cadmium level in the hair analysis is often associated with high blood pressure. Cadmium comes from chemical pollution and cigarette smoking. It inhibits the enzymes that inactivate the catecholamines, adrenalin, and norepinephrine (hypertensive agents). Calcium, magnesium, and zinc are effective in replacing cadmium. Zinc also is flushed out when diuretics are used; it must be replaced. Blood pressures are more likely elevated in areas where the selenium in the soil is low (Pacific Northwest, Great Lakes area, New England, and parts of the South Atlantic region). (Calcium, 1000 mg; magnesium, 500 mg; zinc, 60 mg; and selenium, 100 mcg, would help to compensate.)

Inositol, 1000 mg twice a day, is reputed to be helpful for hypertensives. Bromelain, one to eight capsules a day, is good. Garlic and onions are time-honored remedies for elevated blood pressure, but they probably must be eaten every hour or two. A prostaglandin has been extracted from onions that works to lower blood pressure for an hour or two (worked in rats); some onion and garlic extracts are virtually odor-free (two to five capsules per day). There are indications that a linoleic-acid-rich diet has a beneficial blood-pressure-lowering effect in patients with "borderline" essential hypertension (140/90 mm Hg). (See Coronary Artery Disease.)

Controlling stress seems like an obvious requirement before the blood pressure is corrected. Biofeedback techniques and hypnosis often are successful. The personality type that outwardly remains calm despite obvious stress is no more connected with blood pressure elevation than he is with asthma or ulcers. A number of biochemical, hereditary, and environmental factors are all operating together. The common association with obesity suggests that blood sugar fluctuations, food allergies, and stressed adrenals play a role. Foods that contain tyramine should not be eaten by those receiving therapy with a monamine oxidase inhibitor; elevated blood pressure may occur. It exists in chocolate, herring, yeast, chicken livers, red wine, beer, and all cheese except cream, ricotta, and cottage.

ANASTASIA CHEHAK, my dietician friend, provided me with the following information useful for the hypertensive:

Most herbs, spices, and table wines do not contain sodium, nor cholesterol and fat; they can be used in place of salt as seasonings. You will find that flavoring substances such as black pepper, onion, green pepper, garlic, lemon juice, and vinegar complement and enhance the natural goodness of food.

When using herbs and spices, use them sparingly because a little goes a long way. However, if you use fresh rather than dried herbs, use twice the amount.

To keep a ready supply of seasonings on hand, try using a combination of herbs instead of salt in your salt shaker. You can make your own herb shaker by combining:

½ teaspoon cayenne pepper
1 tablespoon garlic powder
1 teaspoon basil
1 teaspoon marjoram
1 teaspoon thyme
1 teaspoon parsley
1 teaspoon mace
1 teaspoon onion powder
1 teaspoon ground black pepper
1 teaspoon sage
1 teaspoon savory

This will enhance the flavors of meats and vegetables in the kitchen or on the table.

Table wines are fine to use in cooking, but avoid flavoring your meats with "cooking wines" as they contain added salt. As with herbs, a little wine goes a long way. You can devise your own flavorful marinades by using wine, vinegar, and oil, or unsalted salad dressings. Lemon juice, vinegar, Tabasco sauce, or unsalted liquid smoke are also great for adding flavor to meats, soups, and vegetables.

Use onion or garlic powder or celery seed or flakes as indicated in a recipe instead of flavored salts such as onion salt, celery salt, and garlic salt.

Ms. CHEHAK recommends the following flavor enhancers to heighten the taste of the foods. They are all low in sodium.

Beef: Bay leaf, dry mustard powder, green pepper, marjoram, fresh mushrooms, nutmeg, onion, pepper, sage, thyme.

Chicken: Green pepper, lemon juice, marjoram, fresh mushrooms, paprika, parsley, poultry seasoning, sage, thyme.

Fish: Bay leaf, curry powder, dry mustard powder, green pepper, lemon juice, marjoram, fresh mushrooms, paprika.

Lamb: Curry powder, garlic, mint, pineapple, rosemary.

Pork: Apple, applesauce, garlic, onion, sage.

Veal: Apricot, bay leaf, curry powder, ginger, marjoram, rosemary.

Asparagus: Garlic, lemon juice, onion, vinegar.

Corn: Green pepper, pimiento, fresh tomato.

Cucumbers: Chives, dill, garlic, vinegar.

Green beans: Dill, lemon juice, marjoram, nutmeg, pimiento.

Greens: Onion pepper, vinegar.

Peas: Green pepper, mint, fresh mushrooms, onion, parsley.

Potatoes: Green pepper, mace, onion, paprika, parsley.

Rice: Chives, green pepper, onion, mushrooms, saffron.

Squash: Cinnamon, ginger, mace, nutmeg, onion.

Tomatoes: Basil, marjoram, onion, oregano.

Soups: A pinch of dry mustard powder in bean soup; a small amount of vinegar or allspice in vegetable soup; peppercorns in skim-milk chowders; bay leaf and parsley in pea soup.

The following foods are high in sodium, and their ingestion should be kept at a minimum or eliminated entirely from the diet: milk, cheese, puddings, biscuit mixes, cereals, prepared cornbread, muffins, waffles, crackers, pickled foods, instant potatoes, potato salad, sauerkraut, canned and frozen vegetables, anchovies, bacon, corned and chipped beef, luncheon meat, sausage, smoked meats, many canned and frozen stews, hash, pasta, mixes, TV dinners, bouillon, canned soup, soy and steak sauce.

Ms. Chehak recommends to her patients with hypertension, and she says it applies to all of us, that they consume 2000 to 2500 mg of potassium per day from natural sources. This amount is just the average amount needed by the body every day. The following are some of the richest sources of potassium:

Butternut squash, 1 cup, baked	1200 mg potassium
Lima beans, dry, 1 cup, cooked	1200
Spinach, 1 cup, cooked	1160
Black beans, 1 cup, cooked	1000
Soybeans, 1 cup, cooked	970
Pinto beans, 1 cup, cooked	940
Watermelon, 10 by 16″ wedge	900
Navy beans, 1 cup, cooked	790
Almonds, cashews, Brazil nuts, peanuts, 1 cup	780/1000
Papaya, medium size	710
Halibut, 4 oz, broiled	656
Avocado, one half, medium size	650
Raisins, ½ cup	650
Banana, medium size	630
Prune juice, 1 cup	600
Parsnips, 1 cup, cooked	590
Split peas, 1 cup, cooked (but not the canned; too much sodium)	590

Flounder, 1 serving, baked	587
Tomato juice, 1 cup canned (too much sodium)	550
Wheat germ, 1 cup	530
Dates, 10	520
Apricots, 3 medium	500
Orange juice, 1 cup	500
Potato, 1 white, medium, cooked	500
Oatmeal, 1 cup, cooked (poor choice)	130
Whole wheat bread (not too good)	53

Some patients have found that just by cutting back on their intake of caffeine, the blood pressure returned to normal. It is in a lot of drinks:

Coffee, 5 oz cup, drip	150 mg caffeine
Hills Brothers instant	189
Tea, 5 minute brew, 5 oz	20–50
Baking chocolate, 1 oz	35
Dr Pepper, 12 oz	61
Tab, 12 oz	45
Coca-Cola, 12 oz	42
Diet Pepsi, 12 oz	34

HYPOCHONDRIASIS □ Hypochondriacs have symptoms that cannot be verified by the examination, the laboratory, or the x-ray. They use subjective symptoms like "nervousness," or "exhaustion," or "numbness and tingling." Their thyroid function is OK, maybe at the lower end of normal but still in the normal range. The same with the blood count.

But they go on with "I feel irritable," or "I'm forgetful and confused," or "The light bothers my eyes," or "How do you treat inward nervousness?" the doctor has nothing to go on. He can only figure that the symptoms are imaginary. Out of some attention-getting motivation, the patient is exaggerating the normal odd feelings that occasionally come to us all. The symptoms might go away if the patient would just get a job or a hobby and stop being a navel gazer.

The doctor reassures the patient. He threatens to send him or her off to the psychiatrist. Or says, "Do you want to try some Valium?" (Maybe we can trade off the symptoms for a fresh group of complaints.)

The doctor usually remains unconvinced that the body is saying something with these clues. An allergy can do all these things, but the skin tests are nonrevealing. The glucose-tolerance test doesn't always reveal the blood sugar fluctuations consistent with the diagnosis. The rise and fall were not great enough for the doctor, despite the fact the patient got a headache at the third hour, sweaty at the fourth hour, and fell asleep at the fifth hour.

If a patient has leg cramps, how many doctors would make an effort to add up the milligrams of calcium ingested daily? The doctor wants to help, but first to do no harm. He does not want to use a drug to relieve the symptoms, since that would suggest to the patient that he takes it to be a "real" complaint and worthy of attention. He would then have fallen into the trap of reinforcing the neurotic overattention to insignificant squeaks and groans.

The little child with a stomachache from a milk sensitivity may be the adult with colitis. The patient lives in that body, and we must get used to accepting the patient's evaluation of what he perceives.

Most hypochondriacs are sensitive people who are able to notice what their bodies are saying to them. Until laboratory tests are more sophisticated, we may have to stop and listen to the patient's diagnosis.

Remember the epitaph on the tombstone of the hypochondriac: See?

HYPOGLYCEMIA □ Either everyone has it to a certain extent or no one has it at all. A confusion of beliefs about this nondisease has left the lay person still suffering, waiting for help. The medical establishment has encouraged him to give up and become obese, or an alcoholic, or go on Valium, or sit in a dark room, surly and depressed.

The doctors who cannot believe that hypoglycemia is a recognizable clinical entity are probably the ones who never fell asleep during the boring post-lunch pathology lecture, who ate hospital food during their internships and never suffered stress, who have never been able to perceive mood swings in their children.

The problem with diagnosing the symptoms of hypoglycemia is that the doctor is unable to live inside that patient's body and perceive what the patient is perceiving. My wife can tell when I am having a nasty headache—I look gray and pinched. But she has known me for more than three decades. When a new patient comes to the doctor because of feelings of "impending doom," the doctor knows this is crazy stuff, so the patient gets a psychiatric referral or a prescription for a tranquilizer so the brain won't perceive those bad feelings any more.

I remember as a senior medical student having an elderly clinic patient tell me she had a heavy feeling in the lower left side of her abdomen just before having a bowel movement. How simple the body is; it will signal its needs. And what fun medicine is going to be; I thought! My response: "Whenever you feel that way, go to the bathroom and sit on the toilet."

. If only the workings of cause and effect were always so obvious! The "doom" patient might have noticed that her angst happened two hours after her coffee break. She would not have had to see the doctor. Instead, she would have perceived the cause-and-effect relationship and started taking a glass of milk and twenty almonds instead of coffee and a doughnut. She would (or should) have felt stupid saying to the doctor, "I feel tense, anxious, miserable, and fearful two hours after I eat a doughnut with my coffee." The doctor, for his part, would have looked at the patient wisely and responded with, "Maybe you ought not to eat doughnuts and coffee."

The orthodox M.D. is trained to relieve pain and suffering and to do no harm, but he was also trained that diet has only some vague relationship to gas and obesity. That's it, period. The stories that people relate to their doctors are put on a list of "anecdotal evidence" that has nothing to do with clinical proof. Low blood sugar must be low enough to cause some palpable evidence, like coma or a convulsion—*that* gets the doctor's attention. Some laboratory evidence must confirm what is observed; the blood sugar has to drop to below 40 mg/100 ml of serum. That would be a grabber. The doctor might want to do a glucose-tolerance test or follow the blood sugar when the patient is fasting for twenty-four hours. If the level falls too low and symptoms appear, a surgeon will be summoned to remove an insulin-secreting tumor from the patient's pancreas.

Laboratory verification of a biochemical screw-up serious enough to explain these symptoms has come about in the past ten to twenty years and is bringing some cheer to those who were formerly labeled "neurotics" or "hypochondriacs." Dr. William Philpott started out to find the biochemical cause of schizophrenia. He discovered that a few schizophrenics have their distorted perceptions because of hypoglycemia; moreover, he discovered and documented for all skeptics that close to half the diagnosed diabetics and close to half those diagnosed as having epilepsy *do not have these illnesses.* They have their blood sugar patterns and seizures because their bodies are allergic to certain foods or are dependent on certain vitamins and minerals for optimum control of blood sugar.

The brain is the busiest organ of the body, and the brain has no storage capacity for energy. It is dependent on whatever glucose, oxygen, water, vitamins, minerals, and amino acids are floating through it via the bloodstream at any given time. If the supply of any of these nutrients is deficient—

especially the glucose or the oxygen—then parts of the brain will not function properly. Perceptions, thought, feeling, and behavior will alter, sometimes subtly, as in a vague feeling of ennui. Many victims will turn into animals; witness the roomful of snakes and gorillas that teachers have to contend with following the candy orgies of Easter and Halloween.

The Jekyll-and-Hyde behavior in children is quite characteristic. Mood swings, impatience, strong temper, sudden unexplained crying spells, are typical. The off-and-on nature of these feelings and behaviors directly correlates with the food or chemical just recently eaten.

The symptoms described below occur when the blood sugar bounces about—too high or too low for that particular patient.

Fatigue, weakness, or exhaustion would be the most common indicators of an energy problem, not just in the brain but in the muscles. Every tissue needs glucose to function. Mental depression often is seen if the brain is not receiving glucose. Fainting spells and light-headedness suggest a low blood sugar problem. Headaches would occur as a compensatory mechanism; the blood vessels in the head would dilate to increase the supply of blood and its glucose. The pounding, pounding, pounding headache is called vascular. The common factor is that the symptoms are variable; they come and go, sometimes coincidental to environmental stresses, sometimes appearing for no apparent reason—until the diet is examined. I used to get headaches on stress days until I stopped eating a half-pound of cookies daily. The stress triggered the headache, but it needed the two things occurring together—the falling blood sugar *and* the stress. Most people can handle the stresses of ordinary life if they eat properly.

When the blood sugar rises rapidly because of the ingestion of a quick sugar (table sugar, brown sugar, corn syrup, maple syrup, honey), the pancreas responds by producing insulin, perhaps more than is necessary. Down plummets the blood sugar, and a number of responses, usually mental, are produced; the brain's high metabolic rate would dictate that mental symptoms appear first.

Confusion, memory impairment, short attention span, inability to concentrate, are but a few clues that important parts of the brain are not being nourished. That's not all. When the blood sugar falls rapidly, the body assumes that a stress is occurring (enemy attack, severe hunger, falling in love), so it releases adrenalin to help the stressee run or fight or do whatever is appropriate. The adrenalin is also necessary to stimulate the liver to release some of its stored glucose (stored as glycogen). It is this gratuitous adrenalin that creates the other symptoms of nervousness, irritability, apprehension, dread, light-headedness, insomnia, blurred vision, rapid heart, and clammy hands. It is also this adrenalin that explains nightmares, night terrors, some cases of fears and phobias; the adrenalin flows concomitantly with the exposure to the feared object. (See Anxiety.)

A psychotherapist might first assume the fear and withdrawal were due to the situation (animal fears, school phobia, agoraphobia, hydrophobia). However, the fear of the dog, school, the open place, or the water has become a learned response. The attack was due to adrenalin, pure and simple; psychotherapy may be indicated, but, obviously, the diet must be changed.

Similar feelings of anxiety are common in jobs that are inherently safe and free of stress. The coffee, soft drinks, and candy bars consumed by the employees would explain job dissatisfaction. If the boss wants the best from the workers, he or she would do well to ban the junk machines.

Every organ system is capable of having some symptoms when the blood sugar fluctuates. Cravings for food, alcohol, sugar, and salt are common. Dr. Philpott has pointed out that carbohydrate mismanagement is typical in the bodies of these people. It is not just sugar ingestion. Remember the summary by the American College of Allergy: "Anything can do anything."

Diarrhea, constipation, indigestion, gas, frequency of urination, arising at night to urinate (first sign of a slowdown of digestion and food absorption), bed-wetting, premenstrual tension, muscle aches, and allergies are common associative symptoms found in many hypoglycemics. Apparently the body is so busy repairing the damage done by the blood sugar fluctuation that other organs begin to fall apart.

The doctor may note the following findings during the examination: the blood pressure often falls when the patient stands (postural hypotension); skin may be thin and dry; morning temperature (orally) may be below 97.8°, suggesting impaired thyroid function; head hair is thinning; more than average number of cavities; edentulous by age fifty. Many have noticeable lymph glands in the neck; this reflects the allergies and consequent postnasal drip plus the susceptibility to upper respiratory infections. The doctor would not know what to assume from these findings except that the patient has a weak constitution or "poor protoplasm."

The laboratory tests often show that the thyroid function is at the lower end of normal. Eosinophils may be increased in the blood count. The five-hour glucose-tolerance test may not help because the lab did not use the sugar to which the patient is sensitive. (Corn sugar may be the troublemaker, for instance, but beet sugar was used.) The test may *look* OK on paper (80 to 120, back to 80 in three hours), but the one being tested had a headache, rapid pulse, and fell asleep. The perceptions the patient had during the test are more important than the numbers recorded.

If symptoms do not occur during the test, then the patient is not sensitive to *that* sugar. Some doctors will test the levels of cortisol and growth hormone during and after the test. If these levels rise, the patient is a responder and does have hypoglycemia.

I have found that if a patient craves sugar and loves coffee or cola drinks, then he has the sugar problem and we must get him on a more healthful regime. The glucose-tolerance test may be superfluous for these sugar-addicted people, but it may be helpful for the disbelieving adolescent who must see the graph of the sugar values before he will agree to change his habits.

Many "normal" people with symptoms suggesting hypoglycemia will have low levels of blood glucose during the five-hour glucose-tolerance test. These less sensitive bodies can show a glucose level of 35 to 50 mg/100 ml of serum and have no symptoms or signs of any deviated physiology. The answer seems to be that some people are sensitive to these fluctuations and some are not. I have discovered that the sensitive, goosey, ticklish person is the one more likely to respond adversely to these blood sugar variables. Calcium may be the key. Calcium in the blood varies directly with the sugar levels. Most hyperactive, sensitive people are low in calcium. Maybe the calcium prevents the brain from caring if the blood sugar is fluctuating.

The sickest patients have a flat curve in their glucose-tolerance test; it neither goes up nor down. These are the most difficult to treat.

Fluctuating blood sugar may not be the cause of everything, however. The large amounts of insulin may have a direct effect on the brain itself and cause some nerve cells to swell. Brain wave changes in the electroencephalograph when insulin levels are high would suggest another mechanism to explain changes of perception, thought, and behavior. (See Hyperinsulinism.)

I can remember getting brain wave tests on patients who showed episodic odd behavior, thinking it might be psychomotor epilepsy. Some had wave forms suggesting seizures. I prescribed phenytoin, a well-known spell-controlling drug. Some of the patients were calmed. I have since learned that this drug tends to limit insulin secretion. I was probably treating the low blood sugar which was the cause of the deviant behavior. Recently I read that brain waves may change after food has been eaten. The satiety center in the hypothalamus responds to insulin and low blood sugar. When blood sugar is down in lower animals, the "foraging for food" and "feeding" centers are activated. Humans are supposed to be nice about it and say "please." If the higher neocortical centers, where the conscience is stored, are not functioning because of low blood sugar, other varieties of animal response may be set loose—other than just the foraging response.

When blood sugar rises and insulin is released, the type and amount of amino acids in the blood are altered. More tryptophan is selectively allowed to enter the brain, where it is converted to serotonin, a brain chemical known to have a sedative effect on the brain—one reason for the drowsiness after a large meal.

When sugar is unavailable for an energy supply, the body will break down fat. The end products of fat metabolism are acids. This can be tested using the saliva. Normal saliva pH is about 6.6 to 6.8 (slightly acid). When the pH drops, it suggests that acidosis has occurred, and this could interfere with optimum brain function. A teaspoon of sodium bicarbonate may be enough to correct the acidosis and the patient's behavior.

Those patients who have had stomach surgery or peptic ulcer disease may absorb ingested carbohydrate so rapidly that insulin is excreted in large amounts and the blood sugar falls rapidly in two to three hours.

Some prediabetic patients will have hypoglycemia for months or years. These are probably the ones who are reacting to foods. When patients complain of hypoglycemic symptoms despite the high-protein, six-times-a-day nibbling diet, it probably means that they are eating a food to which they are allergic (milk, cheese, wheat, eggs, beef, pork, chicken).

Alcohol blocks the formation of glucose. Alcoholics usually develop hypoglycemia when the glycogen stores in the liver and muscles are depleted.

The treatment of hypoglycemia is to avoid the sugars or foods that cause the fluctuation of blood sugar. The time-honored remedy was the six small protein snacks during the waking hours. It helped but was difficult to maintain. Now the emphasis is on two or three small meals of some protein, minimal fat, and a fairly large amount of complex carbohydrate. Eating all the time stresses the pancreas too much. Dr. Philpott has found that because food allergies are so common, he has patients eat two meals a day and no more than three or four different foods at each meal. The amount of fiber (q.v.) is increased until the stools are slightly sloppy. Fiber may slow the absorption of the simple carbohydrates. The idea is to sneak the foods in, so the body does not notice and overproduce insulin.

A four-day distilled-water fast sounds scary to those who cannot be away from the kitchen for more than twenty minutes, but it is the best way to discover the allergens that might be causing the low blood sugar (see Allergies).

The most difficult job of the health-care professional is to get the whole family to stop eating the foods that are causing the symptoms. These foods are like heroin; there is not just a love of sugar (or eggs, or beef, or chocolate, or corn) but a *craving*. I know patients who are bright and have a normal amount of self-control but who admit to me that they get up three times a night for a dish of ice cream. They will refuse to come to the doctor because they know what the doctor will say: "Don't eat it." They refuse to read health-oriented books because all these say "Stop the junk."

I've had no luck convincing families or the single hypoglycemic patient to stop cold turkey. I've had to accept what they were doing and change them gradually. At least there are fewer discouraging side effects of withdrawal. These people have trouble with self-control because the part of the brain that has conscious control (the conscience) over the lusts of the flesh is the neocortex, and the neocortex is the first to become nonoperative when the blood sugar falls. ("I ate one piece of candy and soon the whole box was gone.")

The trick is to keep the blood sugar fairly even by leaving the two- or three-meal habit the way it is but changing the snacks in between. Depending on routine and cravings, the hypoglycemic is to carry a bag containing whatever he wants of the following: nuts, seeds, "trail mix," raw vegetables, fruit, cheese bits, meat, a hard-boiled egg. Soon the nibbler finds he eats less at the regular meals; he awakens more cheerfully in the morning, has more energy, and even wants to exercise. Exercise makes the body more efficient in handling glucose; less insulin is needed when exercise is done consistently. He smokes less and even cuts down on booze and coffee. He spends less time having his bowel movements. He gets hooked on health.

The B-complex vitamins are especially helpful for those who find the blood sugar fluctuations debilitating. The Bs, especially niacinamide (B_3), seem to hold the blood sugar at an optimum level. Some hypoglycemics can sense an attack coming and will break a 50-mg tablet of niacin in two, place one half on the back of the tongue, and allow it to dissolve. The symptoms are gone in ten to twenty minutes.

Glucose-tolerance factor was found in brewer's yeast and basically is due to the B_3 and the chromium. (Yeast is grown in chrome-steel vats.) Chromium (50 to 1000 mcg per day) and B_3 (100 to 500 mg per day) will prevent the buildup of glucose in the bloodstream and the subsequent release of insulin. Vitamin E (100 to 800 units) helps the storage of glucose as glycogen in the liver and muscles; it tends to keep the blood sugar down. Zinc (30 to 60 mg) and manganese (5 mg) both help to stabilize blood sugar; they are often low in hypoglycemics. L-glutamine goes to the brain where it becomes glutamic acid, which can be used for energy. The dose is 1 to 4 grams a day: use 500 mg three times a day and increase by 500 mg weekly until the effective dose is found.

Remember, you live inside your body; you are the expert. If you notice fluctuations in energy, mood, temper, and ability to handle stress, it is your metabolism, your sugar intake, your response to food allergies. Figure it out. Change your diet. You must live in that body the rest of your life; you might as well be comfortable.

General Rules to Combat Blood Sugar Fluctuation

1. Eat no white sugar, brown sugar, corn syrup, maple syrup. Limit molasses and honey. Some fructose, in decreasing amounts, may be used. Much fructose can hurt the liver. Saccharin and cyclamates taste sweet, but they are chemicals and the liver has to detoxify them; besides, anything that tastes sweet promotes the idea that *everything* must taste sweet. Fruit is allowable. It is sweet but the sugar is inside the cells of the fruit and it takes longer for it to get into the body's bloodstream; it would be prudent to eat some nuts, seeds, cheese, or meat with the fruit. Honey and molasses can be used in cooking for a time to wean the addicted hypoglycemic off his sugar craving.

2. Try to eat complex carbohydrates as an energy source. They have fiber, vitamins, minerals, and energy, but the energy is delivered over a long period of time. They do not make the blood sugar rise and fall so suddenly. Vegetables should be eaten raw or barely cooked—steam or stir-fry by the wok method; more vitamins and minerals will be carried to the body. Carry raw vegetables in pocket or purse. Nuts and seeds can be mixed with a few raisins in a box or bag on the car seat or in the tool or fishing box to nibble during the day. If you must eat out frequently, order hot oatmeal, boiled eggs, fresh fruit salad and cottage cheese, broiled or poached fish. Have fruit and cheese for dessert. Eat the parsley on your plate; in some restaurants it is the only worthwhile item served.

3. Examine your current diet and dump the packaged, processed foods as much as possible. They have sugar, salt, and chemicals. These foods have had the vitamins and min-

erals processed out and require precious vitamins and minerals for metabolism. The body can run on a deficit for only so long. Soon a disease will appear that reflects this deficiency—acne, arthritis, hypoglycemia, obesity, colitis, and other not so obvious problems like depression and insomnia.

Examine your diet for some food (good or junk) that you *must* have every day—milk, corn, wheat, eggs, coffee, beef, or whatever. Any food can set up the allergic-addiction vicious cycle and exhaust the body further. Leaving a favorite food out of the diet for four or more days will make its addictive potency quite obvious when the crippling withdrawal symptoms hit: headache, restlessness, surliness, cold sweats, rapid pulse, insomnia, and muscle cramps.

Usually after discontinuing a food for ninety days it can be eaten once every four to seven days without the syndrome reappearing. As you set up your healthy diet, try to eat each food no more frequently than once every four days. If you eat eggs on Monday, wait until Friday for an omelette. Try to eat only three or four foods at each meal; many find that on this four-day rotation diet they don't need to nibble every two hours; they can eat the standard three meals a day.

4. If you have tried unsuccessfully all the above and the fast and the extra vitamins, you may need biochemical priming from a few muscle shots of B complex. Your intestinal lining cells that do the absorbing may not be functioning properly because they cannot absorb the B vitamins they need. Thyroid (q.v.) may be needed.

5. As a test to see if what I'm saying applies to you, stop the sugar and junk after supper tonight and eat some nuts, seeds, protein (egg, meat, fish) right at bedtime. Then see if you get out of bed better in the morning. Many marital conflicts and job dissatisfactions begin in the early morning because the coffee was not brewed in time to raise the blood sugar.

As a test, ask the next person who gets upset, mad, or

depressed in your presence what they had to eat during the last six hours. Notice your children after birthdays, Easter, and Halloween. If a policeman arrests you for going 56 miles an hour on a clear highway, give him some of the nuts you carry in your car and talk him out of the ticketing mood he is in because he had a doughnut and sugared coffee at the station thirty minutes ago. You cannot reason with a spinal cord.

6. The Pritikin diet prohibits nuts (except chestnuts), seeds, cheese, eggs, and dairy fats because of the damaging effects of saturated and unsaturated fats and oils on the blood vessels. The hypoglycemic can move to the Pritikin regime, but unless there is some compelling and motivating vascular disease, it might be too big a step. Cut the sugar, white-flour processed foods, and cereals out of the diet first, then exercise, then move to Pritikin.

I

ILEOSTOMY □ This is the surgical method of fashioning a new outlet from the intestines through the skin of the abdomen. Usually the patient has had a colon or rectal cancer surgically removed, and there was no way to reconnect the bowel with the anus.

The feces are usually messier because they have not had all the fluid absorbed from them. The digestive juices tend to irritate the skin. The bag to catch the stool may not fit too well. Odors are a problem. This is all stressful to the patient.

Everything noted about cancer would be worthwhile in these cases (see Cancer). Everything to help stress (q.v.) would be appropriate also. Vitamin A (25,000 units) and zinc (30 to 60 mg) would be standard. Too much vitamin C would tend to liquefy the stools too much; find the dose—10,000 mg or so—that just softens them more than usual, then cut back. Vitamin E and selenium should help. B complex might control stress.

If the small bowel near the cecum has been removed, the area that absorbs B_{12} is lost and shots (1000 mcg intramuscularly every two to three weeks) will be needed for life.

Oxalate levels in the blood may rise, so extra oral calcium is given to precipitate the oxalate in the intestines so that it won't be absorbed, move to the kidneys, and precipitate as calcium oxalate in the urine.

Avoid glutens. Raw cabbage juice is soothing.

INFECTIONS □ You may remember that in hygiene class in the sixth grade you were taught that if germs got into you, the white blood cells (good guys) would come running in the nick of time, kill and eat the little beggars. That's about what we got in medical school, too, but now it is known that a wide variety of cells and chemicals are mobilized to defend us—often without our being aware of the minor skirmishes going on all the time. Bacteria, viruses, fungi, and yeasts are all over our skin, up our noses, down our throats, and all through the intestines, just waiting for us to lower our defenses and pop, they're in and eating away.

Several of the defenders have been identified and some can easily be measured. Among them are kinins, complement, immunoglobulins, circulating phagocytes, and the reticulo-endothelial system; all play a role when the bacteria invade.

One of the first events is the release of bradykinin, which increases the ability of the circulating phagocytes to stick to the capillary walls, as well as the permeability of these capillaries, allowing the phagocytes (white cells) to get to the field of action. The bacteria release chemicals which attract these polymorphonuclear leucocytes (PMNs) to them. Antibodies circulating about in the bloodstream recognize the germ as a foreign invader and attach themselves; complement has a similar effect. These two provide a stimulus signal to the circulating PMNs. The PMNs engulf the bacteria and destroy them by manufacturing oxygen metabolites. These active oxygen-carrying molecules include H_2O_2 (hydrogen peroxide), which is formed from oxygen by an enzyme, superoxide dismutase.

Corticosteroids released by the adrenals because of the stress of the invasion have an anti-inflammatory action; they decrease the adherence of the PMNs to capillary walls and slow the movement of the PMNs to the infected tissues. Vitamin C will improve the movement of the PMNs thus interrupted.

B lymphocytes (bone-marrow-derived) develop into plasma cells which produce antibodies (immunoglobulin G) in response to the antigenic material of the bacteria. Inadequate immunoglobulin formation would account for the lethal effects of pneumococcal, streptococcal, and hemophilus infections and other common illnesses in low-protein third-world peoples. Protein-calorie malnutrition, uncommon in our country, may be a factor in susceptibility to infection. Subclinical malnutrition may only manifest itself as six colds a year with three attacks of bronchitis requiring antibiotics. A low albumin fraction of the blood would reflect this protein-poor diet.

T lymphocytes (thymus-produced) release lymphokines when stimulated by antigens from the bacteria. These kines attract phagocytes to the area of infection. Two types of T lymphocytes have been identified: "helper" T cells and "suppressor" T cells. They work together to modulate the production of antibody from the B cells. The effect of nutrition is greater on this cell-mediated immune response than on the B-lymphocyte-immunoglobulin system. The thymus gland is severely atrophied in malnutrition, as are the peripheral lymph nodes, the tonsils, and the spleen. Small tonsils may be a clue in diagnosing impaired cellular immunity. The number of lymphocytes in the blood usually is reduced in malnutrition. These cellular immune defects result in susceptibility to viral, fungal, and protozoan infections. Interferon, an intracellular antiviral substance, is not synthesized as well in the malnourished. Vitamin C in doses of 1000 to 10,000 mg will help overcome this. Vitamin C increases the rate of production of lymphocytes. Intrauterine malnutrition may affect T-cell function; the fetal immune system is susceptible to the mother's poor nutrition.

Since most disorders of the immune system (B cells, T cells, complement, and phagocytes) are genetically determined, extreme susceptibility to infection is usually manifest in the first few months or years of life. Granulocytopenia is a genetic disorder manifested by a low number of circulating PMNs; if the level falls below 500 per cubic mm, the person is likely to succumb to an overwhelming infection. Antibiotics obviously are indicated.

But the phagocytic action of the PMNs in a reasonable well-endowed person can be altered by sugar ingestion (decreases engulfment of bacteria), because the energy for the process is provided by glucose. This is why diabetics have an increased susceptibility to infection. Calcium concentration helps regulate cell movement. Calcium deficiency is common in our country. Cortisone-like drugs will reduce the locomotion and engulfment properties of the PMNs. Those persons on cortisone are the most prone to serious infections. Drugs used for cancer therapy have a negative effect on the number and activity of the PMNs; they can also damage the intestinal lining cells and suppress antibody synthesis. It has been observed that megadoses of vitamin C returned the granulocyte function to normal in a patient with a dysfunction of phagocytosis. Ingestion of food allergens prevents the migration of PMNs (blood sugar drop?).

It is useful to assume that any infection that occurs is a clue that the defense system was inadequate and that the inadequacy should be corrected to prevent a similar, perhaps more devastating, infection from sweeping through the body.

Vitamin and mineral deficiencies usually exist along with the protein and calorie malnutrition. Diet and infection are continuously interacting. One infection seems to lead to another, because the infection is a debilitating event that causes a slight deficiency to become a major one. If a recovered patient does not change his lifestyle, eating habits, exercise program, nutritional support system, he will find himself back in the doctor's office. "You've had this before? You've got it again."

If you have ever been diagnosed as having any of the following conditions, it might be prudent to have the laboratory check the adequacy of your PMNs (the polymorphonuclear leucocytes): pustular dermatitis, lymph nodes that drained pus, recurrent pneumonia, osteomyelitis, liver abscesses, abscesses about the rectum, and attacks of cellulitis.

If you have many bacterial infections, you should have your immunoglobulins tested. Remember that severe iron-deficiency anemia (Hgb less than 10 grams per deciliter) will lead to repeated infections. Iron deficiency affects cell-mediated immunity; the percentage of T cells is decreased in anemia. But if iron therapy has saturated the transferrin (the iron-carrying globulin), the bacteriostatic effect is reduced. Any infection will use protein to help make the immune globulins and the PMNs. The skeletal muscles are used first and most dramatically; full recovery takes several weeks after even a brief infection. All during that time the body is more susceptible. A deficiency of B_{12}, for example, reduces the conversion of folate to the form necessary for DNA synthesis; this would reduce the body's ability to manufacture PMNs, immune globulins, and T-cell-mediated immune response. In malnutrition, the protective effect of the intestinal mucosa against absorption of foreign substances is lost. Lining cells flatten, the mucosal barrier is disrupted, and a decrease in secretory IgA may occur. This could explain the onset of food allergies after a bout of intestinal flu.

Biotin, one of the B-complex vitamins, may be needed by some people as a supplement to help them manufacture some immune system component.

Thus the disease can easily set up the malnutrition that

leads to the disease. Because muscles are used for fuel in acute infections, nitrogen is lost, but also potassium, magnesium, phosphate, sulfate, and a lot of zinc. In infections, zinc falls to 70 percent of normal. The PMNs contain large amounts of zinc; it attaches to the dead virus and is thus excreted. A severe dermatological condition, acrodermatitis enteropathica, clears up when adequate zinc is given. In addition, the zinc therapy enhances the impaired cell-mediated immunity in these patients. Infection uses up albumin (protein) and much vitamin A; vitamin A deficiency impairs protein synthesis and contributes to anemia.

An individual's need for vitamin A varies with the severity of the trauma, the stress, or the infection. The body may use up to 60 percent of its vitamin A. The losses must be made up and the thymus must be stimulated. Children and animals with zinc deficiency frequently have thymus gland atrophy and susceptibility to infection. Zinc and vitamin A work together. Down's syndrome patients usually have a small thymus and an increased number of respiratory infections; they have a diminished number of T cells as well as inadequate immune function of those cells. Large doses of vitamins and minerals have reduced the rate of infectious disease in these patients. B_1 and folic acid levels are low in infection. Infections lower thiamine pyrophosphate by 50 percent. B_6 and pantothenic acid are needed for immunity against some diseases. Intestinal parasites may reduce protein absorption sufficiently to prevent adequate buildup of the immune systems. For every one-degree (Centigrade) rise in the body temperature, there is a 13 percent increase in metabolism. These facts suggest that the seriously ill patient needs more than tea and Jello and an I.V. of glucose and water.

Many conditions, malignant as well as nonmalignant, are being treated with adrenal corticosteroids. Those patients so treated are now known to be immunologically compromised, but those able to control their underlying disease with less than 20 mg per day of prednisone are probably not at significant risk for infection. Larger doses are likely to depress PMN function or cell-mediated immunity. If the PMN count falls below 1000/cumm, be careful; below 500, real danger. The infections these compromised patients get are due to the common bacteria, viruses, fungi, and parasites that normally live on the skin and mucous membranes and in the intestine. When host resistance fails, they invade. Doctors are forced to treat a condition that has resulted from treating a condition. If they improve the immune system, the original disease condition might not return.

It would seem prudent to withhold any treatment with corticosteroids—except for emergencies—until a nutritional approach has been attempted. If it is known that cortisone-like drugs will control a condition, the nutrients that nourish the adrenals should be tried first.

If a person realizes he is having too many respiratory infections, he should get a nose-and-throat specialist to examine him thoroughly. If there are no obvious anatomical anomalies, if his blood test shows no anemia, and if his white cell count is OK and he is not deficient in his IgG, then an allergic workup might be a good move. The patient might also elect to figure it out for himself.

We now know what to do for infections. In doing so we would also be helping an allergy. One can lead to another.

1. Follow the basic good diet. No sugar, no junk.

2. Discontinue dairy products for at least a month and then have them only once every four to seven days.

3. Rotate the diet. Eat no food more frequently than once every four to five days. Eat three to five times a day.

4. Stop any food you eat daily—especially chocolate, corn, wheat, beef. Rotate.

5. Increase vitamin C by 1000 mg per day until the bowel movements are a little sloppy. Use that, or a dose just

short of that, as the daily dose. When an infection begins, take the daily dose hourly until the symptoms subside and then gradually reduce the dose back to the daily amount. When the body is sick, it uses up the vitamin C faster than usual and there is not enough to irritate the intestines.

6. Some people are vitamin A responders. Usually they are those with oily skin, who have had warts, and who notice rough, nutmeg-grater skin on upper arms and thighs. Vitamin A can be taken at 50,000 to 100,000 units per day for a few days along with, or independent of, the vitamin C.

7. A big B-complex capsule, with 50 mg of each of the Bs, two to six capsules a day, would help the body fight the infection and help the enzyme systems that are being stressed.

8. Zinc daily should be at the 30- to 60-mg level.

9. A high-protein diet seems worthwhile.

If a patient finds himself in the hospital, he should insist on a high-protein diet or, if unable to eat, he should be getting amino acids in the I.V. and not just glucose. Vitamin C can be given intravenously for virus infections especially; anywhere from 20 to 200 grams (20,000 to 200,000 mg) of sodium ascorbate or vitamin C (ascorbic acid) plus calcium gluconate. Vitamin C is too acidic by itself, so if used, it is best to add one gram of calcium (as gluconate) to every 20 to 40 grams of vitamin C. One to 3 cc of a B complex can be added to the I.V. drip and could run in over a one- to two-hour period. The sicker the patient, the more vitamin C. It works on poisonings, asthma attacks, bacterial infections, eczema, muscle aches due to low calcium, and many anxiety and stress conditions. Surgeons use this to detoxify their patients from the anesthesia at the end of the operation. It is great for drug addiction.

Thymus gland extract, or the gland itself cold-pressed and dried, has been helpful in controlling infections in some.

Garlic capsules (now come descented), taken daily, work well: five to fifteen capsules a day. Capsicum, goldenseal, thyme, and comfrey are the herbs that help the body with infection.

INSOMNIA □ Insomnia—being unable to fall asleep, waking frequently, or being wide awake hours before it is time to arise—is a common problem in child-rearing. It is often the key motivation that starts drinkers on the path to alcoholism; they drink until they pass out. And when they awaken the next morning, they have the shakes and feel awful, so they have a drink.

Doctors try to help by putting insomniacs on sleeping medicine: "Try this preparation for Seconal. Maybe it will get you in the habit of falling asleep at the proper time." The only habit the doctor gets going is the addiction to sedatives.

For each of us, certain vitamins, amino acids, and minerals are necessary if we are to sleep optimally. Calcium is a great natural tranquilizer. Legend has it that a glass of warm milk at bedtime puts anyone away for a pleasant drug-free eight hours. It does work, unless you are allergic to milk, in which case it might be the worst thing you could do. The allergic reaction would drive the blood sugar down and produce the wakefulness one is trying to avoid. Bad dreams from adrenalin release and a headache in the morning may be the reward for "dairy health." But any food might give this reaction: "Anything can do anything."

Sleep certainly can be influenced by emotions, but it is chiefly affected by biochemistry. The following should be tried after sugar and offending foods are eliminated: Calcium, 1000 mg, about an hour before bedtime. Oyster-shell calcium, calcium orotate, calcium gluconate, and calcium lactate are probably better absorbed than dolomite or bone meal; 1000 mg of vitamin C should help the absorption. I chew up my dolomite with sixteen almonds and swallow all that with a time-release vitamin C. I brush my teeth, pop into bed, sleep my seven hours, and awaken refreshed with very little stiffness, just elephant breath.

Magnesium (as in magnesium oxide or dolomite), 500 mg, should accompany the calcium, as it makes it soluble and cuts down risk of kidney stones. For those deficient in magnesium, sleep is induced rapidly and continues for seven or eight hours without interruption. They awaken refreshed instead of tired. Anxiety and tension are decreased during the day.

Tryptophan is an amino acid found to some extent in all protein. If it can get to the brain it enhances the production of serotonin, a brain chemical that has sedating potential; 500 to 1000 mg about one to two hours before bedtime may help induce sleep; it is best taken an hour after other foods, and accompanied by B_6 (100 mg). Salmon, cottage cheese, and animal meats are good sources of tryptophan. Just eating these protein items, however, is not the answer. Tryptophan has trouble getting to the brain because it is competing with other amino acids for admission. However, if carbohydrate starches (pasta, bread, rice) are eaten in the evening, the insulin thus stimulated will tend to store these competing small-chain amino acids and allow the tryptophan that is floating about to get into the brain and make the serotonin. Carbohydrates at bedtime might help the tryptophan get through during the night for those who awaken during sleep.

If you tend to become drowsy during the day, eat proteins and avoid carbohydrates during the day. The protein will allow tyrosine into the brain, which tends to increase catecholamines (usually with a stimulating effect). If tryptophan gets through instead, due to carbohydrate ingestion, serotonin is produced (calming effect). So the rule is: protein alone to stay awake, and protein and fruits and starchy foods to go to sleep.

Brewer's yeast has niacin and helps many people return to normal sleeping patterns. It works best on those with low histamine levels, since the B complex tends to release histamine from basophils. Calcium can counteract this stimulation. One gram (1000 mg) of niacinamide three times a day will increase the rapid eye movement (REM) sleep by 40 percent. In a recent study, those taking this large amount needed less sleep and were more refreshed.

Other nutrients that work for some are: thiamin, folic acid, B_{12}, pantothenic acid, choline, and inositol (1 gram two times a day). Vitamins A and E, with 1 to 5 grams of C at bedtime, may also be helpful. Valerian root makes many people drowsy; it contains calcium.

Some people sleep better when they quit eating salt. Hops tea and licorice-root tea are very effective sleep inducers.

IRRITABILITY □ Touchy, quarrelsome, negative, ready-to-explode people usually justify their nasty dispositions by saying it's because everyone is against them (paranoid?), or their mother did not love them (was he a brat?), or no one understands them (who can?). It is very difficult to determine if the surly behavior came from not feeling good, or from a misperception of the world that turned him into a short-fused misanthrope.

The bigger problem is to talk these people into trying some nutrients to see if they would become less touchy. *"I'm not the problem; get the world off my back."* If I can find some other symptom to treat—like insomnia, muscle cramps, allergies—and get the patient to try a few things, he begins to feel better and gains some insight into his problem. I can then reason with his cortex.

Daily doses of magnesium (500 mg) and calcium (1000 mg) help the person who is irascible because he feels hemmed in; his space bubble enlarges and he becomes comfortable. B_1, B_6, B_{12}, and folic acid help people to tolerate the world. Zinc can make a difference (30 to 60 mg per day). Restlessness and irritability often point to need for E (400 to 800 units). PABA and GH3 (Gevrital, the Rumanian discovery) make it easier to live under pressure. Pantothenic acid also will help some.

Stress depletes protein, and low protein can lead to irritability. Aluminum and lead poisoning block the action of enzyme systems and cause irritability. A hair test would be revealing. Anemia due to iron deficiency is a possibility.

The knitted, care-worn brow, the forlorn frowner, and the haggard, pinched, picky old man about to hit you with his cane may respond to vitamin C. If you say "Good morning" to a neighbor who responds with "What's good about it?" you fire back, "What did you eat today?"

Low blood sugar can make the touchy one surly. Many edgy people will become gracious and thoughtful, the way humans are supposed to be, if given enough niacinamide (1000 to 3000 mg per day). (See Apathy; Depression.)

If someone gives you a dirty gesture because you got to the parking space first, don't get into a fight. Reminding yourself that he didn't get the nutrients he needed that day will make it easier.

ISCHEMIC ATTACKS, TRANSIENT □ Transient ischemic attacks are temporary episodes of lack of oxygen to areas of the brain due to sluggish circulation, vascular spasm, or clotting of platelets and red cells to the extent that the oxygen cannot get from the red cells to the tissue. No oxygen, no cellular activity. If brain cells controlling memory are cheated, memory is gone, usually temporarily. Little attacks of dizziness, an area of blindness for a few minutes, slurred speech for a moment, all might suggest the problem.

It would be difficult to prove that these are due to slugged blood and not from hypoglycemia or food allergies.

It has been proven that 10 grains of aspirin a day will prevent the platelet cohesiveness that leads to the TIAs. But a safer method to cut this stickiness is the use of vitamin E (400 units minimum to 1600 units maximum). In three months the attacks should be less or gone. Elevated blood pressure is contributory and must be reduced. No sugar and no white flour is mandatory.

J

JUMPING AND JERKING IN SLEEP □ These sudden muscle spasms when least expected while lying quietly in bed fast asleep are usually related to low calcium ingestion. Calcium in 1000-mg doses (500 mg of magnesium makes it work better) taken at bedtime should abolish this problem in about seven to ten days.

Restless legs might respond to vitamin E, 400 to 800 units a day.

If these measures are not helpful, a hair analysis to check the level of minerals might be revealing. Heavy-metal poisoning can make the muscles irritable and twitchy.

K

KIDNEY AND BLADDER INFECTIONS □ Infections of the urinary tract are more common in females than males and have been variously blamed on poor hygiene (wiping from back forward instead of front to back), tight underwear (germs get trapped and multiply), sexual activity (honeymoon cystitis is common), and the short urethra from bladder to perineum. But a lot of women who seldom bathe, and who seem unconcerned about cleanliness down there or the dangers of sitting on cold cement, never get sick. It doesn't seem fair.

I have patients who will get a temperature of 104 and a bona fide kidney infection the day after eating a dairy product. The allergy sets it up. Sugar, too, can cause trouble, because it decreases the ability of the white blood cells to destroy bacteria.

Bacteria grow more easily in alkaline than in acid urine. I have heard from urologists who say that after treating the infection and surgically correcting any physical anomaly present, they have recommended doses of 1000 to 5000 mg of vitamin C daily to promote acid urine and also to improve their patients' immunity.

Cranberry juice acidifies the urine but it must be unsweetened. Cranberries also contain quince, benzoic acid, and other bacteriostatic substances. Try three glasses a day. Other control measures include extra fluid and teas made from uva-ursi, buchu leaves, and chimiphilia.

Take some vitamin C along on the honeymoon. (Helps prickly heat also.)

KIDNEY STONES □ The passage of a kidney stone is supposed to be the most severe pain we can expect to bear. (If I had ever passed one I would leave out the word "supposed.") We all lose about 100 to 200 mg of calcium per day via the kidneys, so it is not surprising to find that 90 percent of kidney stones are calcium phosphate, calcium oxalate, or a mixture. In the urine of those who have a high (alkaline) pH associated with infection, the common one is magnesium ammonium phosphate; 9 percent of stones are uric-acid based, and a few are cystine stones.

Out of motivation to avoid another knifelike attack, kidney-stone makers often stop all calcium intake. But we need calcium daily. The best prevention (of calcium stones) is the following:

1. Drink 1½ to 2 quarts of water daily.

2. Keep calcium at the 800- to 1000-mg level.

3. Magnesium, 100 mg two to four times a day, helps keep the calcium soluble.

4. B_6 reduces oxalate excretion; 50 mg two to three times a day increases the solubility of the calcium.

5. Control infection and use vitamin C, 2 to 3 grams a day; this helps to keep the urine acid, which discourages bacterial growth and helps dissolve calcium. (Cystine stones are more soluble in alkaline urine).

6. Discontinue the oxalates: spinach, rhubarb, and parsley. Reduce the tea, coffee, and chocolate. Slow down on consumption of potato, almonds, pecans, walnuts, and peanuts.

7. Reduce the alkali intake (antacids) and vitamin D.

A milk alkali syndrome is the cause of stones in those consuming much dairy food and taking antacids for a stomach acidity problem. Antacids cause a decrease in phosphates, which increases calcium excretion. The pH rises (more alkaline) and the calcium becomes less soluble. Hyperparathyroidism will bring calcium out of the bones and present so much to the kidneys that stones precipitate out.

Cadmium poisoning may cause kidney stones.

South Carolina natives have a high rate of stones (19/10,000 population) because of the soft water drunk there. There is little magnesium in their diet; it also helps to explain their high heart attack rate.

Diets high in sugar, salt, and protein are associated with hyperoxaliuria and calciuria. A connection with the blood calcium levels associated with hyper- and hypoglycemia (blood sugar fluctuation) is assumed. Diets high in protein result in a severe overall net calcium loss.

On the other hand, a diet very high in vegetable fiber will load the body with oxalates. This coupled with a diet low in phosphate (low in meat) may lead to oxalate crystals in the urine. Orthophosphate will help clear the urine, since it inhibits the precipitation of calcium oxalate.

If a patient has a fat malabsorption problem, the fat in the intestinal tract will bind with calcium, thus freeing oxalates for absorption and possible precipitation in the urine. If the calcium in the diet is increased, it will combine with fats and oxalates and prevent the absorption of the latter.

Uric acid is almost insoluble in acid urine, so the urine must be alkalinized (soda bicarbonate). The presence of uric acid stones means that patient has gout or is eating a diet high in purines. Two to 3 quarts of fluid daily should help make these stones soluble.

Lack of exercise tends to allow calcium to leave the bones and be presented to the kidneys.

L

LABYRINTHITIS □ Labyrinthitis is more properly called a neuronitis of the vestibular apparatus in the inner ear. Vertigo increases over seventy-two hours, forcing the victim to stay in bed because of weakness, nausea, and vomiting. Nystagmus (the eyes snapping back and forth) is obvious. It is caused by a virus, drugs, alcohol, or food allergy. There is no hearing loss or ringing in the ears as is typical of Ménière's disease. It subsides in two days.

Vertigo is the term applied to the sense of whirling, falling, or propulsion; it implies a disease of the ear, the eighth cranial nerve, or the central nervous system. After examination by the ear, nose, and throat specialist, some plan is to be followed to prevent a recurrence.

If an infection is suspected and antibiotics control the disease, the improvement of the immune system is prudent. Vitamins A and C are suggested.

Because allergies can trigger infections and are suspected of even causing vertigo, commonly eaten foods should be discontinued for four weeks to see if improvement is noted. A history of ear infections as a child would lead one to suspect milk as the causative agent even at age forty. Extra vitamin C, calcium, B$_6$, pantothenic acid, and vitamin A should bolster the adrenals.

Fluid accumulation can cause the full feeling and the vertigo and should respond to B_6 (100 to 400 mg per day) and a low-sodium diet. Some show benefit from niacin (B_3); the flush from 50 to 200 mg every few hours is supposed to dilate blood vessels near the inner ear and remove toxins.

LEAD POISONING □ A woman with headaches, weakness, muscle twitches, and poor concentration tried nine doctors, all of whom suggested psychotherapy because there was no clue in the history, the examination, or the lab reports.

A middle-aged doctor noted muscle weakness, overactive intestines, poor memory, skin rashes, and spots before his eyes.

They both suffered from lead poisoning, the great masquerader. The woman was using bone meal to correct a calcium deficiency. Apparently the source was English horses who breathed traffic air (Europeans still use much lead in their gas). The doctor had a colleague who was smart enough to think of the connection between a new house, acid rainfall, and galvanized pipe from the meter into the house. (Copper can be just as devastating.) No particular taste or odor may be associated with the heavy metal.

A Scottish study found a higher incidence of lead poisoning in retarded children than in normal ones. It seemed to correlate with water lead concentrations in the maternal home during the pregnancy. If there is a question, the drinking water in the home should be tested.

Lead poisoning is associated with childhood paint pica: eating the sweet lead-loaded paint that still covers many household walls. But a common source for all of us is the lead spewing out of many cars on our highways. The soil lead level along the freeways is 3000 to 5000 parts per million in the summertime; it does drop to lower levels in the winter after a rain washing or snow run off. Many of us blame headaches and irritability on our spouses and our jobs with no inkling of the real cause.

Many employees who were told their jobs were perfectly safe have poisoned themselves at work and in addition, have brought home enough lead to poison their families as well. An occasional blood test might miss the opportunity to diagnose chronic lead poisoning. Perhaps companies that work with lead should provide a once- or twice-a-year hair analysis for lead storage (lead smelters, storage-battery operations, crystal glass works, demolition work, paint pigment manufacturers, and even shooting galleries).

Anyone can get plumbism, and the diagnosis is difficult because the symptoms are vague and suggestive of neuroses. The absorption and storage of lead and the damage it produces are related to calcium deficiency, which is growing more common in recent years. If calcium is consumed, lead tends to be displaced and is excreted. Some dolomite has lead in it. The calcium in the dolomite may prevent some of the lead from getting into the body. Zinc has a similar effect; up the zinc, and out goes the lead. Children on a good calcium and zinc supplement are less likely to develop lead poisoning.

Lead has been around for a long time, and apparently we are eating and breathing more of it than ever before. If you have contact with civilization you probably are taking in some lead every day. This is one more reason for taking supplements; they will get rid of the lead if you have it and keep it out if you are constantly exposed.

The supplements to be taken are calcium (1000 mg a day), magnesium (500 mg a day), zinc (30 mg a day), vitamin C (1000 to 5000 mg a day), vitamin A (10,000 to 30,000 units a day). Desiccated liver, rutin, and pectin are helpful.

Sulfhydryls chelate with lead; they are found in baked beans and garlic. Algin, or sodium alginate, is a chelating agent; it attaches to lead in the intestinal tract and carries it out of the body. Powdered algin can be used in drinks and food. Lecithin helps the liver neutralize the lead. Potassium iodide has some ability to combine with lead and then get it excreted.

One should not smoke; it can increase your daily intake of lead by 25 percent.

I was worried about the high hair lead level in a patient of mine until he admitted he was using Grecian Formula (which contains lead acetate) to darken his hair!

LEARNING DISABILITIES □ Anyone trying to help a slow-learning child with nutrition realizes that although the difficulty is multifactorial, absorption seems to play a major role. Many of these children cannot absorb the nutrients they eat, and most of the learning disabled don't eat well anyway.

If emotional problems can be ruled out, and if the patient has been checked for lead poisoning and anemia (not just anemia but iron deficiency), a highly nourishing diet with no sugar or junk is the first step. Hypoglycemia (q.v.) or food allergies (q.v.) are the usual cause of learning disabilities if the fuzzy thinking comes and goes—that is, is coincidental with blood sugar fluctuations and, presumably, with neocortical function.

If you had some difficulty during your school years—everyone said you were bright but not working up to your potential—then the following may still be of some benefit:

B_6, pyridoxine, plays a role in the functioning of serotonin and catecholamine in the brain, with calming and stimulating effects respectively; 100 to 400 mg of B_6 a day would be especially helpful in those learning-disabled persons who also have trouble recalling their dreams. Too much B_6 can interfere with magnesium absorption, so 500 mg of that mineral would help.

Calcium is a common deficiency if restless, hyperactive behavior (q.v.) is interfering with learning ability; 500 to 1000 mg a day, depending on dairy product intake, should help. Calcium and magnesium usually are taken at bedtime.

Learning disabilities often are associated with lead and cadmium poisoning, so the hair test might be valuable. Low lithium is another characteristic. Zinc, calcium, and vitamin

C should help replace bad minerals with good. When pregnant animals are low in zinc, their offspring have difficulties learning. Furthermore, it is reported that 30 percent of the children in Iran and Egypt are slow learners. In these countries zinc is difficult to absorb because of the high amounts of phytates in the unleavened bread that is a staple food.

Acetylcholine is another nervous-system chemical needed for thinking, functioning, and learning. Good sources are lecithin granules, 2 to 3 tablespoons a day, or choline (250 mg) one to three times a day.

Those with a long history of allergies, and especially those who needed many formula changes in infancy, may have a milk allergy. The B vitamins help, 100 mg of each, with emphasis on B_1 and B_{12}. Niacin (or niacinamide if the flush produced by niacin is too uncomfortable), at 1 to 3 grams per day, should made some difference in just two to three months. Pantothenic acid, 100 mg two or three times a day, should ease an allergic problem. Vitamin E, 400 to 800 units a day, will make oxygen more available to learning areas of the brain.

Glutamic acid increases GABA, a brain chemical that inhibits neural fatigue, but will take about a month to make a difference.

Vitamin C, 2 to 4 grams a day, helps the brain and the body work. It can allow the brain to think more clearly because it increases the pain threshold and permits the user to pay less attention to incoming stimuli. Also, if one is exposed to an allergen, 2 to 4 grams of vitamin C at the moment of exposure usually will preclude an allergic reaction that could manifest itself with a learning, memory, or thinking failure.

Daryl Maseck of Kinsman, Ohio, described to me a simply contrived experiment in which one half of a class took daily doses of vitamin A (5000 to 10,000 units), vitamin D (500 units), and the B complex (10 to 20 mg of each). In a few weeks the supplemented children gained more than four months' worth in measurable additional skills. In addition absences went down, and the kids paid closer attention and showed less anger and forgetfulness.

A nutrition program for learning could still work for you, even if you are getting too old for the classroom. If you can read this, you are probably not beyond redemption.

LUPUS ERYTHEMATOSIS □ This is considered to be an autoimmune disease. Somehow, through a stress, an infection, or a biochemical screw-up, the body manufactures antibodies against its own tissues. We are set up to make antibodies against foreign bacteria and viruses, and—in the allergic—to produce an itch or sneeze or wheeze. But when the body reacts to itself, it clearly cannot differentiate between self and nonself.

Lupus affects young people, especially females, on the skin of the face first. The cheeks become red, then the heart, kidneys, joints, and muscles become inflamed. The progress is irregular; it may go into remission for a few years.

Rheumatic fever, with its joint and heart damage; glomerulonephritis, which scars the kidneys; dermatomyositis, which hurts the vessels in the muscles and skin; and the devastating ulcerative colitis are all considered to be in this group of autoimmune diseases.

All these conditions have been controlled or modified—but not cured—by cortisone drugs, whence comes the idea that they are superallergies. The problem with cortisone drugs is the side effects: calcium loss, moon face, ulcers, hypertension, and alteration of immunity.

By using cortisone hormone precursors, it is possible to help a victim's adrenal glands make their own cortisol and perhaps even control these autoimmune diseases in a more natural way. Some have tried large doses of vitamin E—1200 to 1600 units after a slow buildup. Selenium is felt to help; 100 to 200 mcg. Pantothenic acid is a cortisol precursor; calcium pantothenate, 5 to 10 grams a day, might push the body into manufacturing enough cortisol to handle the problem. Vitamin C should be increased to 4 to 10 grams a day.

Manganese is low in the bodies of lupus victims, as it is also in the bodies of those with connective-tissue problems (for example, rheumatoid arthritis).

Contraceptive pills will exacerbate lupus. PABA cream is the best protector for the sun-sensitive face.

I have given I.V.s of calcium (1 gram), C (10 grams), B complex (1 cc), plus magnesium (0.5 grams) and some B_6 (100 mg), and these people say they had a more comfortable few days. But we have to go on hoping and searching for something better.

M

MALE HORMONES ☐ Zinc is a key mineral for sexual and genital function. The prostate normally contains a high concentration of zinc. The joke about eating oysters to improve sexual functions is no joke; oysters are the most zinc-laden food known. But zinc would only help if the zinc in the body is low. When men were given a diet deficient in zinc, in two months the sperm count fell from a normal of about 300 million per ml to less than 50 million in some, and to less than that in *all* subjects after fourteen months.

Sperm count is not entirely correlated with desire, ability, mental attiude, or even an erection at the appropriate time. If a man is aware of a nocturnal erection, it means that the nerves and blood vessels are operative. The brain now needs to be involved. B vitamins and an all-purpose mineral supplement, along with a sugarless diet, should allow him to get his act together. I have given B-complex shots to many elderly (even young) men whose chief complaint was impotence. Somehow the shots permitted the brain to tell the genitals what to do, and they responded.

Zinc is usually used at the 30- to 60-mg amount daily. Eggs, onions, and sunflower and pumpkin seeds are rich in zinc. Meat and poultry may have diethylstilbesterol in them; it is a growth stimulant in animals, but because it is a female hormone it may reduce a male's potency. Smoking and alcohol reduce a male's ability to perform. Cold sitz baths can stimulate the male's genitalia. Ginseng is supposed to work wonders.

Some set the alarm for a half-hour earlier to catch the erection at its most tumescent.

MEMORY IMPAIRMENT □ I used to think that my poor memory for people's names was due to narcissism, that I had no energy to remember anyone but myself. I must have picked this up by reading psychiatry texts. But I like people, and this poor memory for names, I now believe, is more likely a genetic defect. My dad was the same way.

In 1979 Dr. Marie Gibbs summarized her memory research findings. Memory formation starts with a change in the electrical properties of the nerve cell membrane. The change is followed by activation of the sodium "pump" in the affected cells, which leads to changes in proteins made by these cells in the brain. Enzymes, which need vitamins and minerals and a good diet, will provide the protein.

Minerals, vitamins, and amino acids can help the brain do as good a job as possible with what it has to work with. The following supplements are all helpful. Give them a try for at least a month.

B_6 is the chief memory vitamin; 50 to 300 mg a day may be necessary. It is usually increased until there is good dream recall. Many learning-disabled persons (q.v.) do better as soon as they get sufficient B_6.

Magnesium is low in some individuals with memory defects; it is also needed if B_6 is used in large amounts. B_1 and B_{12} and folic acid help some. Possibly those who are helped by the latter two were on the borderline of pernicious anemia. Low iron storage may be responsible for poor memory. Lecithin has choline, and choline in the brain can help the enzymes produce acetylcholine, an important chemical that serves the memory skills.

If those are ineffective, manganese (5 to 10 mg a day), may be useful. But remember, if a symptom is hard to understand, an allergy or a heavy-metal poisoning (aluminum or lead) should be considered. Dr. C. Orian Truss ponts out that memory loss is one of the most common symptoms of yeast infestation (q.v.).

One authority stated that more than 15 percent of our population cannot visualize mental images. Their minds are blank. This phenomenon is supposed to be a result of a high histamine level. Calcium and methionine might modify this. L-glutamine has been demonstrated to improve retention among students.

MÉNIÈRE'S DISEASE □ The symptoms are debilitating: vertigo, feeling of fullness in the ear, hearing loss that comes and goes, and tinnitus or ringing in the ear. The cause is still unknown. One sensible hypothesis is a buildup of fluid in the space of the inner ear. Cellular debris ordinarily is transported to a sac from which it is absorbed into the general circulation and disposed of. If the sac distends and irritates the balance center, imbalance and dizziness would be noted. If it lies close to the cochlea, ringing and fullness would be the chief symptom.

Others believe that an imbalance in the autonomic nervous system (due to allergy, virus, or hormones) causes an oversecretion of this endolymph. Microsurgery has been useful to create a shunt away from the area. Medical management is not satisfactory, because the attacks may occur every day for a while and then be gone for a year. The patient (and doctor) may believe that the last treatment was the answer.

On the chance that an infection or an immune deficiency allowed this distressing condition to appear, and because cortisone-like drugs may relieve it, one should try all the nutritional tricks in addition to what the doctor might do. If diuretics and a low-salt diet are helpful, then B_6 might be a safer alternative; 100 to 400 mg a day may suppress a neuritis as well as release fluid. If food allergies are in the family, a water fast may help. Niacin, up to the flush response, is supposed to improve circulation inside; some doubt about that remains, however. Vitamin E helps vascular problems and diseases related to poor oxygenation (400 to 1200 units).

One woman used a water extract of fenugreek seeds; a cup or two of this daily cut the noises in her ears.

(See Dizziness.)

MENOPAUSE ☐ A woman at the menopause must make a tough decision. If she elects to use estrogen-replacement therapy to cut out the hot flashes and to normalize the dry vagina, she runs the risk of breast and uterine cancer. If she decides to go without, she has a 4 times greater risk of ischemic heart disease. Osteoporosis seems to be more common and severe in the older woman (q.v.). Extra calcium seems prudent (1000 to 2000 mg of calcium daily). Exercise will slow the calcium loss and calm some of the menopausal symptoms.

The decision might be easier if her uterus has already been removed, but estrogens should be used cyclically and only in the dose that barely suppresses the symptoms.

If she takes ovarian extract, vitamin E at the 800- to 1200-unit level, vitamin C up to bowel tolerance, and black cohosh, she should be safe and comfortable. Wheat-germ oil and bioflavonoids calm the hot flashes. Food allergies are known to produce all the symptoms of the menopause.

If her morning temperature is consistently low, she could use some thyroid hormone also. B-complex injections every week or so will make the symptoms tolerable.

MENSTRUAL DISORDERS ☐ Menstrual disorders are difficult to evaluate because "normal" is so varied. Medical authorities feel comfortable with the following:

Menarche occurs between age 9 and 16½.
Menses last 1 to 7 days.
Menstrual cycle varies between 21 and 35 days.

Total blood loss should be less than 2½ ounces; the average is 1 ounce.

Perhaps when a woman settles into *her* routine about two years after her menarche, she knows what normal is for *her* body and a change would be a clue of disease, stress, or nutritional fault. I'm sure most women would prefer to have regular periods lasting but forty-eight hours with a half-ounce of blood. Shouldn't a woman try for less discomfort?

Cycles that don't fit the twenty-eight day phases of the moon may be normal. Mothers and daughters often will have the same number of days per cycle. It is not unusual for girls in dorms to arrive at a mean after months of living together. Cycles are optimal when the body and mind are harmonious. A good diet, lack of stress, and extra B vitamins (50 mg of each per day) plus extra B_6 (100 to 300 mg per day) should help the body form and metabolize the hormones at the right time.

Many women assume they are supposed to feel rotten for a few days before their periods. On a good diet (no sugar), extra B complex, choline, and inositol, most women have no clue about the onset of their period. In one study, the length of flow was cut to three days from the "normal" of five days. Fibroid tumors disappeared.

Sixty percent of women have *dysmenorrhea,* or painful periods, sometimes with excessive bleeding.

Painful periods may be relieved with calcium (1000 mg), magnesium (500 mg), zinc (30 to 60 mg), and vitamin E (400 units); it takes at least thirty days to show some results.

Abnormal uterine bleeding is usually a complication of pregnancy. Hypothyroidism and liver disease are often possible causes. If no organic reason can be found, it may respond to good-sized doses of vitamin A (10,000 to 60,000 units). After a month of this amount of A, the bleeding should be less and the dose can be lowered for maintenance. Vitmin E (400 units) and zinc (30 to 60 mg) should make the A more efficient. The contraceptive pill increases the A in the blood;

when the pill is stopped, excessive bleeding occurs. A yeast infection (q.v.) is more likely to show up if vitamin A is deficient. Infertility is associated with low levels of vitamin A. Vitamin C and the bioflavonoids would reduce capillary fragility.

Amenorrhea, or absence of menstrual flow, is most commonly due to pregnancy. If a mature adolescent girl never has had a period, a gynecological exam is obviously mandatory.

Girls who exercise vigorously may become amenorrheic, especially if they lose considerable subcutaneous fat. Eighty percent of the women in the first year at West Point and Annapolis were amenorrheic, but only 20 percent in the second year. Stress and strenuous activity could explain this response. Some message gets to the brain that turns off the pituitary hormones responsible for the menstrual cycle. Mother Nature does not want these girls to become pregnant. Anorexia nervosa will produce the same effect.

Low thyroid function, hypoglycemia, stress, and inadequate nutrition will alter the menstrual pattern. Prolonged allergen exposure can cause missed periods.

Nutrition will help to normalize and stabilize menstrual function, but an examination plus blood tests to rule out the presence of infection, tumors, and anatomical displacements is mandatory.

Menstrual cycles are often the first bodily function to change if a systemic disease, stress, or nutritional fault occurs.

MULTIPLE SCLEROSIS □ This progressive wasting condition is probably a number of diseases.

It seems nihilistic to me to do nothing until the "cause" is discovered and the "cure" can be definitely planned. I like Dr. Frederick Klenner's idea that the disease is a chronic virus (like measles or influenza) that slowly nibbles away at scattered parts of the nervous system, creating widely diverse symptoms and signs, including double vision, poor urinary control, paresthesia, loss of skin temperature sense in some, and muscle weakness. Once the nerves have died, functions associated with those nerves are permanently lost. If the disease can be controlled or reversed before the nerve damage, the patient may have a remission and the diagnosis may be in doubt. It is probably the toughest diagnosis for the neurologist to make in the early stages because it is all too subjective.

An autoimmune process may be involved in the progression of M.S. An initial viral infection may cause injury to the myelin (nerve covering). The products of this degeneration then act as antigens, and the immune response they induce in local cells perpetuates the nerve damage.* Dr. Kenneth Johnson, at the University of California at San Francisco, has found that the ratio of immunoglobulin G to albumin is fairly characteristic in the spinal fluid of M.S. patients. All the work points to an abnormality of the immune system. Dr. Klenner uses vitamin therapy to help convert that imbalance back to normal.

Others have hypothesized the viral connection.† A T cell immune defect is hypothesized. It would fit Dr. Klenner's ideas. Dr. Roy Swank, of the University of Oregon Health Sciences Center, Neurology Department, believes that fat plugs up the tiny capillaries that nourish the nerves. This also would explain the widespread nature of the lesions. He has some success with a no-sugar, no-fat, high-vegetable diet.

Dr. Marshall Mandell has found that a number of patients have been able to make their M.S. symptoms come and go by changing their diet. Inhalation of molds can make some sensitized patients develop a full-blown case of M.S. Freedom from the allergens relieved the symptoms again.

Dr. Hal Huggins has "cured" M.S. patients by removing their amalgam fillings and replacing them with gold. The

* Trese, "Multiple Sclerosis."
† Brody, "Epidemiology."

only clue was that the symptoms appeared within three to twelve months after the fillings were put into place. This is not exactly a mercury or silver poisoning; rather, a sensitivity or an electrical change takes place in the mouth that seems to create some nervous system imbalance.

Less than the normal amount of lecithin has been found in the brains of M.S. victims. This might mean there is less than the normal amount of choline or of nerve covering. But is this a cause or an effect? Hair analysis (for what it is worth toward solving this problem) showed that copper, iodine, manganese, and sulfur were lower in M.S. patients, while selenium was higher.

Dr. Klenner has a regular protocol including vitamin C, thiamin, pyridoxine, and niacinamide intravenously two to four times a week. Intramuscular injections of these plus B_{12}, riboflavin, and crude liver are given daily. Orally the patients get pantothenic acid, lecithin, vitamins A, E, C, folic acid, and choline and mixed minerals plus all the Bs in large amounts. The less time the patient has been ill with M.S., the more rapidly will he go into remission. It is safe and effective, but it doesn't work in every case. The treatment is based on the idea of helping the body develop a better immune system.

Naturopathic physicians believe that most M.S. patients have a gluten intolerance and need pancreatic enzymes; they are often deficient in lipase.

Suggestions: Essential fatty acids should comprise 3 to 10 percent of the caloric intake (from cold-pressed soy oil—3 to 5 teaspoons a day). Selenium, 300 to 500 mcg per day. Copper, 2 to 4 mg per day. Lecithin, 2000 mg per day.

Orotic acid (in liquid whey) has been useful. Raw brain tissue should be tried. Physiotherapy, swimming, and hot mineral baths are helpful, of course.

MUSCLE SYMPTOMS □ Muscles can feel painful, cramped, tight, or tender. Weakness and fatigue are common symptoms. Some symptoms are specifically related to nutritional defects: calcium (1000 mg) and magnesium (500 mg) with some vitamin D are used for cramps, shin splints, and charleyhorses. A manganese deficiency can cause pain; try 5 to 10 mg per day. Those muscle cramps that get you straight up and out of bed like a knifing usually are solved with the above, although B_1, B_6, vitamin E, and potassium may be needed.

Tightness and tenderness in the calves may be relieved with thiamin (B_1). Stiff muscles may be relieved with large doses of C (5 to 10 grams).

Muscle fatigue may be reversed with pangamic acid. Magnesium (500 mg per day) helps muscle weakness and improves stamina. Some weakness is due to low potassium; 3 to 5 grams should relieve it right away. B_6, 100 to 200 mg, may relieve muscle weakness. Vitamin E (400 to 800 units) and selenium (100 to 200 mcg) help muscle performance, probably by improving oxygen utilization. Because E improves glycogen storage, it also prevents disturbed sleep due to restless legs (ill-defined creepy, crawly sensations, and jerks in the muscles). Folic acid makes a difference (1 mg a day). And no more caffeine.

Vitamin E may prevent some muscle wasting; it might improve the circulation that nourishes the muscle tissue.

Dr. Emanuel Cheraskin has been following the symptoms of hundreds of professionals (doctors and dentists) as related to their nutrition. The higher the use of refined sugar, the more muscular complaints noted. Higher doses of C, B, and E were associated with fewer musculoskeletal symptoms.

MUSCULAR DYSTROPHY □ This is a general name for a variety of muscular wasting diseases, usually starting in childhood. The muscles deteriorate, sometimes rapidly, until there are not enough left for function.

Nutrition can slow the progress, but once the muscles have atrophied and scarred, recovery is nil. We try to identify the disease early and apply what has been helpful. I have two patients who were identified by neurologists and biopsies as having muscular dystrophy; one is functioning normally and the other has an arrested case with minimal involvement.

The basic help seems to come from wheat-germ oil. It contains octacosanol, which somehow helps repair the damage. Vitamin E also is useful. Lots of B vitamins and brewer's yeast contribute. Vitamin C also makes a difference.

Muscular dystrophy can be caused by a diet deficient in sulfur-containing amino acids, vitamin E, and selenium.

MYASTHENIA GRAVIS □ This is now felt to be another autoimmune disease (see Lupus) in which antibodies block acetylcholine receptors at the nerve-muscle junction. The motor neuron endplate secretes the neurotransmitter, acetylcholine, but the receptor sites are unresponsive; the nerve cannot tell the muscle to contract. This is especially noted in the head, neck, and diaphragm muscles.

Treatment includes use of drugs that have an anticholinesterase activity (cholinesterase is an enzyme that metabolizes acetylcholine), thus leaving more acetylcholine at the neuromuscular junction to stimulate the muscle. Removal of the thymus has helped some because of its relation to immunity reactions.

Manganese has been reported to help. Vitamin C and the B complex could help the body function properly and possibly overcome an autoimmune disease. Vitamin E shows promise; the 400-unit dose is increased every few days to 800 units and even higher than 1600 units in some.

Prostaglandins help this autoimmune disease; use an unsaturated fatty acid mixture with about 70 percent linoleic acid. Brewer's yeast is helpful, as are arachidonic acid (cereal grain oils), liquid lecithin, calcium, and vitamin D.

N

NAILS □ Healthy nails are hard, firm, pink, and smooth. Examining the nails is part of the reading-the-body routine that we all owe ourselves. What some nails show us:

Ridges running lengthwise probably mean a protein deficiency or a vitamin A deficiency. Nails that peel easily probably are low in vitamin A. Flattened or dished nails are usually due to an iron deficiency, which also accounts for thin and brittle nails. White spots on the nails are most often due to a zinc deficiency, but low thyroid function can do the same thing. Calcium and magnesium supplements toughen brittle nails, since these are often a sign of a calcium deficiency. Brittle nails that peel easily need silica. Drinking horsetail tea daily will improve this. If the nails are whitish and opaque, it suggests too much copper; zinc will help this. If a woman sees a white line running across the nail, it means that she is high in copper and low in zinc at the time of each menstrual period. Poor nail growth as well as slow body growth may be due to poor zinc absorption.

Both hair and nails need sulfur-containing amino acids to help keratin growth. Split nails may mean sulfur amino acids are low in the diet. Vitamin C, 3000 mg a day, will often help control split nails. Try this one: to 6 ounces water add 3 teaspoons protein powder, 1 teaspoon unsweetened gelatin, plus a little Vegesal for flavoring; drink daily.

NARCOLEPSY □ These sleep attacks are irresistible and may occur at inappropriate moments. Usually the sleep is accompanied by extreme fatigue. Those afflicted have to take daily naps, and they feel tired and dragged-out in between. Some disorder of the sleep center is obviously at fault. Because Ritalin is almost a specific for narcolepsy, and because this drug potentiates the brain chemical norepinephrine, it suggests that a supportive therapy might involve giving the patient enough B vitamins to help him make his own.

The triggering mechanism seems to be sugar or allergen consumption. (See Hypoglycemia.) I have had luck with B-complex injections; the patient gives himself a shot every week. It cuts the need for Ritalin.

NAUSEA ☐ This symptom can be associated with anxiety, depression, virus disease invasion, pregnancy, food allergy, and bad news. It is an exhausting symptom since it usually is accompanied by weakness, light-headedness, and sweating.

The pregnant woman used to be told that her nausea was the symbolic rejection of the unwanted child. We now know that her excess hormones at this time are creating the problem. She must remember her high metabolic rate and eat every two to four hours night and day and take extra B complex, especially B_6 (50 to 200 mg a day). Some require B-vitamin injections.

If nausea is the first clue that a virus illness is about to overwhelm the queasy one, he should begin to take about 1000 mg of vitamin C (orally if he can choke it down) every hour until the illness calms down. Muscle shots would be an alternative choice.

Vitamin C, along with calcium and B_6, usually can reverse a food allergy reaction if taken on ingestion of the offender. Once the nausea begins it may be too late, but is worth trying.

Anxiety is frightening because of the adrenalin that accompanies the anxiety (or causes it), but this evoked chemical reaction could be assuaged—if one thinks of it and can get it down—by some protein, B complex, and sometimes a niacin pill (50 to 100 mg) held until dissolved on the back of the tongue.

Sometimes throwing up solves the problem. Persistent nausea should be investigated with at least an x-ray barium meal.

(See Abdominal Discomfort.)

NERVOUSNESS ☐ This can mean anything from a slight twinge of shakiness when you almost got run over by a car to an attack of overwhelming panic for no good reason. Everyone has different perceptions of what is frightening.

Some cannot go anywhere because they fear an anxiety attack.

These inappropriate yet scary perceptions of the world are due to a faulty screening device. Calcium and magnesium are helpful in permitting the nervous person to feel the world as less close and threatening. Vitamin A also has calmed the nervous.

Hypoglycemia (q.v.) and food allergies (q.v.) can keep people on the edge of "scared to death" because of the constant flow of adrenalin stimulated by falling blood sugar. All the B-complex vitamins are helpful here; B_1, B_3, and B_6 especially seem to keep the taker cool and comfortable.

(See Anxiety; Depression; Fatigue.)

NEURITIS □ Nerve inflammation can be due to trauma, viral infection, heavy-metal poisoning (see Hair Analysis, Chapter 4), and vitamin and mineral deficiencies. When you hit your "crazy bone" and feel the tingling and notice the numbness, you are suffering from a traumatic neuritis. But you also know it will soon be gone. The carpal tunnel syndrome (q.v.) is a neuritis that does not go away until the constricting ligament is cut or the person takes B_6 to get the nerve back to normal.

Numbness and tingling can be due to a neuritis caused by muscle or bone pressure on a nerve coming from the spinal column. All the B vitamins are used to treat neuritis, but B_1, B_6, and B_{12} are the primary ones that help. Calcium can calm the muscle spasm and perhaps slow down further loss of bone from the osteoporotic (q.v.) spine. A daily B_{12} shot (1000 mg) intramuscularly for five to ten days often stops the symptoms.

If one is using over 2 grams of B_6 a day for any condition, numbness and tingling of fingers and toes could appear, possibly because folate is being displaced. Also, large doses of B_6 cause a relative magnesium deficiency.

Bell's palsy is a facial-muscle paralysis due to an infection or trauma of the facial nerve. If the nerve has not been severed, B_{12} and the rest of the B complex, especially pantothenic acid, may help restore function.

Painful neuritis may be helped with large doses of manganese, 80 to 150 mg a day for a few days. Calcium will help neuritis; 1000 mg a day should do it.

Pins-and-needles sensations in the legs may be solved with folic acid and B_{12}, best as muscle injections; it may be the first clue of incipient pernicious anemia.

Burning or "electric feet" (the sensation of small electric shocks) usually respond to pantothenic acid. Tingling of the lips is usually due to low magnesium.

Chronic acidosis and toxemia will trigger neuritis. Constipation is a stress.

Acupuncture is very effective for neuritis.

NIGHT BLINDNESS □ Trouble seeing in the semi-darkness usually is associated with vitamin A deficiency. Vitamin A needs zinc to function properly, and a protein deficiency will aggravate a borderline A deficiency.

Vitamin A deficiency is often associated with hyperkeratosis, warts, acne, excessive bleeding in menses, and respiratory infections that do not respond to vitamin C.

The recommended daily allowance of A is only 5000 units, which 20 to 40 percent of our population is not getting. For night blindness, one aims at about 20,000 to 50,000 units daily for three to five weeks, and then the dose is lowered to about 10,000 to 20,000 units for maintenance.

(See Eyes.)

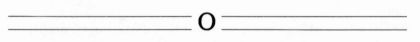

OBESITY □ It seems logical to assume that in a condition so obviously related to diet as is obesity, simply reducing the calorie intake would solve the problem. This was our teaching in medical school forty years ago. This is the reason your doctor may curl his lip at you when you tell him that you tried; he knows you didn't follow his directions. This upsets him because he needs to feel successful and you are wrecking his statistics.

Whenever lay people organize into therapeutic groups, it indicates that orthodox medicine has failed. TOPS, Weight Watchers, Alcoholics Anonymous, all indicate that doctors have had a poor success rate with weight reduction and the control of alcoholism. (No ex-pneumonia or post-appendectomy societies have been formed; these patients are either well or gone.)

Because obesity is such a depressing problem to have and so frustrating to treat, a great deal of research has been accomplished, some of which has filtered down to the discouraged overweight individual. The popularity of weight-reducing programs and best-selling diet books attest to the great desire of a large number of our citizens to lose weight and feel more energetic. The many different methods of losing weight suggest there are many different causes.

From all the investigations—biochemical, psychiatric, genetic, and anthropological—a few generalizations can be made.

Primitive people who exercise and get no sugar or processed food are rarely overweight.

It is hard to be fat on a vegetarian diet. The sheer bulk of the usual vegetarian diet precludes a calorie overload. Vegetarians feel stuffed before they get enough calories to gain weight.

If both parents are obese, 80 percent of the children will be heavy. If only one parent is so disposed, only 40 percent of the children will be so touched. If both parents are thin, only 10 percent of the children will have the tendency to overweight. Heredity obviously plays a role here, but it is not clear-cut like the inheritance of blue eyes. Dr. William Sheldon stumbled on one explanation of how genetic factors can promote overweight. In the 1930s while doing autopsies, he noticed that the characteristics of obese people included a long intestinal tract (40 feet), short tapering fingers, and thick lips. The skinny ectomorphs, on the other hand, had 20 feet of intestines for absorption, long thin fingers, and thin lips. The assumption is made that the endomorphs are fat-suscep-tible because they have twice as much area for absorption; they pick up every last calorie. And this probably is a factor.

The consistent biochemical abnormality that overweight people carry with them from their chubby childhood is a high circulating level of insulin. Insulin, a hormone secreted by the beta cells of the pancreas, is essential in carbohydrate metabolism. The insulin molecule binds to receptor sites on cell membranes. This initiates the metabolic process of con-version of glucose into energy or else the process of storing it as glycogen (in liver or muscle cells) or as fat in adipose tissue.

It is known that early feeding of quickly absorbed sugary foods will "induce" the enzyme that secretes insulin. In rats, at least (and humans are somewhat comparable), if food is given in small amounts early in life, obesity is rare in later life no matter what amounts of food are given. Studies of adults whose mothers were subjected to famine in Holland and Leningrad during World War II reveal that if the calorie restriction was confined to the last half of the pregnancy, few of these infants developed obesity as adults. The assumption is made that they developed fewer adipocytes (fat storage cells). The adipocytes proliferate from birth to age two years and again in puberty. Obese children tend to have increased numbers of these fat cells. And once the cells have been filled with fat, they seem more ready to balloon up with fat again, even after weight loss.

The social factors of obesity are very real and compel-ling. Generally, the higher women are on the socioeconomic scale, the less apt are they to be overweight. However, Mid-dle European families show the opposite trend; the higher up on the socioeconomic ladder, the more obese they become. The longer families have lived in the United States, the less likely it is that the children will grow up obese.

If obesity sets in before six to eight years of age, it is more likely to be a lifetime problem, defying treatment. If it sets in just at the beginning of puberty, it is easier to treat. Studies of identical twins reared in different environments revealed a striking similarity in their weights. Genetics plays a big role.

No consistent, pervasive psychological profile has been found in the obese. Immaturity, dependency, frustration, depression, and anxiety are thought to be secondary to the poundage. Obese adolescents usually are inactive. They isolate themselves, feel sorry for themselves, are rejected by their peer group, become depressed, and then eat because of their depression and misery. The heavy parents cannot seem to help because they frequently have the same problem themselves. The most typical pattern in the obese teenager is to eat no breakfast or lunch and then to snack on high-energy, sugar-laden foods from supper to bedtime. Mealtimes for the heavy child or adolescent are stressful because someone is usually lecturing about food and diet; the youngster prefers to eat somewhere else and often chooses junk.

After the school years are over, energy expenditure is less but calorie intake may stay the same. Most of us pick up 20 pounds in the twenty years from marriage to middle age. We are not exercising enough. (I see people *standing* on the down escalator.) Just ingesting 100 calories a day more than is expended will add 36,500 calories in a year—that's 12 pounds of extra stored energy (fat). We get those 100 calories in one bottle of pop or beer, or one slice of bread with a little butter, or just 1½ ounces of steak. A common cause of obesity is the slowing of metabolism with age. Many of use continue to consume the same amount of food as we age; instead of burning it up, we store it.

A "glandular" disorder is rarely the cause of obesity.

Low levels of thyroid hormone excretion due to a thyroid disease usually produce dry, thick skin, slow heart rate, constipation, feeling cold when others are comfortable, but almost never obesity. If a person has warm, moist palms, the thyroid is usually working well. Cold, dry palms are more likely an indication of low thyroid function (see Thyroid Problems). Some have an insulin-secreting tumor that produces hunger and fat storage. A few lack an enzyme that completes the metabolism of carbohydrates; the energy is stored as fat. Some rare endocrine disorders complete the list.

If a mother is exposed to severe calorie restriction in the first half of her pregnancy, that infant she is carrying has an increased chance of becoming obese. The Dutch and Russian women who were subjected to famine in World War II while pregnant had low-birth-weight newborns. If the food restriction was in the first few months of pregnancy, the study suggested that damage occurred to the developing nervous system of the infant. Under such conditions, the hypothalamus apparently is not put together properly and will not respond to satiety or biochemical cues in later life. Obesity is common in those thus hurt.

Early feeding of solid food and the increased use of formula (cow's) milk has been felt by some to program the child's biochemistry for future love of sweets, the need to feel full, and the desire to eat when frustrated, tired, or anxious. Breast-fed babies quit when they feel full, and they tend to suck frequently day and night. The amount of protein in human breast milk is low compared to that of other mammals that nurse their infants less often. (Human milk, 3 percent protein; rabbits' milk, 13 percent protein—bunnies get nursed once a day.) We may have set up a child for future fat by telling the mother, "What a cute, chubby baby" and paying extra attention to the weight gain in those early months. Bottle-fed babies often are urged to finish the last ounce or two.

Hilde Bruch has stated that if parents offer food when the baby is fussy for nonhunger reasons, the learned response is "Eat when upset." The infant becomes unable to differentiate between hunger and fullness; every discomfort, physical or emotional, is now a cue to eat.

Pediatricians urged solids down the reluctant babies' throats to preclude the milk anemia so common with babies fed on cow's milk. I'm embarrassed to remember that I told mothers to get the rice cereal down the baby at two to three weeks of age—all in the name of good preventive medicine. We thereby set susceptible babies up for a lifetime of allergies and opened fat cells for future use.

The foods that went down the easiest, of course, were the puddings, gelatines, ice cream, and soft drinks. As the child grew, he would eat little unless it tasted sweet. TV advertising and fast-food restaurants promoted and catered to this tilted taste. School cafeteria cooks know that if they put out vegetables, they are going to get vegetables back. Luncheon menus are sugar-, starch-, and salt-laden because that is what the children will eat.

Allergies enter into the picture also. Eighty percent of people with food allergies have hypoglycemia. That is, when a person eats a food to which he is allergic (milk, corn, wheat, eggs, nuts), his metabolism deals with the food in such a way that the blood sugar rises and falls and the glucose from that food is stored as fat. When the blood sugar falls, the victim feels a craving to eat more. The cortex of the brain usually is not functioning too well when the blood sugar fluctuates, so self-control is lost and the craving is satisfied. This leads to obesity.

THERE ARE SOME suggestions that might prevent the accumulation of unwanted fat:

Do not allow sugar in your house. Sugar may be the most important factor in fat accumulation because of its stimulation of insulin secretions. It is also the major substrate for alpha-glycerophosphate synthesis, essential in fat production. Glucose supplies the 2-carbon fragment (acetyl-coenzyme-A) that is built into fatty acid chains. Glucose also supplies the hydrogen used in fatty acid synthesis. The availability of quick carbohydrate is the major facilitating factor in the release of insulin and the accumulation of fat. When insulin levels are low, fat can more easily be used. White and brown sugar, corn syrup, maple syrup, molasses, and honey are the offenders. It would be best not to use saccharin, cyclamates, or other artificial sweeteners, because they promote the idea that things must taste sweet. This policy would be especially important in those families that have a high incidence of diabetes, obesity, alcoholism, hypoglycemia, mental illness, hyperactivity, and allergies. There are biochemical connections.

During any pregnancy try to avoid sugary foods and empty calories (for example, white bread, boxed cereals, processed food). Pregnancy is a stress, and extra B vitamins, folic acid, calcium, iron, zinc, trace minerals, and vitamin C are needed in abundance and not in RDA amounts. One should aim for a 30-pound weight gain. The foods should include protein, complex carbohydrates, roughage foods, some saturated and unsaturated fats. Try to nibble; eat six small meals a day. The idea is to keep the blood sugar level as even as possible. Avoid drugs, even aspirin and antihistamines, if possible. You are going to rear this child; if a child is healthy and cheerful, he or she is easier to love and care for. Don't let the doctor give you a prescription for a diuretic; you need this extra fluid so you can nurse the baby. Try to eat common foods only every fourth day. (See Pregnancy.)

Nurse the baby for at least a year; two is better, if possible. But even two weeks of nursing is better than none. Nursing cuts down the chance of a food allergy, which often goes hand-in-hand with hypoglycemia. If the baby seems colicky, do not stop the nursing, since the distress is very probably due to an allergy to something the mother is eating. She should alter her diet. (Extra calcium, magnesium, vitamin C, and the B complex for the baby, might control the crying.) Delay solid foods until close to the first-year birthday. Babies fed on cow's milk should have an iron supplement; the only reason for starting solids is to prevent iron-deficiency anemia. Breast-fed babies rarely become anemic.

The growing child should be checked periodically for a too-rapid weight gain in relation to the increase in linear growth. The pediatrician has growth charts that will tell, but physical inspection ("Does he or she look fat?") and a quick check of skin-fold thickness will reveal the problem. It is probably better to cut down the rate of weight increase than to try to get a child to reduce. Weight reduction during the growing years is difficult and potentially dangerous to overall health.

If the adolescent has been overweight from infancy on, treatment is very difficult but possible. Treatment is easier if the youngster acquired the excess weight in puberty. Motivation is all-important. The whole family should be involved. Behavior modification, exercise, and attention to the types and quality of food are important. Crash and fad diets are to be discouraged. Aiming for a vegetarian diet is worthwhile. The trick is to sneak enough food in for body function without the pancreas suspecting what is happening, so that it won't overproduce insulin. Energy would come from the fatty acids mobilized from fat.

The diet must fulfill the following criteria: (1) all needs of the body must be met except the high calorie demand; (2) the food habits must be catered to; (3) fatigue and hunger must be minimal; (4) the foods must be easy to obtain and not appear too different from "ordinary" food.

Nibbling—eating like a grazing animal—may be the best approach for most dieters who get that "all gone" feeling when they attempt to cut calories. Eating one meal a day not only increases the cholesterol level in the blood but reduces the infrequent eater's glucose tolerance. One- and two-meal-a-day eaters are likely to be fatter than four- to six-meal-a-day eaters.

If the 24-hour caloric requirement is consumed in one half-hour time period (like eating one meal a day), the capacity of the liver to store glycogen will be exceeded. The glucose floating about stimulates the production of insulin, and this glucose is stored in the adipocytes as fat.

But the body needs energy during the remaining 23½ hours, so it more conveniently turns muscle protein into energy. Each day a little more fat is laid down and a little more muscle protein is lost. These people become fat and tired. Exercise is difficult when they are so weak.

Excess fatty acids in the bloodstream may exceed the ability of the liver to store them. The blood level remains high and the adipocytes have another source of fat. The ingested amounts must be reduced, the efficiency of the liver increased, and an exercise program launched.

Exercise is a helpful part of the total plan. It must be fun, consistent, and convenient. For aerobic exercise to burn the fat in muscles, it must be strenuous enough to get the pulse elevated for twelve to fifteen minutes at a level close to this formula: 180 minus the age in years equals the pulse rate to maintain. Doing this every other day would be ideal. To become fit, one must really use the major muscles in the calves, thighs, and lower back. *Use* them, that is, not massage or vibrate them. An hour of jogging burns 900 calories. Walking at four miles an hour consumes 200 calories. Walking daily for an hour will take off about 20 pounds in a year; it will also decrease cholesterol levels.

Fat is burned by muscles, so heavy people must exercise, though they usually find it difficult and uncomfortable. They should push up to their capacity: until they are just short of breath. That's the exercise level that is burning the fat.

The protein of the muscle cells is the chief user of fatty

acids, so most authorities recommend a diet that spares the body's protein. Starvation is not an efficient way to lose, because to maintain energy levels the body will mobilize protein and turn it into glucose to be burned. When humans are starved, 35 percent of the weight loss comes from fat tissue and 65 percent from muscles! The muscles must not be allowed to disappear; they are needed to burn fat, and fat is mobilized and burned more easily when insulin levels are low. This is why a nibbling, low-carbohydrate, high-protein—or at least high-complex-carbohydrate—diet is essential.

My estimate for a 900-calorie diet is that 35 grams of high-quality, complete protein would be the minimum amount to hold a 150-pound (70-kg) normal-weight adult together; 150 grams of carbohydrate and 20 grams of fat (half saturated and half unsaturated) would make the food palatable. Many people have trouble counting calories, so this would translate into the following: a piece of protein food about the size of an egg six times a day; about a tablespoon of corn, peas, potatoes, six times a day; the fat allowed is equivalent to 1½ tablespoons of butter. Cheese and meat would already have enough fat in them to satisfy the 20 grams. If a heavy person needed 2500 calories to maintain the weight and used a 900-calorie diet per day, in a week this deficit of 1600 calories a day would amount to 11,200 calories, or about a 3-pound loss of fat.

The following diet limits carbohydrates even more (down to 50 to 80 grams per day) and would encourage fat utilization for energy because the body would not be encouraged to secrete insulin.

Breakfast: 1 egg (or equivalent amount of fish, meat, cheese); one-half slice of whole wheat toast and butter; piece of fruit.

Snack: 1-inch cube of low-fat cheese; piece of fruit.

Lunch: One chicken leg, broiled or baked, no skin;
          green salad with 1 ounce vegetable oil; raw
          vegetables: celery, cauliflower, carrots.
Snack: wheat cracker with old-fashioned peanut
          butter.
Dinner: piece of fish; low-carbohydrate vegetables,
          steamed; green salad with ½ ounce of vege-
          table oil.
Bedtime: 6 almonds.

Some believe that unsaturated fat helps oxidize stored fat. If the Pritikin method is used, the dieter may not get enough of the essential fatty acids. (Linoleic acid [EFA] is needed to produce prostaglandins.) Primrose seed is almost all essential fatty acid. Soy oil is 75 percent; safflower, 55 percent. Two to 3 tablespoons per day is about right. Vitamins must be added: C, B complex, folic acid, kelp tablets, some potassium supplement, as well as calcium (1000 mg) and magnesium (500 mg).

Sometimes a loss doesn't happen because with calorie restriction the metabolism slows. This may be counteracted with thyroid medication so that the serum thyroid levels are held in the upper part of the normal range. An easy home assay of thyroid function is to take the oral or axillary (armpit) temperature in the morning, before arising. According to Dr. Broda Barnes, it should be 97.8 to 98.2° and not under, if thyroid function is normal. If thyroid medication is needed, it may not be necessary after normal weight is achieved.

If a heavy person got that way because he or she had been eating sugar, white flour, and empty calories, that person is probably low in B-complex vitamins. The Bs are absolutely essential for carbohydrate (and all) metabolism. Many people when trying to reduce find that large doses (50 to 100 mg of each of the Bs) are essential. These vitamins are the first to be depleted in times of stress, and they are involved in the glucose-tolerance factor. They help the body get the fat out of storage so it can be burned. They help with the energy level. Vitamin B complex shots often are needed at the beginning of treatment to "prime the pump." Folic acid may be a key vitamin because it is essential in intestinal absorption. Taking the B vitamins after eating may prevent appetite stimulation.

Lecithin is helpful to some. In powder, granules, or capsules, it seems to have some effect on fat metabolism. A daily intake of 2 to 5 tablespoons of the solids stirred into a drink, or five to ten capsules, would be about right.

Lipotropic factors, methionine, choline, and inositol metabolize fats. These have methyl donors that help the liver metabolize wastes. Suggested: choline, 1000 mg; methionine, 1000 mg; B_6, 100 mg; B_{12}, 30 mg; iodine, 225 mcg (kelp); magnesium, 100 to 500 mg. Herbs that help: taraxicum, chelidonium majus, Russian black radish beet leaf.

Many people tell me that the vitamins gave just enough boost to their energy level that they could exercise a little and be more cheerful. The exercise made their bodies more efficient. It increased the oxygen supply to the tissues, which improves metabolism.

Behavior modification attempts to change the actions that lead to food consumption. Thin people usually cannot eat when angry; obese people find that food calms their emotions. The visible cues that suggest food must be minimized. Slow eating allows ingested glucose to get to the brain's appetite control center and signal "full" before too much has been consumed. As a base line, the heavy person must write down when, where, what, how much he ate for an average week. This person must then plan to eat six small meals in the same place in one room. No TV, no reading—just eating slowly in the company of compatible people. Many people eat while watching TV. If this association is carried on for some time, watching TV will signal a hunger sensation. Overweight people eat twice as much if the clock is turned ahead to fool them into thinking it is supper time. Obese people will eat less if only one sandwich is served (and the others are stored in the refrigerator) than if three are placed before them. Eating the protein first uses stomach acid digestion more appropriately; chew slowly and lovingly, putting the fork down after every mouthful. Starches, fruits, and vegetables should be chewed to a soupy pulp before swallowing.

Drinking eight to ten glasses of water a day helps the dieter. No caffeine-containing drinks should be allowed, since they promote insulin secretion, which puts the fat into the cells.

You may call the above paragraphs the Lendon Smith Diet if it helps you to stick to it. Motivation is important in any weight-control program. No one has ever motivated a fat person to lose weight by frightening him or her with statistics about the association of overweight with diabetes, hypertension, coronary artery disease, gallstones, fatty liver, and thrombo-embolic problems. (The increase in morbidity occurs only in those who are 20 percent overweight or more. In those persons 30 percent overweight, the mortality is up 35 percent.) Falling in love may help, making the team is good, so is feeling good about oneself because of landing a great job—but these may not last. People with high anxiety levels rarely lose much weight (the anxiety, however, could be due to the adrenalin released when the high insulin level rapidly reduces the level of blood sugar). Weight Watchers is helpful as a support group; dieters easily get discouraged. Medical Diet Service provides psychological support also.

The overweight patient and the doctor—or the support group—must establish working relationships and some realistic goals. For example, 4 pounds of weight loss per month and a 40-pound loss per year.

Nutritional education is a must. (What is a protein?) Drug therapy is a dangerous crutch. Thyroid medication can be used with safety to encourage the metabolic process. With some patients whose fat clings tenaciously, I have had luck with the nibbling diet accompanied by vitamin B complex shots given every other day intramuscularly. This seems to help some enzyme system work better along the metabolic pathway, but most importantly, it helps the patient's resolve by inducing some system in the brain to make some chemical that tells the patient, "You're OK; you can do it."

If everything has been tried, the patient may find the pounds fall off when he stops eating the particular food he loves. Sugar is not the only villain; dairy products, soy, corn and beef are common allergens, and allergens will produce the metabolic screw-up the discouraged person is trying to avoid. Remember, anything can do anything.

ODORS, BODY □ Give me a good, honest, sweaty smell anytime. Most of us are so used to the nonsmell of the other humans about us that now, when we get a whiff of someone who had to run through traffic, we are shocked—even though the smell is normal.

Sometimes a patient comes along who is getting complaints from friends and relatives and even from a few strangers. The odor is unmistakable. It hits with a force that makes the smeller stop midbreath. It is full and overpowering.

"It's there within an hour after a good long bath. I've changed soap ten times."

Magnesium is the answer. In about a week of 500 mg a day, the odor is gone. Magnesium is present in chlorophyll; alfalfa tablets can be used. Zinc deficiency can be responsible for disagreeable body odors, especially smelly feet. Some have an unwashable skin odor when reacting to certain allergens.

The skin acts as an organ of elimination. Constipation, with its autointoxication, can be the cause of smelly skin. A dry-brush rub will help to take off the outer layers of dead skin so it can act as a pathway for elimination.

(See Abdominal Problems; Breath and Breathing.)

OSTEOMALACIA (RICKETS) □ It is hard to diagnose rickets in an adult until the soft bones in the legs begin to bow, or the spine bends and pinches nerves, or the teeth fall out. Caused by a decreased intake of vitamin D, it is prevalent among residents of smoggy North American cities and especially among blacks (because of the pigment protection).

Weakness, limping, and aches and pains in muscles and bones characterize osteomalacia. Calcium and phosphorus are at low levels in the blood, and the enzyme indicating bone activity, alkaline phosphatase, is elevated. (These tests are normal in the osteoporotic patient—q.v.). This represents a loss of calcium from the protein matrix of the bone and is caused by malabsorption of vitamin D, calcium, and phosphorus, as well as by chronic liver disease and kidney failure. (If phosphates are not absorbed adequately and vitamin D is administered, calcium is absorbed, and in the presence of low phosphate calcium moves out into the urine to possibly produce stones. Vitamin D activity depends on adequately functioning kidneys.) Osteomalacia is easily treated with calcium, phosphorus, and vitamin D (500 to 1000 units/day).

Almost everyone living indoors or in sun-poor areas should take some Vitamin D in the winter. A teaspoon of cod liver oil a day would provide 500 units of D, 5000 units of A, and some of the essential fatty acids. Vitamin D will not be effective without calcium; if you cannot stand dairy products, take a supplement. Magnesium helps the calcium stay soluble. (Calcium, 1000 mg a day; if rickets is present, double the calcium for a few weeks; magnesium, 500 mg.) Phosphates are necessary for bone structure if rickets is present. Meat eaters usually have enough. Brewer's yeast is a good source; it's full of phosphorus.

OSTEOPOROSIS □ It is somewhat embarrassing when dentists are the ones to diagnose a body condition first. A simple question asked of the thirty-year-old might have saved him or her the loss of all the teeth at age fifty and a broken hip at age seventy. For people destined to have osteoporosis, it is known that once the skeleton gets well fixed and established at age twenty-five, if no calcium is added, 1 percent of the calcium will wash out of the skeleton in these susceptible people every year. By the age of seventy-five, one-half of the skeleton is gone. In most people the skeletal mass is maintained effectively from age twenty-five to fifty. After the menopause and presumably because they have lost the calcium-retaining properties of estrogens, women "normally" lose about 1 percent of the skeletal mass every two years. In men this loss occurs after age sixty to seventy. Loss of 2 to 4 inches of height in fifty years is not uncommon. X-rays diagnose the condition only after at least 30 percent of the calcium is leached out. A blood test for calcium is usually at 8 mg per 100 ml of blood; the blood will continue to pull calcium out of the bone to maintain an optimum level in the blood.

If the doctor had only thought to ask just a couple of questions about the diet! "How do you get your calcium?" "Do you take vitamin D?" "What is the amount of phosphorus (meat and soft drinks) ingested compared to the calcium?" The trick is to be suspicious that something is wrong with the balance of minerals in the body and to take some remedial action early.

Usually the first symptom noticed by the calcium loser is chronic low back pain. X-rays and examination show the doctor nothing. Stress is diagnosed and a muscle relaxant is prescribed. A chiropractor can sometimes tell by the feel of the tight muscles that it is due to a low calcium condition. A few questions at this point would have helped indicate the source of the difficulty. Clues are a history of milk allergy or low intake, growing pains, restless behavior, foot jiggling, hair twisting, thumb sucking, insomnia, muscle cramps, inadequate calcium and vitamin D intake.

In the fourth decade the teeth may start to loosen; pyorrhea allows the support structures of the teeth to degenerate.

Stress has something to do with this. Poor oral hygiene and an inadequate diet are also responsible. Sugar and soft-food intake prevent proper jaw bone exercise. Tissues need exercise or they atrophy. Deposits about the teeth will make the gum slough. Some preventive-minded dentists will use a nutrition approach to prevent further loss of the bone supports; they are treating the whole body to save the teeth. Some doctors take an x-ray of the middle phalanx of the little finger and compare the density of that bone with a standard. It can indicate how much bone has disappeared.

By the fifth decade the osteoporotic calcium loser notices more stiffness on arising, occasional muscle cramps, some difficulties going to sleep, and more aches and pains. The teeth are going. These people begin to shrink by the sixth decade due to the vertebral column compressing; the bones of the spine are constricting. A dowager's hump begins to show. The low backache may have moved all up and down the spine. The pain and stiffness often require bed rest, which further contributes to calcium loss. The skin becomes more translucent. All of us have these things happen to us. We all should know why. We all should be reminded by our doctor that we have to take our supplements.

Males at age twenty-five have 25 percent more bone density than females, perhaps related to the female's childbearing role and less vigorous exercise. But even at that early age, 10 percent of the surveyed population, male or female, had less than optimum bone density. For a time it was thought that osteoporosis was an inherited condition, because it seemed to run in families. Blacks in general have heavy, sturdy skeletons and are less prone to osteoporosis. Oriental women are very susceptible to calcium loss, as are Scandinavians and Northern Europeans. Notice the short, hunched-over, bow-legged people in the stores shopping; notice also what they have in their shopping carts.

But the genetic connection has not been proven. Life-long diet patterns may be more important. If a large amount of dense bone can be established by the age of twenty-five, the onset of osteoporosis could be delayed or prevented. The type of diet followed over the years may play the most important role. Vegetarians, for example, lose only 18 percent of their calcium from age fifty to ninety. Meat eaters lose almost twice as much (35 percent) in the same space of time. Meat is full of phosphorus, and if calcium is not consumed at an equivalent rate (about 1 to 1), the low ratio of calcium to phosphorus in the body triggers the secretion of parathyroid hormone, which decalcifies the bones, and the calcium and phosphorus will run out through the kidneys. A diet deficient in calcium or high in phosphates will have this decalcifying effect. The high intake of phosphoric acid in soft drinks further imbalances the disturbed calcium/phosphorus ratio. A soft drink and a hamburger is about the worst diet for an adolescent; he or she should be getting calcium, vitamin C, and folic acid. Calcium retention is best with a low-protein diet and poorest with a high-protein diet. The fat in meat protein combines with calcium in the intestinal tract and prevents its absorption.

But vegetarians, in general, have trouble with oxalates and phytates in vegetables and grains. These substances combine with iron, zinc, and, of course, calcium to form insoluble salts; the body cannot absorb them. In countries where most of the grains are eaten as unleavened bread, the problem is magnified. Yeast—which most of us get in leavened bread—releases phytase, which degrades the phytic acid, and the minerals are then free to be absorbed. It has been found that some short, immature Eastern Mediterranean types were low in zinc; the diet high in phytates prevented the zinc and other minerals from being absorbed. Rickets is not uncommon in Pakistanis and East Indians because of their heavy use of unleavened bread.

Vitamin D is obviously a factor; it promotes the absorption and distribution of calcium and phosphorus. An hour a day of sunshine is considered sufficient. Those living in northern smog-enshrouded cities will have trouble. The Bantus in Africa have almost no caries, rickets, or osteoporosis on a diet of 200 to 300 mg of calcium a day. This is about one-third to one-half of what is considered an adequate amount for Americans. Cod-liver oil in the winter and some summer sunshine should help.

Osteoporosis affects trabecular bone (ends of long bones, vertebrae, and supportive gum tissue) rather than cortical bone (shafts of long bones). This explains the alarming number of spontaneous fractures in those over age forty-five. Five million of the 6 million fractures occur in women. "Grandmother just stepped off the curb, fell, and broke her hip." Grandmother probably stepped off the curb, broke her hip, and *then* fell. It could be that she was drinking coffee and cola, ate meat at each meal, had one bit of cheese a day, stopped exercising years ago, had all her teeth removed as they were falling out anyway, takes antacids to handle the heartburn from sugar ingestion (aluminum and magnesium antacids may overalkalinize the intestines, so that the phosphates are bound and malabsorbed), and needs a laxative because of the low-roughage diet (and the laxative makes calcium run through faster).

Although it seems obvious that calcium is needed to toughen up the bones, the rate of new bone formation only seems to be able to match the rate of bone dissolution. The decalcification can be slowed, that's all; maybe 10 percent of the 30 to 50 percent loss can be made up. Prevention seems to be the best answer.

Sodium fluoride, 40 to 60 mg per day, is believed to prevent calcium resorption. Some feel it only hardens the outer plate, not the weakened trabeculae inside. It's a scary, controversial therapy; let a few more thousand try it before you do. If you do use it, try to imitate Mother Nature. Always have it with calcium and magnesium; maybe stick to 1 or 2 mg a day.

The lowering and finally the depletion of the estrogen levels plays a role in the calcium loss. Taking 0.625 to 1.25 mg of conjugated estrogen daily may aid in preventing rapid bone atrophy, but it is not proven that its use will increase bone mass. There are a number of real and potential side effects, so no one is highly enthusiastic about this approach. Androgens (male hormones) and calcitonin (a hormone that prevents resorption of bone) are expensive and unproven as yet. Walking three miles a day and swimming are safe exercises for the person with already decalcified bones. Riding a stationary bicycle would be safer than being out on the bumpy, risky streets.

Another condition of lowered calcium called osteomalacia (q.v.) (softened bones) will lead to spontaneous fractures. It is an adult form of rickets.

Some minimal effort must be made to discover any underlying disease that would lead to softened bones. If kidney, liver, and malabsorption problems can be ruled out and if the blood tests are normal, osteoporosis can be assumed to be present and then the diet changed and supplements added—something that should have been done for the patient a long time before.

A RECENT STUDY indicated that osteoporosis was improved if dibasic calcium phosphate (capsules) and vitamin D along with cheese were used as treatment. The calcium-bearing foods combined with calcium compounds seemed to enhance the absorption of the calcium.

Since excess dietary phosphorus may accelerate the rate of bone loss, we should aim for a ratio of calcium to phosphorus of at least 1 to 1 and better 2 to 1. Examples of calcium and phosphorus in some foods (100-gram or 3+-oz portions):

Food	Calcium	Phosphorus	Ratio
Beef liver	8 mg	352 mg	1 : 44
Hot dog	32	603	1 : 19
Whole-wheat flour	41	372	1 : 9
Eggs	54	205	1 : 4
Almonds	234	504	1 : 2
Cottage cheese	94	152	1 : 1.6
Cow's milk	118	93	1 : 0.8
Cheddar cheese	750	478	1 : 0.6
Turnip greens	246	58	1 : 0.2

Meat eaters probably need calcium and magnesium supplements.

Age twenty to thirty: Check your daily calcium intake, using the accompanying table. The average American gets only about 400 to 500 mg per day. Remember, 200 mg runs out in the urine, 150 mg is lost in the stools, the skin excretes 30 mg a day, and at best absorption is only 30 to 35 percent. So just to accommodate the losses one needs 800 to 1000 mg per day. Add it up. Try to keep the phosphorus at less than 1000 mg a day. (Remember, there is phosphorus in lecithin, brewer's yeast, and bone meal.) Remember, too, that stress and smoking will cause calcium depletion. Be sure some sunshine hits your skin every day; when it doesn't, take 400 units of vitamin D; this is the daily recommended dose. Special conditions would require more than 1000 units per day. Cut out the fats in the diet, because they interfere with calcium absorption. If you *have* to have a hamburger, make it just once a month: too much fat and phosphorus. If you are allergic to dairy products, take calcium supplements. Calcium orotate is absorbed well, but oyster-shell calcium and the gluconate and lactate forms are good too. Dolomite is calcium and magnesium at the right 2-to-1 ratio but is poorly absorbed. Best to take these minerals at bedtime, since they have a calming effect. Vitamin C, 1000 mg, taken with the minerals, will promote absorption.

If you are a female and anticipating a pregnancy: The baby needs about 400 mg of *your* calcium every day from the fourth month of gestation on, and breast-feeding demands 300 to 700 mg a day. Irritability, aches and pains, low back pain, and insomnia suggest insufficient calcium (and possibly magnesium). Pregnant and lactating women should try for 1500 to 2000 mg of calcium per day. If you are full of allergies, it would be best not to consume dairy products daily—only once every fourth day.

Age thirty to fifty: Check your eating habits, your calcium intake, your dental health, your exercise routine, your weight. It's not too late. Do you have aching in the lower back not necessarily related to exercise? Do you have some trouble dropping off to sleep? Does your dentist say your teeth are loose and gums receding? You should know what to do. Increase your calcium by 50 percent. Cut down on heavy animal meats. Try a touch of vegetarianism. Remember that high-protein weight reduction programs are high in phosphorus and low in calcium and potassium.

Age fifty on: Your stomach acid is less and you will absorb your minerals at a lower rate. Take at least 500 to 1500 mg of calcium daily and 400 to 1000 units of vitamin D daily, depending on your dairy product ingestion. Add hydrochloric acid, two tablets with each meal. Add vitamin C, 1000 mg, each time you take calcium and magnesium.

If you already have osteoporosis because of a compression fracture in your spine, if you are edentulous, have a terrible backache, a hump back, and are shorter than you used to be, you should take, with the advice of your doctor, 2000 mg of calcium daily, 50,000 units of vitamin D (calciferol) one to three times per week, and try fluoride (at least for a while). I have given people with these conditions I.V.s of calcium gluconate (1000 mg), vitamin C (5000 mg), magnesium sulfate (500 mg), and a B complex (1 cc) with great relief of the symptoms. I assume I am getting around their poorly absorbing gut. I repeat these injections every few days until their bodies work well enough that they can absorb these nutrients by the oral route.

You and the doctor must decide about the pros and cons of estrogen replacement. (See Menopause.)

The program must be continued forever. The use of magnesium and vitamin B_6 (100 mg per day) should preclude the formation of calcium kidney stones in those so predisposed. Some doctors want to be more accurate with the evaluation of the minerals in the body and will get a hair analysis. Most of the patients with muscle and bone complaints have low calcium levels in their hair. If, however, the hair test shows that calcium and magnesium levels are high, it means there is too much phosphorus and too little calcium in the diet, and that this imbalance is causing an increase in the parathyroid secretion, which, in turn, is pulling calcium and presumably magnesium out of the body.

Phenytoin, a medication prescribed for convulsions, has an effect on calcium metabolism; it can lead to osteomalacia and low calcium and a possible increase in the seizures it was prescribed to reduce. Lead poisoning can do the same thing. People on calcium supplements have less absorption of lead.

Calcium is lost more rapidly from the body in diabetes, thyrotoxicosis, sarcoidosis, and prolonged bed rest. Cortisol and derivatives promote calcium losses.

Manganese and zinc are important for bone structure and should be included in an all-purpose mineral supplement; we don't get enough of them in our vegetables any more. Seventy-five percent of the body's copper is in the bones, which suggests that this mineral is important; most of us get enough without a supplement.

High levels of aluminum in the hair analysis are associated with many of the symptoms of osteoporosis; aluminum poisoning often allows spontaneous fractures.

Silicon, which can be obtained from the horsetail plant, is good for skin and bone integrity. Comfrey also has beneficial properties.

Pancreatic enzymes improve absorption of the minerals. Hydrochloric acid acidifies the minerals and thus improves absorption. Vitamin C would help also, but more than 6 to 10 grams of C a day might facilitate the removal of some of the minerals.

Exercise is just as important as diet. Without stimulation the bones decalcify; walking around just a little will help you retain calcium.

P

PAIN ☐ Doctors are supposed to relieve suffering but, first, to do no harm. We'd love to have everyone feeling good and suffering no pain. Why not, then, give everyone some good drug? Because in our enthusiasm to be helpful, we inadvertently get the patient addicted to that drug. The doctor must realize that in prescribing a drug he is merely treating a symptom. He needs to find the reason for the pain and to search more diligently for a safer way to relieve the symptom.

We all make our own endorphins, which act in the body like a narcotic. We can help our bodies handle our own little aches and pains by increasing our intake of vitamin C, the key nutrient responsible for endorphin manufacture. The aches and pains of adolescent growth could be solved to a large extent by the ingestion of extra vitamin C.

B_1 has the reputation for raising the pain threshold; the brain is less responsive. The pain of the demineralized backbone can be subdued with calcium and magnesium.

Acupuncture can work wonders in suppressing pain, supposedly by stimulating the release of endorphins. Hydrotherapy helps control pain. Manipulation, physiotherapy, and relaxation techniques are all valuable.

PALLOR ☐ Since we associate this sign with anemia, the blood must be tested. Iron, copper, folic acid, B_{12}, and a smidgen of molybdenum all may be necessary to get the blood back to normal.

Still, many people are pale and washed out and their blood shows no signs of anemia. A condition called tension-fatigue syndrome (q.v.) often explains the pallor.

Those suffering from hypothyroidism may be pale and puffy with a bit of a yellow waxy look. It is amazing how pink-cheeked and cheerful a face can become after a month or so of 1000 to 3000 mg of niacinamide. Many people simply do not feel good, and the existing tests cannot lead to an answer. The B vitamins, especially B_3, seem to make people feel and act better.

PARANOIA □ The feeling that everyone is against you is something we all sense every once in a while. However, if this perception controls a person's every action; if his face is expressionless, if he feels persecuted and perhaps hears voices, it is called a psychosis. (See Schizophrenia.)

The perception that some force, person, or thing is determined to "get" one is a dysperception. It is now believed that poor parenting skills cannot make a person grow up to be paranoid. Almost all authorities feel that it is multifactorial in origin and that treatment therefore may have to employ a variety of modalities.

Low blood sugar, copper and lead poisoning, food allergies, and yeast infection are all possibilities that should be explored before antipsychotic medication is used—or at least together with that approach.

Some patients need magnesium, B_3, B_6, B_{12}, vitamin C, and other vitamins and minerals. The problem with nutritional therapy is that it takes a while for some improvement to show. These patients are, of course, suspicious, and as a consequence are not always compliant in following the diet and taking the numerous pills required.

PERIODONTAL DISEASE □ A receding gum line, inflammation about the gum edge, and loose teeth are the giveaway that the whole skeleton is decalcifying. Dentists can see the devastation in the mouth long before the patient's regular doctor suspects something is amiss. This is why many dentists are heavily involved with a nutritional support system for their patients. They know, for example, that too much meat with its phosphorus tends to displace calcium; bone is resorbed from the jawbone and the teeth loosen. The patient feels a few aches and pains, loose teeth, some insomnia, some stiffness on turning, long before the doctors can diagnose by examination or laboratory tests. They need calcium, magnesium, manganese, zinc, and vitamin C especially. (See Osteoporosis.)

PHARYNGITIS (SORE THROAT) □ If you still have your tonsils, this disease is called tonsillitis.

A doctor in Alabama told me that he has never seen a strep throat that was not related somehow to dairy food ingestion. I see the connection, but it is more circuitous than his observation suggests. Milk is the most common allergen. Daily ingestion could set up an immune deficiency and a mucous-membrane susceptibility that would allow a strep to grow more easily.

Tonsillectomy and adenoidectomy usually are done to remove obstructive tissue and eliminate a focus of infection. Milk allergy plays a role in stimulating those tissues to grow. If an adult has tension-fatigue syndrome (q.v.) or chronic sinusitis and loves milk, my first question is "Did they remove your tonsils and adenoids?" The answer is usually "Yes." Then I know that a milk allergy is still operating.

Repeated sore throats or other respiratory infections suggest that an allergy is causing the susceptibility. One must stop the food that is most loved. (See Allergies.)

Vitamin C, 1000 mg and increasing by 1000 mg daily until the bowel-tolerance dose is found, is the daily dose. When a scratchy throat appears, one is to take the daily dose hourly until the soreness subsides. Then the dose is tapered off to the maintenance level.

Rheumatic fever is more common in green-eyed red-heads and blue-eyed blonds. Allergies are more common in these people. Could a milk allergy have allowed a strep to invade these fair-complexioned people? Strep is the infection that precedes rheumatic fever. Should all fair people take extra vitamin C and strop drinking milk?

PICA ☐ When you see this word you think of little children eating dirt. But you would be surprised at how many sane adults there are who also eat nonfoods. Adult pica is almost invariably associated with iron-deficiency anemia. Ice-eating is a common form. Many adults *must* eat a certain food every day, and iron therapy stops the compulsion. Some will eat clay but can be moved over to laundry starch. Salt lovers, those who salt all their food vigorously before even tasting it, are "looking" for some mineral, like iron or zinc, or some vitamins, like the B complex. Best to put Vegesal or kelp powder in the saltcellar.

PIGMENTATION ☐ Some unwanted brown spots on the body will be less noticeable if folic acid (2 to 5 mg) and B_{12} (1000 mcg) are used. Senile keratosis and moles are affected only by surgery. Any mole that changes, bleeds, or itches should be harvested.

POLYPOSIS ☐ Polyps that grow in the large bowel, sigmoid colon, and rectum are considered precancerous. They can be removed surgically but 3 grams of vitamin C a day will wipe them out in a few months. It suggests that a healthy dose of C daily might cut the cancer rate; it does help make interferon.

PREGNANCY ☐ Almost every sickly, allergic, or hyperactive child I've seen came from a woman who was sick, stressed, or deficient in some way during the pregnancy. With a little advance thinking and nutrition planning, a couple can bless themselves with a cute, healthy, reasonably bright, and well-behaved child.

Doctors and accoucheurs have been forced to use drugs and surgery more and more, due to the decrease in general health of modern mothers and the problems they have with delivery. The age of the mother influences the baby's health; the years between age twenty and thirty-five seem to be the best for childbearing. Between twenty-eight and thirty-two the woman is mature and usually has figured out what is best for herself and her family. The spacing between pregnancies is considered important by primitive peoples; two to three years is the minimum time they believe compatible with a healthy child.

Stress—or the pregnant woman's perception of stress—is a key factor in the future health of the child. I asked the mother of a very allergic child if she had stress during the pregnancy. She said, "Well, I was fourteen at the time." Stress apparently exhausts the baby's adrenals as well as the mother's. The high incidence of allergic phenomena would seem to be a logical consequence of this adrenal exhaustion.

Dr. Thomas Brewer has devoted his entire professional life to trying to debunk the orthodox thinking that says a pregnant woman should not gain more than 20 pounds during pregnancy. Most M.D. obstetricians have believed, until recently, that a large weight gain would invite toxemia. Now it has been well established that toxemia does lead to weight gain, but it is excess-fluid weight gain and not protein body tissue and rich blood.

The pregnant woman has to increase her blood volume by 25 percent or more. This extra blood volume must be filled with protein, water, salt, blood cells, vitamins, and minerals. If adequate nutrition is not provided, the blood will not nourish the baby and, because of poor osmotic properties, fluid will leak into the mother's tissues and brain, producing toxemia.

The woman cannot have alcohol or drugs during pregnancy. The water pill (diuretic) is dangerous; she needs some extra fluid in her body so she can handle the stress of the delivery and have fluid available to nurse the baby. She needs protein and salt (to taste). (Read Gail Brewer's *What Every Pregnant Woman Should Know*, and check with SPUN, the Society for the Protection of the Unborn through Nutrition.) She needs the basic food groups daily and some desiccated liver each week. Because the vitamins and minerals are not in sufficient supply in good foods, supplements are mandatory to provide the baby with just the adequate amounts to make him healthy.

Dr. Frederick Klenner has pioneered the use of large doses of vitamin C. Dr. Irwin Stone has seconded this emphasis, and Dr. Linus Pauling has told us why. Dr. Robert Cathcart has told us how to figure the dose by pushing it to the point of bowel tolerance. Dr. Klenner recommends 4 grams of vitamin C daily in the first trimester, 6 grams in the second, and 10 to 15 grams a day in the last three months. Vitamin C has many benefits for mother and child: it detoxifies chemicals; it has antifatigue potential; it helps build collagen and maintain the elasticity of the perineum; and it aids in the metabolism of protein and the absorption of minerals, especially calcium, magnesium, and zinc. In addition, labor is reduced by two hours on an average. There are fewer miscarriages, less bleeding, and less tooth decay in the mother.

Iodine (as in kelp and seafood) cuts down the chances of having a low-thyroid baby. Zinc is an important pregnancy mineral; it is especially helpful if the woman is diabetic. The strange tastes and food demands of pregnant women usually are due to a zinc deficiency; 30 to 60 mg a day should suffice. Low-zinc diets have been associated with learning disabilities, increased incidence of miscarriages, syndactyly, hydrocephaly, scoliosis, allergies, and immune-system inadequacies. Magnesium and vitamin deficiencies have been associated with malformations in the rat (at least). If selenium is low in the third to twenty-fourth week of the pregnancy, the child is a candidate for cystic fibrosis; 50 to 200 mcg, plus B_2, plus vitamin E, 400 to 800 units, should solve that problem, since they are needed for an important enzyme, glutathione peroxidase.

Some women have a diabetic tendency because of the demands of pregnancy. B_6, 100 mg per day, brewer's yeast with chromium, and small frequent meals should help. Manganese, 10 mg a day, also helps.

The troublesome nausea associated with pregnancy should disappear with the following: B_6, 100 mg two or three times a day; frequent meals (set the alarm and eat some cheese at 4 A.M.); zinc, 30 mg; and manganese, 5 to 10 mg a day. Metabolism is so rapid in pregnancy that even a well-balanced supper will not preclude a "starvation" acidosis by 6 A.M.

Cramps in the first three months of the pregnancy suggest an incipient miscarriage; magnesium, 500 mg a day, should forestall the loss.

The most common deficiencies in pregnancy are iron, folic acid, calcium, and vitamin D. The usual recommended prenatal vitamins are OK but usually are not sufficient in these four. What is swallowed may not be absorbed. Twenty to 30 mg iron daily is usually required.

If a woman has been on the contraceptive pill and soon after its discontinuance becomes pregnant, she is most likely to be deficient in B_6, folic acid, and B_{12}. Deficiencies of all of these easily lead to fatigue, depression, irritability, and forgetfulness. These symptoms should alert someone to treat the woman; shots would be more effective, because the baby is suffering also. The pregnancy may not appear stressful to an outsider, but if the woman feels miserable because of a deficiency, that is stress enough to cause a loss of the very nutrients she needs. A Catch-22!

At the time of labor, use of extra calcium should ease the pain; 1000 to 3000 mg of calcium (dolomite, bone meal, or gluconate) when labor starts is about right. One to 5 grams of C also. Do not go to bed during labor. Labor is prolonged and pain is increased when the mother is supine. Also, the use of forceps is more commonly associated with bed rest. Remember, too, there is *no drug* that has been proven safe for the unborn baby.

It is possible to have a child reasonably free of allergies if: (1) allergic parents don't have children; (2) the pregnant woman uses the rotation diet as much as possible; (3) stress is avoided; (4) children are spaced at least three years apart; and (5) calcium, vitamin C, B_6 and pantothenic acid are taken during the pregnancy. I see many infants allergic to milk who grow up to have hay fever and asthma. I believe that many were sensitized to milk while still in the uterus. It would be prudent for a mother who knows that allergy is all through her family to drink milk and eat dairy products only every fourth day (Monday, Friday, Tuesday, Saturday, etc.). She needs calcium, however, so 1500 to 2000 mg a day on the nondairy days would satisfy that need. The more the exposure to a food, the more likely it is that an allergy to that food will develop.

Once the potentially allergic baby is born, nurse "forever"—well, aim for eighteen to twenty-four months. Give the baby vitamin C powder, 100 mg a day, and cod-liver oil as the only supplements. Continue to use the rotation diet yourself, because the food or milk that you eat will go to the baby and set up the allergy. Do not begin solids until the baby is beyond nine to ten months and then only one thing at a time. No dairy products, wheat, citrus, egg, or corn until over one year of age. Keep the room free of dust, rugs, wool; no animals with fur or feathers in the house in the first year. (Frog or salamander as a safe pet?)

(See Breast-Feeding.)

PSORIASIS □ Some evidence suggests that psoriasis is an autoimmune disease. A specific immunoglobulin antibody is found in the active lesions and is directed against an antigen in a layer of the skin. Slight trauma allows the antigen-antibody reaction to occur. This damages the skin; an infiltrate appears which further damages the skin, exposing more antigen. Cortisone-like drugs have been used, but the side effects are worse than the original disease. The fact that heredity plays a role suggests an enzyme deficiency. Enzymes can be made to work better if the patient is supernourished. Stress can trigger an exacerbation.

The epidermal cells in psoriasis proliferate rapidly, completing a cell cycle every one and a half days, compared with nineteen days for normal skin. With this understanding, drugs have been used that suppress cellular division; Methotrexate is an example. Psoralens plus UVA (black light) photoreacts with nucleic acids, leading to inhibition of epidermal DNA synthesis; skin production slows and the lesions clear. It works, but the risk of cancer and cataracts is real.

Some claim equally good results with vitamin A, 50,000 units (retinol palmitate), plus vitamin E, 100 units three times a day.

One researcher used 3,000,000 units of vitamin A per day. He followed patients with liver-function tests and asked about headaches. In two to four weeks the skin became red and peeled off, taking the psoriatic scales with it. Skin calmed down and seemed normal for some months afterwards. The A was discontinued when the skin became red or some other toxic effect was noted, whichever came first.

Folic acid works on some.

Lecithin, three capsules three times a day, or 4 to 8 tablespoons a day, can be helpful to some, although it takes five months for the benefits to appear.

Zinc helps the skin, but it is not as important in this condition as vitamin A. Sulfur helps; so do eggs, garlic, and onions.

Naturopaths find that "cleaning out" the liver helps; lecithin, five to ten capsules, choline, 1000 mg, inositol, 1000 mg, are recommended for this. No soap should be used on the affected skin; the areas can be cleansed with non-allergic oil and cotton balls. Ingestion of sugar, salt, and corn must be avoided. Pancreatic enzymes improve digestion. Essential fatty acids help to some extent. Exercise improves the condition. Citrus juices seem to cause the condition to worsen.

R

REFLEXES □ When the neurologist taps below your kneecap and on the Achilles tendon, he is checking reflexes. If they are sluggish and you are cold and dry, your thyroid may be at fault (q.v.). Some borderline hypothyroid patients may help themselves with iodine, as in kelp tablets (five to ten daily for a month). B_1, 100 mg a day, helps the nerves function better.

If the reflexes are hyperactive and there is no demonstrable disease of the central nervous system, it may be the stimulation from too much caffeine (tea, coffee, chocolate, cola drinks). If restless legs accompany the brisk reflexes, vitamin E may calm this: 800 to 1000 units (d-alpha tocopherol); some use up to 2000 units if the blood pressure is OK.

Calcium, magnesium, vitamin C, and potassium might soothe the active reflexes.

RESPIRATORY SYMPTOMS □ We all breathe, and in consequence we are subject to a variety of conditions, because the air we breathe is not just oxygen, carbon dioxide, and nitrogen. Dirt, lead, pollens, carbon monoxide, fuel, perfumes, and germs in the air are just a few of the hazards of breathing.

Given all this smog entering our bodies, why aren't we all wheezing and coughing? Genetic differences would explain a few things, but susceptibility to infection could be due to a poorly functioning immune system, and that may be dependent on nutrition. Allergies frequently manifest themselves by a drippy nose, sneeze, throat clearing, croup, cough, or wheeze. This phlegm produced by the body to dilute the invaders seems to be a grand medium in which germs are able to grow. Infection can weaken the body, and this stress aggravates the allergy.

And not every respiratory symptom is due to some irritant floating by that particular area. Just inside the nostrils, on the septum, is a bit of tissue that responds to hormones, and not a few ear-nose-throat doctors have diagnosed pregnancy when the woman came in for "sinus trouble." I know a surgeon who constantly sniffs as if there were a bit of phlegm running out of his nose. He wears a mask so the patient's health is not jeopardized, but it drives the operating-room nurses crazy. It is one of the symptoms and signs that constitute tension-fatigue syndrome (q.v.), a well-recognized, usually pediatric diagnosis that includes a sniffing, throat-clearing, zonking sound these people make, as if they were trying to dislodge a bunch of rubber bands from the back of their nose and throat. It is almost always due to a food allergy, most likely milk. It is as bothersome to their loved ones as a drippy faucet. "Blow your nose, for God's sake." "I did." "Weeelll."

The common cold is a boring drag but not, in general, a necessary part of life. There are people who have grown up, worked hard, and died with nary a trace of a cold or respiratory virus, indicating that freedom from this irritating problem is possible for most, if not all, of us.

Allergies frequently weaken the protective mucous membrane that lines the nose and throat, allowing a cold virus to invade. Keeping the animals outside and changing to synthetic bedding may help. Special filters that precipitate dust out of the air can be installed. Babies fed breast milk have fewer colds, but adults may have a supply problem. Discontinuing *all* dairy products for at least three weeks may eliminate the sinus congestion, the surface phlegm, or the postnasal drip that attracts the virus.

Most of us who have adopted a healthier way of life have noticed fewer respiratory infections as a bonus after energy has returned. That fact suggests that previously the body was so busy trying to keep its basic metabolism operative that the peripheral defenses were weakened. Health is *not* a matter of taking the proper drug; health means that you don't need drugs, because the wisdom of the body is in charge.

It is well known that ingested sugar (white, brown, corn syrup) will reduce the ability of the white blood cells to entrap and destroy bacteria. It is well known that stress depletes the body of vitamin A, which is essential in maintaining the integrity of mucous membranes. And it is well known that vitamin C enables the body to produce interferon, a natural intracellular antiviral substance.

Those of us who treat our patients with large doses of vitamin C for a variety of infections cannot understand the negative reactions that we get from the more orthodox M.D.s. I know—or try to believe—that they are not the tools of the big pharmaceutical companies who stand to make more from selling drugs. I know they are taught that anyone who uses vitamins as therapy is a quack, and they do not want to be so labeled. But Linus Pauling is right: vitamin C does work—although various articles in "scientific" journals would suggest otherwise.

About four years ago, the *Journal of the American Medical Association* reported a large double-blind (patient and doctor did not know who was getting the vitamin C and who the sugar pill), crossover (patients on placebos now got vitamin C and vice versa) study. The results showed minimal help against the common cold when humans took vitamin C. Of course I was disappointed, because I *see* improvement with the C. Maybe the subjects did not take enough? The daily dose was 500 mg; that should do *something,* I thought.

Then I reread the protocol. "Of course, we did not use anyone with allergies." That's it! Those with allergies are much more susceptible to the virus. And those are my findings. In many cases, when the allergy or the stress that precipitated the allergy is minimized, the body can fight off the infections. The cold, cough, and wheeze is the body telling you that something is stressed. Either we unstress it, or give it the nutrients we know will help the body handle that stress.

Dr. Robert Cathcart is our leader when it comes to vitamin C therapy. He gives big amounts early and then tapers off. The sicker the patient, the higher the dose. He has given as much as 200 grams (200,000 mg) of vitamin C intravenously to patients severely ill with virus pneumonia. (He uses sodium ascorbate in distilled water, 500 ml, letting it run in over a one-hour period.) The fever falls overnight, pain is assuaged, cough slows or loosens, sleep is fairly comfortable, and energy returns. The patient may or may not need another I.V. in the succeeding days, but he is usually able to handle the convalescence with oral vitamin C, 20 to 50 grams per day, then tapering down to a daily maintenance dose.

Dr. Cathcart can now guess by the physical exam just how much C will be required. "This influenza is a 20-gram job." "This mononucleosis will take 100 grams a day for three days." In ten years, he has not yet needed to hospitalize a patient with a virus infection.

I used to treat a woman, thirty years old, named Polly, who had repeated attacks of either bronchitis or asthmatic bronchitis, or bronchopneumonia or virus pneumonia. Antibiotics were required, but despite their benefit she was stuck with diarrhea, weakness, and a vaginal yeast infection.

I was anxious to try Dr. Cathcart's method, but failed to evaluate the extent of her illness and gave her only 20 grams of vitamin C. The next day she was back. "This is faster than the antibiotics. I have more energy, but I am still sick. I am taking 3 grams of vitamin C by mouth every hour or two." And no diarrhea. Her body needed the C to help with the immune system. The C was absorbed before it could cause loose bowels. I did another I.V. with about the same amount of C and she was essentially well the next day. She tapered off to her bowel tolerance dose, 5000 mg per day.

Now her husband gives her a vitamin C and B complex (Darby/Rugby #7) injection every week, she drinks no milk, and she has been well for about a year. Not everyone needs to do all this; just those of us who want to stay well.

My obvious enthusiasm for vitamin therapy is motivated by my own improved health on this regime, and also by the rather disturbing research by Dr. C. Orian Truss. He has detected a large group of people in our country whose immune systems have been compromised by the frequent use of antibiotics, cortisone, poor foods, and oral contraceptives. All these factors, plus stress of course, permit a yeast overgrowth. This yeast growing in the intestinal tract makes the body respond as if to a foreign substance and the patient becomes fatigued. A variety of bizarre physical and mental symptoms follow which defy diagnosis. (See Yeast Infections.)

Vitamin A plays an important role in the control of respiratory infections, since it has a specific beneficial action on mucous membranes. Many people have found that they need to increase their A when they are sick. C does a good job but the A makes it better. One way to discover if A is indicated is to consider these factors: past or present history of warts would suggest a need of more than the recommended dose of 5000 units; past or present history of hyperkeratosis, the feeling of rough, nutmeg-grater skin on the back of the upper arms and the front and sides of the thighs; a stressful life; history of past or present smoking; history of acne; history of cortisone use (vitamin A counteracts the bad effects of cortisone); and, of course, a poor-protein diet, which prevents the liver from manufacturing a vitamin-A-binding protein (see Vitamin A, Chapter 7).

Zinc could be a missing ingredient in those most susceptible to respiratory infections since vitamin A needs zinc in the liver to permit its release. White blood cells contain large amounts of zinc. It combines with dead viruses and is excreted; in acute infections zinc in the serum falls to 70 percent of normal.

Iron-deficiency anemia (hemoglobin less than 10 grams per decaliter) usually leads to repeated infections. A poor-protein diet may have the same consequences.

I would like to suggest a regime for those with repeated respiratory infections, including sore throats, ear infections, laryngitis, bronchitis, asthma, bronchopneumonia, viral pneumonia, lobar pneumonia: if the victim has any of these and does nothing about his diet, his lifestyle, or his vitamins, he is going to get it again. My suggestion for nutritional support is hinged on the basic premise that any reader who feels qualified for this already has had a good examination by a reliable doctor who found no obvious active tuberculosis, low serum albumin, bean up the nose or peanut down the bronchial tube, heart failure, low thyroid, or other condition that should be corrected medically or surgically.

If he wants to help by putting you on antibiotics prophylactically or on cortisone for long periods of time, shouldn't you at least try some safe, albeit slow, nutrient therapy first?

If you sniff, snort, sneeze, and find your finger near your nose a lot, you probably have an inhalation allergy and should follow the adrenal-gland support system (see Allergies). At least make an effort to cut down on the allergic load from inhalants (animals, blankets, house dust, smoking). Many have found that their hay fever disappeared when they stopped some food to which they were allergic. (If they drank milk, they could not use a feather pillow.) Removing sugar from the diet will stop some allergies because the adrenals are able to function more efficiently.

If the problem is frequent colds, coughs, and sinus infections with no obvious allergy as a trigger mechanism, then the following should be done before the next attack: (1) avoid stress; (2) try to eat good nourishing food six times a day; (3) increase the daily dose of vitamin C by 1000 mg daily until your bowel movements are just a little soft. That will be the daily dose (usually 4000 mg to 10,000 mg). Then, when you feel that stinging in the nose and throat, the creepy skin, the tightness in the muscles in the neck, the headache and soreness all over, don't wait to see what it's going to be; instead, take the daily dose of vitamin C every hour. Usually in eight to twelve hours the symptoms are less rather than more severe, and you can use that dose every two hours. If you are overtreating with C, the looseness of the bowels will tell you. If you are on target, you will notice less stool action, because the vitamin C is being absorbed and utilized in the anti-infective action so fast that there is little left to exceed the bowel's tolerance. Taper off the dose for the next few days until you are back to your daily maintenance dose.

If you are worse overnight, get some professional help. You may need an antibiotic along with the vitamin C. This is not cheating. You don't have to be a purist; drugs and vitamins are not incompatible.

Suppose, despite your efforts, you come down with the "virus that's going around" and you now have a chesty cough and chartreuse-colored phlegm but your fever is down. Keep on with the vitamin C while adding vitamin A to help clear up the remainder; take 100,000 units of A daily for a few days. Vitamin E (400 units) will make the A work better. If you have ever had warts, acne, or hyperkeratosis, you are probably vitamin A dependent and should have started the big doses of A with big doses of C. I use 25,000 units of A along with C to suppress infections, occasionally moving up to 100,000 units. (See Vitamin A, Chapter 7.)

The green or yellow junk you cough up represents a secondary infection and suggests that an antibiotic would help, but if your fever is down and you can drag around, you can wait. The point is, you should be getting better every day. If not, see your doctor. This nutrition doesn't work on everybody. Now, at least, you have something the doctor is trained to treat.

If you have done all the nutritional things and you still get sick, an allergic workup with skin tests would be prudent. If you have been getting sick all your life, you may have an immune deficiency disease. There are reliable tests for those.

S

SCHIZOPHRENIA ☐ The term *schizophrenia* has been used as a label for a wide variety of symptoms and signs in an attempt to codify or simplify a mental illness whose chief characteristic is a dysperception. If a person perceives a telephone pole to be orange and threatening and acts as if that were true, he is considered to be schizophrenic. He is unable to tell whether the changes he perceives in the world are real or not. Because of these dysperceptions, his thoughts, feelings, and resultant behaviors are strange, bizarre, and inappropriate.

Schizophrenics usually have a poor or distorted sense of humor and a flattened affect, which means they display a blank, staring face; no emotions show. They may be paranoid (q.v.), have feelings of depersonalization, hear voices, be aloof, indifferent, shy, withdrawn, and often depressed. Anxiety, fatigue, and insomnia are frequently present.

Fifty years ago, if a person showed these symptoms it was suspected that he had pellagra, a fairly common disease due to lack of niacinamide, or vitamin B_3. It often was associated with diarrhea, a skin rash, distorted sensations, and odd bodily complaints. When pellagrins were given the newly discovered niacin, half the mentally ill could be discharged from the hospitals as cured. Some of the others were discovered to have central-nervous-system syphilis. But nothing seemed to help the catatonic, the paranoid, the delusional, and the wildly aggressive schizophrenics. Many psychiatrists tried to fit the psychodynamics of the illness into the framework of an emotionally or environmentally produced distur-

357

bance, which produced a great deal of guilt in the parents of these children. Couch or talk therapy was of no benefit.

About the time that Thorazine was synthesized (1950) and proved helpful in controlling the most disturbing symptoms, Abram Hoffer and Humphry Osmund discovered that large doses of niacinamide—3000 mg or more per day— would calm the patient with dysperceptions. The megavitamin approach did work, but the response was usually slower than with the various drugs that were being marketed.

Over the past thirty years a lot of research, controversy, and trial-and-error treatment has left us with the following well-documented facts:

Schizophrenia is a number of mental diseases manifesting themselves as dysperceptions.

Strong genetic factors are operative. Since genetic factors express themselves through enzyme dysfunction, it is an easy step to assume that some psychotic people cannot convert food into the appropriate brain chemicals. Without the proper or adequate neurotransmitters, one part of the brain cannot tell another part of the brain what is going on, either with inside-the-body messages or with messages from the environment. Dysperceptions occur.

We have learned through the study of deficiencies like pellagra that mental health is a function of a number of chemical factors operating together, and that some people, because of a genetic fault, have dependency needs for certain chemicals, vitamins, minerals, and amino acids. Some defective enzymes can be induced to function almost optimally if megadoses of the enzyme factors are provided.

Nicotinamide adenine dinucleotide (NAD) is an essential enzyme necessary for cellular metabolism. Some schizophrenics do not have enough of this in vital areas of the brain. Tryptophan, niacin, and pyridoxine (B$_6$) are needed to produce NAD. Two percent of ingested tryptophan turns into niacin, and a fair amount goes to the brain to become serotonin. If an enzyme (an amino oxidase) does not metabolize tryptophan, an overload becomes harmful, creating changes in perception and mood in normal people. A large amount of niacin (niacinamide is less effective)—2000 to 5000 mg per day—is the mainstay of the treatment of most schizophrenics because it provides the essential ingredient of NAD.

The tranquilizers and antipsychotic drugs used to calm the agitation, stress, and restlessness of the disturbed schizophrenic block dopamine receptor sites in the brain. Vitamin C has a similar effect; if these nerves are not overloaded with incoming stimuli, the brain perceives the environment as less threatening. Vitamin C is given in doses of 3 to 10 grams a day to help control anxiety. If we increase the amount of vitamin C orally, more will go to the brain, where it will be stored; it will not just wash out through the urine. Many schizophrenics do not show even a trace of vitamin C in the urine until the oral dose gets above 4 to 5 grams. Some have to take 30 grams of C a day before it will show in the urine. With these high doses they can walk in the streets again; they are less paranoid. Calcium or sodium ascorbate would be a better form. Could public libraries, where these people often come, serve C and B_3 as a snack? Librarians do not like to have their facilities used as a psychiatric dayroom. Apparently a dependency, not a deficiency, is operating here.

Vitamin B_6, pyridoxine, is a precursor to, or coenzyme with, at least fifty enzyme systems of the body. Many psychotic patients need 500 mg a day of B_6 just to help these metabolic functions work adequately. Most folk need but 2 to 5 mg a day, easily obtained from a reasonable diet. We *are* all different.

Dr. Carl Pfeiffer of the Princeton Brain Bio Center has found at least two subgroups of schizophrenics. One is called *histadelic;* they produce large amounts of histamine and have allergic symptoms. They would respond better to the following daily program: 2 grams of C, only 200 mg of niacin, 200 units of E, 1 gram of calcium lactate, and some methionine, zinc and manganese.

The *histapenic* are the low-histamine, low-allergy group. Their doses would be at this level: 3 grams of C, 3 grams of B_3, 200 mg of B_6, 2 mg of folic acid; 1 mg of B_{12} (weekly injection), 200 units of E, and a high-protein diet.

About one-third of schizophrenics have a substance called kryptopyrrole in their urine. It is associated with a higher number of beta waves in the EEG. Kryptopyrrole complexes with B_6 and zinc; 30 mg of zinc twice a day would control these psychotic symptoms.

Schizophrenics have less zinc in their brains than do normal people; low zinc in the hair test often is associated with high copper. Copper poisoning can produce psychotic symptoms. Zinc-deficient people often have taste and smell dysperceptions. Zinc and manganese are useful for those with high histamine levels and suicidal depression.

Pantothenic acid is useful for anyone who perceives the world as stressful; 100 to 500 mg a day would help the adrenals function optimally. More than half the elderly psychiatric patients are low in folic acid; vitamin C is needed to convert the folic acid into a usable form. Low B_{12} is found in many depressed, agitated, and hallucinating patients; cystine and biotin can help regulate the level of B_{12} in the body. A deficiency of B_1 (thiamin) may cause irritability, confusion, memory loss, depression, and increased sensitivity to noise. If someone wears ear muffs in the summer, we would think him strange. To the sufferer it all seems logical. Look at his diet, however. It might give away the reason.

Magnesium deficiency has been reported in paranoid psychosis. Amino-acid imbalance can lead to depression, apathy, or desire to be left alone. The relationship of leucine and isoleucine demonstrates how some people have genetic faults that force them to be very careful about what they eat. Schizophrenics who have been controlled with B_3 will become psychotic overnight if they are given leucine; if they take isoleucine and extra B_6, it will not happen.

The neurotransmitters dopamine, epinephrine, and norepinephrine are metabolized to adrenochrome. In some schizophrenics, adrenochrome will become adrenolutin, a toxic substance. (In the normal person it becomes leucoadrenochrome, a harmless substance.) Sufficient vitamin C, cysteine, and glutathione will help produce the benign metabolite. Adrenochrome disrupts synaptic transmission. Some forms of senility and Parkinsonism are caused by this. B_3, E, and selenium would help control this effect.

Psychiatrists are the usual consultants for the long-term help these patients need. Antipsychotic drugs are their first choice to quickly control the out-of-contact, violent patient. Once some calmness and order have been established, a nutritional support system must be used to help the brain produce the appropriate neurotransmitters. A hair analysis would be the minimum laboratory workup. Some assessment of the dysperceptions can be arrived at by using the Hoffer-Osmund Diagnostic Test and Experiential World Inventory. The higher the score (greater the dysperception), the better the response to orthomolecular therapy. Giving B_1, B_2, B_3, B_6, pantothenic acid, C, and E in the doses suggested above—along with the drugs a doctor might have prescribed—is a good start.

Dr. George Watson has identified other subgroups that require different therapeutic emphasis. One group he called slow oxidizers of carbohydrates; they did better on fats and certain amino acids. The other group, called fast oxidizers, did better on different vitamins and foods.

A water fast for at least four to five days would uncover the schizophrenic who has a food allergy. It is well known that wheat, milk, and beef bother many people and make them temporarily psychotic. Dr. William Philpott has biochemical tests to verify the truth of the psychogenic aspects of food allergies. Many psychotic people consume huge volumes of one food—really a giveaway that they have the allergic-addictive syndrome.

Hypoglycemia can produce psychotic symptoms. The brain is affected by the body.

One can easily see how the odd behavior of these people, reacting to their dysperceptions, makes the rest of us treat them in a fashion commensurate with *our* perceptions. We would tend to reinforce in them the idea that they are crazy. How much more helpful it would be if we relabeled schizophrenia and called it "cerebral dysmetabolism."

SEBORRHEA □ What is called a bad case of dandruff in an adult is called cradle cap in a baby. Many of these infants were delivered of mothers who had nausea and vomiting. This all ties together, because a B_6 deficiency often is to blame for each of these symptoms.

If a person has dandruff, scaly red-rimmed eyes, cracks behind the ears, a groin rash, and poor memory, it would have to be a B_6 deficiency. I have cured some seborrhea-dandruff cases by discontinuing the dairy-product intake. But it may also need the following: 100 to 300 mg of B_6, best balanced with 50 to 100 mg of the other Bs; B_2, 100 to 200 mg; zinc, 30 to 60 mg; and the essential fatty acids, as in safflower oil. Cod-liver oil with A and D and some essential fatty acids might make a difference. Shampoos would help. A dermatologist may be needed to name the disease, since psoriasis and eczema can mimic seborrhea.

Biotin is needed for fatty acid metabolism; a biotin deficiency may lead to a fine, scaly dermatitis, nausea, vomiting, and depression. An I.V. of biotin (5 mg) will control seborrhea dermatitis almost overnight.

Some have taken lecithin for seborrhea and seen it improve. PABA, 30 mg twice daily, stops the itch and scaliness of some dandruff patients.

Jojoba shampoo will help.

SENSITIVITY □ Sensitive people may be built that way. We are all different. Some mothers of more than one or two children say they can notice a difference in their children's response to noise and movement (and even intestinal gas) while the children are still in utero. The hyperactive child sometimes can be diagnosed before birth. It may not be a genetically determined sensitivity to the world, however; it could be a nutritional deficit in the mother that is affecting her child. They are connected, and if she is low in calcium (muscle aches and insomnia), the child might be sensitive to the confinement of the womb and kick more.

On a ticklish scale of 1 to 10, hyperactive children—and adults—rate 7 to 10+. They notice things more; their nervous systems cannot disregard incoming stimuli.

Increased sensitivity to light and pain may be controlled with vitamins B_1 and B_3. Those sensitive to noise do better with B_1 and magnesium. A hyperacute sense of smell would respond to B_3. And hyperesthesia in general is solved with B_3. Potassium may be low in those who seem indifferent to stimuli.

Exquisite tenderness to a light touch—the burning-foot syndrome—is supposed to be due to a pantothenic acid deficiency. One really has to be on a poor diet to be low in pantothenic acid. To do: eat good food and take pantothenic acid, 200 mg three or four times a day.

SHINGLES □ This is a dreary, painful, aggravating condition because it just sits there like a knife, stabbing away. It is the same virus that causes chicken pox, so it often shows up in grandparents in January after a visit with the children who looked a little spotty at Christmas time.

The virus erupts the skin following the distribution line of a nerve, usually around the chest on one side from spine to breastbone. If it hits a facial nerve it can hurt the eye. Early treatment will slow the progress.

Try a daily dose of B_{12} (1000 mcg) intramuscularly for five to ten days. Use vitamin C, perhaps up to bowel tolerance—somewhere at the 1000-mg level every waking hour or two. Continue for two weeks then taper off. Vitamin E locally and orally is soothing and might cut down the chance of scarring.

SINUSITIS □ As I travel about the country, I find that almost every community claims the right to be Sinus City or Sinusitis Valley. They blame it on mold, dust, smog, dampness, wind, no wind, dryness, and, of course, on stress and unemployment. The claimants are probably all correct, at least for *them*. But lots of other folk live in those places who never have to blow their noses. I believe these sinus sufferers are allergic and that they do not have the correct nutrition to help the body withstand the irritation of breathing. The extra work that the mucous membranes perform must weaken them enough to allow an allergy or infection to appear.

Many do not realize how common the connection is between food and phlegm. Hay fever is usually easily recognized because of the unignorable itch and sneeze and clear mucous that flows so copiously. If, however, the phlegm is clear, or gray, and is accompanied by much honking, spitting, and throat-clearing, it suggests an allergy to some food, milk most likely. It takes three weeks of no dairy-food ingestion to rid oneself of the last remnants of the allergen. It is usually the food that one loves the most. Snoring is often a related sign.

If upon blowing the nose one sees that the phlegm is colored (green, yellow, chartreuse), it means that a secondary infection has become superimposed atop the allergy. I use a series of dead-bacteria shots to teach these people how we can fight off infection.

The allergy-control program with C, A, B_6, and pantothenic acid should do some good. No sugar, obviously. (See Allergies; Respiratory Symptoms.)

SKIN PROBLEMS □ The skin is a flag that often signals some internal tilt. Topical ointments just treat the surface; usually we have to treat the whole body in order to help the skin clear up.

Nevertheless, topical treatment is a good place to start. The dermatologist has thousands of diagnoses filed in his brain and is eager to show off his skills, but his treatment may be limited to "Let's try this sample and call me back."

If he suggests a cortisone shot and you are really not that sick, beg his indulgence and try the slow but safe adrenal-gland-support system. When the doctor makes a diagnosis and his training indicates to him that cortisone (a synthetic hormone patterned after one of the secretions from the cortex of the adrenal glands) would be helpful, he is telling *you* that your adrenal glands have failed.

Eczema (see Allergies) is a good example of poorly functioning adrenal glands; otherwise the skin would not have broken down. The skin is waving its flag, and it wants us to do more than prescribe an ointment.

The failure could be due to one or all of the following: genetic tendency, stress, inappropriate nutrition experienced by the mother during the victim's gestation, stress at delivery or premature birth, multiple sicknesses in the past, recent physical or emotional trauma, overwhelming allergic load, "enough to bother anyone."

Example: Your mother has to have chocolate on the day prior to each menstrual period (suggesting the allergic-addictive syndrome), she ate a lot of chocolate in the pregnancy with you, you have a history of touchy skin (diaper rash as an infant, pimples on buttocks when you wear synthetic underwear, some nasty adolescent acne requiring antibiotics, irritation when you use some perfumed soaps). You work hard all afternoon shoveling snow. When you relax in the evening with a cup of hot chocolate, suddenly you are a mess: swollen lips and eyelids, arthritis of the joints, and giant hives that make you limp to the emergency room of the local hospital. A shot of adrenalin helps and the cortisone tablets you take provide sustaining relief. You are grateful but you wonder what will be the next devastation. You have heard of fatal reactions.

Most of these dermatological emergencies can be averted by implementing available nutritional knowledge. But the patient needs someone smart enough to see the connection between the adrenal gland "exhaustion," or allergic overload, and the need for the nutritional supports.

Vitamin A and zinc work together to help the skin maintain its toughness, elasticity, and ability to heal when injured. Skin ulcers caused by confinement to bed or by other sources of pressure heal faster with vitamin C (1 to 5 grams a day), vitamin A (25,000 units a day), zinc (30 to 60 mg a day), and a good protein diet. Vitamin A needs protein and zinc to work. Vitamin A in big doses (50,000 to 100,000 units) for three to five weeks should help warts fall off. Patients taking these doses must be observed for toxic signs, but those who have warts usually can stand big doses; they have a need for A or they wouldn't have gotten the warts in the first place. Dry, red skin that peels off like sunburned skin may indeed be sunburned, but it also could be due to a vitamin A overdose. A little bit of this drying effect could be therapeutic for hyperkeratosis, psoriasis, and acne. Sebaceous cysts respond to the drying effect of vitamin A. Vitamin E makes the A work better.

Fatty deposits or whiteheads on the face may represent deficiencies of B_2, B_6, and folic acid. Bloodshot eyes, veins showing on the cheeks, and cracks in the corner of the mouth are usually due to a B_2 deficiency.

Puffiness about the face may be due to hypothyroidism, an infection, venous obstruction, low protein levels in the blood, kidney disease, allergies, and trichinosis.

Lecithin is of benefit for psoriasis, dry skin, eczema, scleroderma, senile atrophy, seborrhea, and sometimes acne. Also, dry, cracked, scaly skin that leads to hair loss usually is improved with linoleic acid, lecithin, and B_6. If the problem is in the dandruff category, extra magnesium (500 mg a day) should help. PABA, 30 mg, once or twice a day, can stop an itchy, scaly scalp.

Sunburn and poison oak are calmed nicely with vitamin E internally and locally. Soaking in water hot enough to be uncomfortable sometimes can stop the itch of poison oak for hours. Contact rashes suggest that the adrenal glands are slipping, so C, calcium, B_6, pantothenic acid, A, and zinc should help. To protect from sunshine, use a lotion with PABA in it before exposure. Vitamin C internally and aloe vera externally will soothe and speed healing. Ice helps any burn. I have known people to put a raw onion on small burns; it is soothing, and healing is rapid. Vitamin E, locally, helps hangnails heal. Sore nipples on a nursing mother heal faster with vitamin E locally and internally. Vitamin E and iodine (as in kelp) are effective in preventing wrinkles, but are minimally effective for established wrinkles. For athlete's foot, E topically twice a day is good; the contents of a capsule rubbed in well should help.

Striae, or stretch marks, are small tears in the skin that usually form with sudden weight gain (puberty, pregnancy, and obesity) but do not disappear with weight loss or delivery of the baby. They mean that the involved person is low in zinc (try 60 mg a day), B_6 (100 mg a day), E (400 units a day), and vitamin C, which helps the body make collagen. During the pregnancy 4 to 10 grams of vitamin C daily should prevent their appearance. Another read-your-body clue.

Zinc is good also for acne, and for a rare mess called acrodermatitis enteropathica.

Bruises are less noticeable and disappear faster with vitamin C, fatty acids, and bioflavonoids. Boils that keep recurring might be controlled with a better diet and supplements of A, C, zinc, and silicon.

Taking brewer's yeast or B_1 (50 mg every two to three hours) affects the smell of the skin in such a way that mosquitos are discouraged from biting. If they do bite, vitamin C would help the inflammation disappear more rapidly. It also works on prickly heat, heat cramps, heat stroke, and heat exhaustion. It is best to take the C before going into the heat.

When all else fails, an itchy skin without rash may be due to an iron deficiency.

Dr. Emanuel Cheraskin and Dr. W. M. Ringsdorf followed the symptoms of over a thousand professionals (M.D.s and D.D.S.s) and their spouses for a number of years. They found a significant high correlation between sucrose ingestion and dermatoses.

Dr. A. M. Kligman, of the University of Pennsylvania, feels that our skin does pretty well until age fifty and then begins to deteriorate. He has patients look at the underside of their upper arms; that's the way the skin of the face should appear. If the skin of the face and hands becomes blemished and worn, it is due to wind, rain, soap, cold, but especially sunshine. Heat and sun destroy the collagen and elastin of the skin, and this causes wrinkles. Vitamin E and iodine might slow this process. Dr. Kligman feels that even some premalignant skin lesions will fade if sun is excluded.

Lanolin and petroleum jelly—the greasier the better—are protective for dry skin, which cracks and wrinkles faster than oily skin.

The anal itch that drives many of us mad, or at least to distraction, is often caused by a food allergy—milk, citrus, and coffee being the most common. A little bit of the fecal material gets stuck at the opening and a "contact" rash begins. Colored toilet paper can do it too. The bidet seems a civilized way of eliminating the problem. Washing the anal opening with wet tissue or a little Balneol or vitamin E oil should calm the maddening pruritis.

SPOILED BRATS or SURLY ADULTS □ Crabby, selfish, spoiled, snippy, smug, sassy people may not feel good. Some years ago someone put together the following potion: 1 drop of Lugol's solution (potassium iodide) and 1 teaspoon of apple cider vinegar in a glass of fruit juice;

taken daily, it could change someone nasty into a sweet, compliant human being.

What this suggests is that these undesirables are suffering from an absorption problem. The extra acid in the potion would make calcium, magnesium, and zinc more absorbable. The iodine would be helping the thyroid function, and thyroid is needed to get the nutrients into the cells.

(See Aggressive Behavior.)

STRESS □ I see a great number of babies who are sick. They are formed properly, the birth weight was 6 to 7 pounds, and they seem to be developing OK, but they have colic, insomnia, ear infections, diaper rashes, stomach flu, hay fever, pallor, sunken eyes, and often a worried look. The exhausted parents bring them in to get them well and on a normal schedule. The parents themselves are falling apart.

I have learned to ask about any stress that may have occurred during the pregnancy, slight though it may have been. Sometimes a whole flood of emotional and physical traumas come pouring out; car accident, overdrawn accounts, husband in the service, glumpy in-laws, move to another city, death of a parent, flu, kidney infection, on and on. Some will deny any upsetting experience, but *something* they did or experienced in that nine-month period was a stress to the baby. Booze, drugs, exposure to allergens, chronic hay fever, and asthma are other possibilities.

I now ask questions that tell me how much prenatal stress or malnutrition the baby experienced in utero; the answers to the questions give me some clues about the mother's needs and what part nutrition is playing in the baby's difficulties.

"Did you drink milk every day?" Daily ingestion of good-sized amounts of any food is asking for an allergy—in mother and baby too.

"Did you have nausea and vomiting?" A positive answer here means low B_6 intake and possibly hypoglycemia. I give the mother extra B vitamins, especially B$_6$. I also give the baby 0.3 cc of a B complex mixture intramuscularly; usually the symptoms are assuaged overnight. It is a therapeutic trial; if he is better, he needed it.

"Did you have aches and pains, stiff back, or sore muscles?" This is the clue for calcium deficiency. I up the mother's calcium intake (1000 to 2000 mg—somewhere in that range if she is nursing) or give an I.V. of 1000 mg of calcium gluconate (usually combined with magnesium, C, and B complex). If she has had these symptoms despite a quart or so of milk a day, I know some milk allergy or malabsorption is going on that is interfering with the calcium on its way to the cells. Similarly, I am aware that the baby probably is also suffering from a calcium deficiency, so he or she will get some dolomite, bone meal, or calcium/magnesium down by mouth (about 100 to 300 mg of calcium orally would be about right as a daily dose); in a few days the baby should be easy, cheerful, and sleeping better.

The reason I go into these details is only to emphasize how we are all at the mercy of our mother's diet, thoughts, traumas, and both our parents' genes. These factors will set up a physiological weakness that may prevent the offspring from handling stress well. The critics of our use of diet, vitamins, and minerals to help maintain homeostasis assume that we are all equal, come from an ideal pregnancy, are endowed with good genes, and have all the good food we need.

One of the biggest problems I see is that once we slip, because of stress or an inadequate diet, it takes megadoses in many people just to get back into shape or to achieve homeostasis. If you get mononucleosis in college, you can blame the kissing at the fraternity-house party, but it might also be the stress of almost flunking plus the dorm food plus the weekend boozing. Why didn't everyone get the mono? Your body was doing you a favor. It told you you had slipped; stress and nutrition depletion had lowered your defenses to the point where a virus that was lying around was able to invade and set up a family.

Stress of any kind will deplete the body of the following especially: C, A, E, calcium, manganese, magnesium, zinc, and protein. Animals who can manufacture their own ascorbic acid will produce 4 to 29 times their resting level. Stressed humans should increase their intake proportionately (at least 1000 mg a day and on up to 20 grams a day for a biggie).

Vitamin A is depleted with stress, especially burns, temperature changes, and respiratory stress; 10,000 to 50,000 units a day would be close to a replacement dose. Ulcers may be prevented with A.

If vitamin E is not taken during stress the muscles will atrophy faster, because muscle protein is used as energy during sickness and fever. When protein is depleted and is not correctly replaced, an imbalance of amino acids occurs. Depression, apathy, irritability, and a desire to be left alone could appear. The approximate dose of E would be 400 to 1200 units daily—more if a vascular insult is superimposed. Calcium should be taken—1000 to 2000 mg a day for a week, then cutting back to the maintenance dose. Zinc should be increased to 60 to 90 mg for a couple of weeks before dropping back to 15 to 30 mg. Zinc is important after an infection because it chelates with the dead virus and is lost in the urine. Low levels of zinc in the body allow the adrenals to be hypersensitive to stress. An adolescent with acne might get mono and then be too nervous to take his finals. Manganese should be increased to 15 to 20 mg for a week or so.

The B complex usually is increased with any stress; 50 mg of each of the Bs would be the minimum. If the urine stays fairly yellow, one is probably taking about the proper amount. Stressed rats made to swim in cold water died if not given nutrients, B vitamins especially. Brewer's yeast was a good source, but desiccated liver really allowed them to survive that dirty laboratory trick.

Heat, cold, insulin, adrenalin, and forced muscle work lead to enlargement and hyperfunction of the adrenal cortex and atrophy of the thymus (the key organ in immunity).

It is impossible at the present level of biochemical and physiological knowledge to see the direct cause and effect of stress and blood pressure, coronary heart disease, cancer, psychosis, and other psychosomatic disease. Dr. S. Wolfe wrote in 1968, "The stress accruing from a situation is based in large part on the way the affected subject perceives it." Coping daily with the problems of living slowly eats away at all of us. Most of us have trouble closing the breach between overwhelming, omnipresent reality and our individual desires.

When we perceive a stress or the anticipation of a stress, the cortex of the brain sends messages to the thalamus, which relays them to the hypothalamus. The adrenocorticotropic hormone is secreted, which stimulates the adrenal glands to provide the hormones that further mobilize the body to respond to the perceived stress. Glucose formation is one response, but fat and cholesterol also are increased with stress. I can see the relationship between stress, increased cholesterol and fats in the bloodstream, and the eventual vascular damage. The type-A heart-attack-prone person may *think* he is under pressure, because he cannot screen out the world. His poor filtering system may be genetic or the result of his mother's diet during her pregnancy with him. In primitive man the glucose and fats might have been used in running or fighting.

If the resolution choices are limited, a disease may appear, depending upon genetics and organ susceptibility. A condition of relative depletion would allow all this to happen, and the stress of the superimposed disease would create a further exhaustion which would make that tissue or organ more susceptible.

I notice that ticklish, touchy kids and adults are more likely to be allergic. Allergic people are more likely to have secondary infections. You have to be healthy to be healthy. If we are on tilt a great deal of the time we need supplements just to barely maintain homeostasis. Three balanced meals a day are adequate if you get no mail, have no children or in-laws, and your phone never rings.

But remember, if you are alive you will have some stress. Getting married may be as stressful as getting divorced. If you feel stressed, you are. You can help restore homeostasis with nutrition, but try to climb out of the ice water too.

STUTTERING ☐ The "I-I-I-I-am-am-am going" speech of the three-year-old who seems stuck in neutral gear is often eliminated in a week with but 10 mg of B_1 (thiamin) daily. Best to give all the Bs.

I have had no experience with adult stutterers, but I assume that the B complex would help the biofeedback and hypnosis that sometimes correct it.

SURGERY ☐ Surgeons are supposed to know that burn patients will get out of the hospital in half the time if zinc levels are kept up; 60 to 90 mg a day seem about right. Zinc is necessary to an enzyme in the skin that manufactures protein essential to healing. Zinc is lost rapidly with stress (q.v.), and surgery is a stress.

Poor healing of wounds is directly related to the levels of zinc, vitamin A, and vitamin C. The C is reduced in white blood cells postsurgically. It is found that postoperative infections can be reduced with vitamin C; 3 to 5 grams a day for a few days preoperatively seems prudent. Some surgeons give C (5 to 7 grams) intravenously at the end of surgery to metabolize the anesthesia; the patient is awake, alert, and can walk back to the bed in about 60 seconds. No recovery-room time is necessary. In general, the I.V. should have amino acids to replenish the protein lost with the surgical stress. I.V. sugar water is rarely enough. Protein in the I.V. or orally usually will prevent discouraging wound separation. If vitamin C and amino acids are provided, collagen is easily synthesized to strengthen the wound.

Vitamin A is needed for healing; 25,000 to 50,000 units a

day for a few days before and after surgery would help and is not a toxic dose. Vitamin E helps the A work. E prevents the platelet aggregation that could lead to thromboses, a not uncommon surgical complication. Rubbing vitamin E on the wound three times a day usually prevents the ugly keloid scarring. Bioflavonoids and rutin would reduce capillary leakage and enhance vitamin C benefits. Folic acid, 1 mg a day, helps enzymes make tissue protein. The B complex makes the liver do its job better; the liver is the chief architect for protein assemblage. An injection of 1 ml of a B complex intramuscularly should be routine. B_{12} shots weekly or monthly forever are given to the patient who has had parts of the intestine removed.

Dentists give vitamin C (5 grams), calcium (1 gram), and B complex (1 cc) to patients who are about to have restorative work. This is I.V. and orally two times in the week before oral surgery and once or twice after. The patients have little or no trouble with appliance failure. Usually they have osteoporosis (q.v.), or they would not have needed the restoration in the first place.

Bring your sick friend in the hospital some protein drink and vitamin C; no wine and no chocolates. Some hospitals have improved to the point where they no longer serve white bread and red gelatin all the time.

SWEATING, EXCESS □ I was told that if someone sweats when exercising, it is a sign of good health. No sweat in a warm environment suggests low thyroid function. But excessive sweating when everyone else is not doing the same thing may mean a magnesium deficiency. If so, 500 mg a day should suffice.

SYNCOPE □ Syncope (fainting) is the momentary loss of consciousness due to a decrease in brain function. Heart abnormalities must be looked for; if the heart does not supply blood to the brain for ten seconds, syncope will occur.

Dehydration, bleeding, and adrenal insufficiency will prevent sufficient venous return to the heart.

Ordinary fainting usually is due to reflex dilation of systemic arterioles; too much blood goes to the body and an insufficient amount arrives at the brain. Stress, pain, or a sudden upright posture following prolonged bed rest or illness can do it. Hot weather, anxiety, or hunger will make a susceptible person more likely to keel over. The pregnant woman sends so much blood to her uterus that her brain sometimes gets cheated. Some have orthostatic hypotension; when they stand, the blood pressure falls whereas normally it would rise. Arteriosclerosis of cerebral arteries will reduce blood flow.

Seizures can mimic fainting, but the seizure victim does not know, usually, that something is amiss. The fainter senses the oncoming blackout.

If all these are absent, then anemia (q.v.) or hypoglycemia (q.v.) would be the most likely cause of syncope.

T

TASTE □ Someone found that when zinc-deficient people are given 50 mg of zinc daily, their ability to detect sweetness in food was enhanced.

Zinc is necessary for the taste buds to function adequately. The people who must salt everything before they even try the food on the plate usually are the same ones who *must* put sugar in their coffee. (Rats, also, will eat increased amounts of salt if they are zinc deficient.) Zinc-supplemented people get the sharpness without needing all that added salt.

Vitamin A and zinc work together. Thyroid may be at a low level of functioning because its hormone is needed to synthesize the zinc protein used by the taste buds.

B_6 and B_{12} seem to help the brain notice what the taste buds are saying. A dulled sense of taste may be improved with B$_3$; a persistent taste of salt in the mouth may be corrected with the same B$_3$.

Other mineral deficiencies may be associated with alterations in taste and smell. A balance between zinc, copper, and nickel seems to be important. Many claim that their sense of taste disappeared with the last bout of the flu; this is logical, since zinc chelates with the dead virus and runs out in the urine.

TEMPOROMANDIBULAR JOINT DYSFUNCTION

□ A variety of aches, pains, muscle spasms, and stress symptoms are now felt to be due to malfunction of the jawbone joint (just forward of the ear hole). Originally, the symptoms were thought to be due to malocclusion (overbite, crossbite), causing abnormal pressures to be applied to the joint when food was chewed. Now it is known that teeth-grinding and tension in the chewing muscles due to stress (and low calcium and magnesium) will cause similar symptoms.

What the patient may notice to indicate that the symptoms have something to do with this joint:

1. Popping, snapping, cracking noises from the joint when chewing.

2. Clenched teeth; nocturnal teeth-grinding; morning headaches; jaw painful or locked in morning; tongue edges scalloped; tongue slips between teeth when swallowing; difficulty moving jaw sideways, forward, or backward; unable to open mouth more than an inch; eye, ear, corner of mouth higher on one side.

3. Headaches, sinus pain, pains in shoulder, neck, and back, numbness in arms and fingers.

TMJ dysfunction frequently is seen in the edentulous or in those who have had extensive dental and bridge work;

many have had orthodontia. I am convinced it is more likely to be found in those people who were not breast-fed as infants. But emotional tension, too, can cause the jaw-muscle spasm that hurts the joint. Thus the vicious cycle begins.

Usually a bite plate is made which these people wear all night and much of the day. The appliance takes the pressure off the joint but also seems to have a calming effect on the nervous system. Reduction of stress and its perception would help. (See Anxiety; Stress.)

TENSION-FATIGUE SYNDROME □ The symptoms and signs of this condition are a giveaway for a food allergy, most likely due to milk (see Allergies). It is more often seen, or recognized, in the light-skinned, blue-eyed blond or green-eyed redhead because the dark skin of the lower lids is in sharp contrast to the pale cheeks. They look and act tired. They have frequent head- and stomachaches. All tests are normal. The clincher to the diagnosis is the snorting or zonking noise these people make to clear the phlegm that hangs down the back of the throat like a bunch of rubber bands. It takes about three weeks of no milk (or whatever) to get rid of the symptoms and restore normal facial color.

THROMBOSIS □ Blood that clots in a blood vessel and occludes the passage of blood is a thrombosis. A coronary thrombosis is a heart attack and may be fatal. Diabetics may get clots in the vessels of the feet and toes; the resulting gangrene could require amputation. Some clots in the leg veins of the bedridden may break off and lodge in the pulmonary vessels; these are called pulmonary emboli.

Vitamin E acts as a preventive, since it reduces platelet cohesiveness and keeps blood from clotting where it is not supposed to, that is, inside the vessels. (When we are cut, we need the blood to clot.) A good starting dose is 400 units of E, although that is probably not enough for a diabetic in a polluted area. If a thrombosis has already occurred, immediate large doses might be protective or prevent propagation of the clot. High-blood-pressure patients must increase the dose carefully—400 units for a few days, then 800 units, then 1200; 1600 units a day may not be too much for some.

THYROID □ More people are being treated with thyroid medication who do not need it than those who need it and are not getting it. The treatment of hypothyroidism seems to depend more on the doctor's philosophical orientation to medical management of patients than on the principle of "prove the existence of a disease, then treat it." This all started decades ago when the Armour Company began making pills out of steer and pig thyroid. This organ therapy was a boon to the harassed doctor trying to help patients who were tired, listless, depressed, who had aches and pains, who could not remember or concentrate—the neurasthenics. The medicine helped many who were obviously hypothyroid and made others feel that something at least was being done.

Various tests have been devised since then to help the clinician be more accurate with his diagnostic suspicions. However, he still has to keep the thyroid near the top of the list of problems whenever patients report any oddball symptoms.

The following are the classical symptoms of low thyroid function (the blood tests to verify hypothyroidism are probably not necessary): cold when others are warm, always need a sweater and a blanket when spouse doesn't; wear socks to bed; constipation; hoarseness; weight gain; never refreshed after eight to ten hours of sleep; no interest in fun activities, depressed, everything seems an effort; loss of hair; brittle nails; dry skin; never have sweaty palms; puffy eyelids.

Here are a few of the other symptoms that documented hypothyroid patients have displayed: irritability, dislike of crowds or closeness to others, slowness in comprehending new material, taking inordinate amount of time to do simple tasks (eat or dress), inability to concentrate, forgetfulness, deafness or noises in the ear, poor muscular coordination, depression, sore joints, odd skin sensations (prickling, tingling, numbness, creepy-crawly feelings), dizziness, light-headedness, suspiciousness even to the point of paranoia, nightmares, hyperactivity (which seems odd since low thyroid would be expected to slow them down). Many elderly people show the effects of low thyroid function, which doctors and family attribute to "aging." Menstrual disorders were one of the most common reasons for giving thyroid medication in the old days; irregularities of the menses and sexual misfunctions are common complaints of the hypothyroid patient. A lumpy uterus has been linked to thyroid malfunction. Remember, however, that all these symptoms could be due to anemia, hypoglycemia, food allergies, heavy-metal posioning, yeast overgrowth, a rotten marriage, or a boring job.

Thyroid hormone is needed by every cell in the body. Without it children fail to grow and will have a permanently stunted intelligence. The incidence of hypothyroidism increases after age thirty and is 5 to 10 times more frequent in females. The diagnostic picture is extremely complicated.

The following illnesses increase the risk of low thyroid function: insulin-dependent diabetes, hypoparathyroidism, pernicious anemia, vitiligo, rheumatoid arthritis, myasthenia gravis, chronic hepatitis. Zinc deficiency is common in thyroid deficiency and in many of the above diseases. High lithium and iodine doses can cause a hypothyroid state. Infections are more common in low-thyroid patients. Thyroid deficiency is connected to adrenal deficiency, and that is connected to allergies. Rheumatic fever is more likely to develop in low-thyroid patients. High cholesterol blood levels and persistent high blood pressure are associated with low thyroid levels; low cholesterol usually is seen in those with normal thyroid function. The thyroid helps regulate liver function; hypoglycemic patients usually have less trouble with sugar when on proper thyroid medication. Hypoglycemic and hypothyroid patients share similar symptoms. Thyroid medication may help clear stubborn acne.

I see a number of people with symptoms suggesting hypothyroid function who respond to vitamin B, C, and kelp therapy. Many people have poor intestinal absorption for vitamins and minerals, so the thyroid gland does not get nourished properly. And, of course, thyroid secretion is necessary to allow the lining cells of the intestines to absorb the vitamins and minerals so the thyroid gland can work properly. A few vitamin B injections intramuscularly (two times a week for three weeks) are usually sufficient to improve the absorption and to make the body (and the thyroid gland) function adequatley. B_1 deficiency will cause hypothyroidism.

Dr. Broda Barnes has found that the patient's morning oral or axillary temperature before rising helps to establish hypothyroid function more accurately than the laboratory. After five minutes the thermometer should read 97.8° to 98.2°. If it registers consistently below this over a period of two weeks, thyroid replacement therapy should be tried for the symptoms. (It would be nice if the lab tests agreed or were at least suggestive.)

If you ever had a swollen, tender thyroid, were treated for hyperthyroidism with radioactive iodine, or had thyroid surgery, a full-scale laboratory investigation of your defects should be launched.

Biochemical testing is becoming more accurate and sophisticated. It is now known that the following is going on: iodide in food is transported to, trapped in, and concentrated by the thyroid cells. Iodide is oxidized and combines with tyrosine. These intermediate iodotyrosines couple and become thyroxine (T_4), and triiodothyronine (T_3) within the thyroglobulin, the principle protein of the thyroid gland. The gland has a large reserve store of T_3 and T_4. The control of the level of circulating T_3 and T_4 depends upon the thyroid gland and the thyroid-stimulating hormone (TSH) of the anterior pituitary gland. Increased levels of T_3 and T_4 will suppress the flow of TSH. But TSH is also influenced by the hypothalamus in the lower brain, which secretes thyrotropin-releasing hormone (TRH). T_3 and T_4 circulate bound to protein. Thyroxine-binding protein (TBG) is the most important because of its strong binding action to T_4. Only about 0.05 percent of the total T_4 in the circulation is free, and only this free thyroxine (FT_4) is available to the tissues for its metabolic effect. FT_4 levels are more closely correlated with the hypo- or hyperthyroid clinical states. The total thyroxine in the serum cannot be considered without the effect of unsaturated binding protein. When these rise (as in pregnancy or use of oral contraceptives) more FT_4 is bound. With less FT_4 flowing, the TSH is activated and more FT_4 is liberated from the thyroid gland. The total amount of thyroxine in the blood of normal humans may vary considerably due to the various levels of binding proteins, which fluctuate because of individual physiological changes. If a pregnant woman has an abnormally high T_4, she may still be normal-thyroid because her TBG is elevated. All the above has not indicated the considerable effect of T_3. This hormone is found in the serum at only one-seventieth the level of T_4. Some feel it is more active than T_4; T_4 may be converted to T_3.

There are several possible tests the doctor may order:

T_4, *total thyroxine:* 4.4 to 9.8 mcg/100 ml serum.

TBG, thyroxine-binding globulin: 10 to 26 mcg T_4 per 100 ml of serum (as T_4 binding capacity). In normal conditions only one-third of the TBG sites are saturated; thus the bound T_4 is about 8 mcg per 100 ml. In normal individuals the ratio of bound T_4 to TBG is fairly constant. In hyperthyroidism the ratio is increased; in hypothyroidism the ratio will fall.

TBG is increased in women after giving birth, with use of estrogens or contraceptive pills, and with heroin and marijuana. It decreases with age, stress, illness, and steroid (cortisone) therapy. Phenytoin (Dilantin) increases the liver's thyroid-hormone metabolizing function.

FT₄, free unbound thyroxine: 1 to 2.3 ng/100 ml serum. More reliance has been placed on this test because of the variability of levels of protein binding capacity. (Some patients have high thyroid symptoms and others have hypothyroidism with normal T_4 values.)

T₃, triodothyronine: 110 to 230 ng/ml serum. This hormone may be more active than T_4. In hyperthyroidism the proportion of T_3 is much higher relative to T_4. The measurement of T_3 is useful in the early diagnosis of hyperthyroidism but not in hypothyroidism, since the T_3 may be normal. Low T_3 is the rule in almost all serious illnesses; the lower the level the more serious the problem.

RT₃U, the resin T₃ uptake test: 10.0 to 14.6 percent. An index of the unsaturated thyroxine-binding globulin fraction of serum. In cases of hyperthyroidism a relative decrease in the unsaturated TBG will show a high uptake of the resin. An increase in the unsaturated TBG (as in hypothyroidism) results in a low T_3 uptake by the resin. This test may help clear up confusing cases.

TSH, thyroid-stimulating hormone: up to 10 microunits/ml of serum. The principle use of this test is to differentiate between hypothyroidism that is due to thyroid dysfunction and that due to a pituitary inadequacy. The TSH would be elevated if the problem is primarily in the thyroid; with no thyroid hormone feedback, the pituitary would increase its output in an effort to get the thyroid going.

The reliability of thyroid-function tests is notably poor in liver disease, spreading cancer, heart failure, renal disease, and serious pneumonia; the thyroid cuts down its secretion of T_3, probably in an effort to conserve energy.

I have wanted to point out the difficulty and complexity of diagnosing hypothyroidism biochemically in order to emphasize the concept that you, the patient, are the one who must live inside your body, imperfect though it may be. Your evaluation should be the deciding factor in determining what your disease is and how it should be treated. The laboratory tests are not sophisticated enough yet for the doctor to say, "This is it." Test figures can vary fivefold and still be in the normal range; your test may be at the low end of normal, and because your symptoms are not typical enough or not severe enough, the doctor is reluctant to treat you. He doesn't want to be trapped into treating a psychogenic condition that should have been referred to a psychiatrist.

The next question, "Does your hypothyroidism require thyroid replacement?" The disease is usually permanent, so thyroid hormone is to be taken for a lifetime. Those on thyroid hormone for other than well-documented hypothyroidism will recover the function of the pituitary-thyroid gland relationship within 5 weeks of discontinuing the therapy—which is reassuring if you and your doctor elect to try some thyroid for a while. Women who develop hypothyroidism after childbrith would become euthyroid again within six to ten months.

Most doctors recommend synthetic preparations such as Levothyroxine (T_4). Using desiccated thyroid or combinations of T_3 and T_4 may lead to high T_3 levels. The patient would be the best judge of the response; the dose is gradually increased every two to three weeks until the patient, the doctor, and—finally—the laboratory are satisfied.

Some thyroid glands will function satisfactorily if they are supplied with enough iodine. If an iodine supplement does not work, and if you get acne from the iodine, try something else. In some patients, iodine has a suppressive effect.

The following foods, if eaten frequently, could interfere with iodine uptake and cause poor thyroid function: cabbage, kale, brussels sprouts, cauliflower, broccoli, kohlrabi, turnips, rutabaga, rapeseed, and brown (Indian), black, or white mustard. The milk from cows that have been grazing on these plants would have a similar effect. Garden cress and radish could do the same. Soybeans and the skins of peanuts, almonds, and cashews have a suppressive effect. If they are consumed frequently, iodine should be taken as a supplement; 100 to 150 mcg daily is the suggested dose. Try an all-purpose mineral supplement from the health store. Nitrates could interfere with the tyrosine-iodine linkage that produces thyroid hormone.

Copper is necessary for the production of TSH from the pituitary. Enzymes containing copper and zinc in the proper ratio are required for the peripheral cellular metabolism of T_4. Most of us get more copper than we need because of the extensive use of copper piping.

TICS, TWITCHES, AND TREMORS □ These are all signs of calcium and magnesium deficiencies, but low levels of potassium, zinc, and vitamin E could be related. Neuritis might make the muscles twitch, but usually skin sensations predominate. B_6, B_{12}, and B_1 are sometimes needed to calm down nervous tics.

TINNITUS □ Ringing in the ear is often the precursor of deafness. The nerve is dying and the activity of the nerve is perceived as a ringing sound. The cause should be sought, although it is rarely found. Food and inhalant allergies could cause a swelling in the nerve. (See Ménière's Disease.)

High doses of bioflavonoids have helped in some cases. Manganese helps nervous tissue; 5 to 10 mg a day for a month or two might help.

TONGUE □ If the tongue looks glossy, red, or inflamed, B_{12} should help. If it is coated and the surface looks like a road map, a food allergy is the most likely cause. If it is white-coated with a crack down the middle and a red tip, a B_3 deficiency is suspected; scalloped edges also indicated a need for B_3. A magenta tongue is usually due to a B_2 deficiency. A swollen, tender tongue may be due to a pantothenic acid deficiency. Sore tongue and mouth mean B_6 is needed.

(See Taste.)

TOOTH DECAY □ The tooth is mainly calcium phosphate, but the mineral content must be laid down before the tooth erupts from the gum. The diet of the pregnant woman is important for the baby teeth, and the diet of the child in the first six years is important for the permanent teeth.

Teeth need protein, calcium, phosphorus, magnesium, molybdenum, and vitamin B_6. Try an all-purpose mineral supplement for a while. Many parents give their children a powdered earth dug up in the Nevada desert; it has all the minerals needed for body function. Fluoride does help, but only in trace amounts. Most authorities feel it should not exceed 0.25 mg a day in the first year. Magnesium phosphate is a good choice. Phosphate is generally oversupplied by the high meat and soft-drink diet of American children. Dolomite might be better because it is calcium and magnesium. Calcium from oyster shells is better absorbed, however.

A shift in mineral concentration may cause a more acid saliva, which would promote growth of cariogenic (cavity-making) bacteria. More calcium would buffer the acids. Acid saliva also comes from hypoglycemia, which could follow from sugar ingestion. Adequate mineral ingestion will discourage cavities. The hair of those whose teeth are full of cavities usually shows high calcium, low phosphorus, and low magnesium. Magnesium by mouth would help to balance this discrepancy. Zinc deficiency also is associated with cavities.

Dr. Herbert Fleege quotes a study: "A survey was once done with fifty children, in which they were fed an average meal: 50 percent of the children were given an orange cut into four pieces, and the other 50 percent brushed their teeth. Researchers discovered that the children who had eaten the orange had teeth 35 percent cleaner than those who had used a toothbrush. Thus the indication is that there is less pollution to the oral ecology of the mouth through the use of coarse calories rather than soft calories. As an observation: we all know children have very poor manual dexterity, so coarse calories do a better job than a toothbrush."

One suggestion about flossing: chew up a 400-unit vitamin E, swallow it, and then floss.

Don't eat sugar, of course.

(See Periodontal Disease.)

U

ULCERS: STOMACH AND DUODENAL □ The present treatment for peptic ulcers involves using a drug, cimetidine (an H_2 receptor antagonist), which cuts acid secretion. Some doctors are still advising the use of cream and milk despite the fact that for ten years it has been known that although milk does cut the pain it actually increases the acid secreted. Its buffering ability has been oversold. An occasional glassful seems to be OK, but the total therapy lies elsewhere. Cimetidine is to be used for a short six to eight weeks.

The causes of the peptic ulcer are unknown. When food hits the stomach, the stomach lining pours out acid and pepsin. There is no alteration in the concentration according to the type of food; a marshmallow gets the same amount of acid as does a cube of meat. The acid overwhelms the first item, and whatever is left over lies about to work on the lining or to run out into the duodenum if no more food is ingested. Acid digestion of the lining is worse with protein deprivation, aging, aspirin ingestion, smoking, and excessive cortisone therapy. Emotional stress allows it to happen, but it is not the cause.

Duodenal ulcers are common in children with chronic allergies. Histamine may be contributing to the ulcer as well as to the allergy. Calcium counteracts histamine, and the fact that many of these children crave milk means either that they are allergic to it, that it solves the immediate pain, or that they are searching for calcium.

Dr. Thomas Latimer Cleave found a low incidence of stomach ulcers among German soldiers in a stressful situation on the Russian front in World War II. The soldiers had little sugar or white flour or processed food. Their chief diet was raw fruits, vegetables, a piece of stolen duck, whatever was available, and eaten mostly raw. He believed that stress would probably cause an ulcer in the susceptible person, but that a nourishing diet would protect the stomach from its own acid. Raw and natural whole foods have a buffering capacity to neutralize stomach acid that processed food does not.

The only recognized gastric irritants are alcohol, drugs, caffeine, coffee, tea, cocoa, black pepper, and chili powder. Decaffeinated coffee causes as much acid stimulation as regular. There is no evidence that roughage or coarse food can scratch or irritate the ulcer crater. Celery, fruit skins, nuts, and seeds are all OK, and would be better foods to eat.

Antacids that contain magnesium and aluminum should be used sparingly. Magnesium may cause diarrhea (not the hydroxide, however, which is virtually nonabsorbable). Aluminum can accumulate in the brain and cause a dementia or increased bone aluminum concentration and demineralized bones. The calcium in antacids can cause hypercalcemia, and that can stimulate gastric acid secretion. Antacids can help in the healing of duodenal ulcers; best taken at the end of meals.

Nutritionally, three to five medium-size meals a day would be the best plan. No sugar, white flour, or junk is allowed to be swallowed. Salads, beans, meat, cheese, fruit, and vegetables are the standard. A hair test may show a copper deficiency; 1 to 2 mg for two months might be enough. Vitamin A is helpful for all mucous membranes, 20,000 to 30,000 units; L-glutamine is supposed to help things heal. Cabbage is the old favorite and does seem to work. Vitamin C, vitamin E, and a little zinc should complete the list of helpful nutrients.

Stress ulcers may occur after burns or injury. The doctor should have his patients on C, calcium, A, B complex, and zinc anyway.

Stomach ulcers are occasionally cancerous.

V

VARICOSITIES ☐ Varicosities, varicose veins, and varicoceles are all related to hemorrhoids in that they have a common etiology: venous back pressure has dilated the vein walls to the extent that the valves in the veins do not make contact efficiently. Venous blood puddles. Because they are so rarely found in people with bulky, easy-to-pass bowel movements, these dilated vessels are felt to be due to straining at stool.

A roughage diet and avoidance of milled flour and dairy products, which constipate most people, seem prudent measures to prevent the progression of the vein-wall weakness. Many sufferers have found that vitamin E (400 to 1200 units) can help make these swollen veins shrink back to a normal size. Vitamin C has a collagen-building effect, so big doses would soften the bowels as well as firm up the vein walls.

VASCULAR PROBLEMS: Chilblains, Buerger's Disease ☐ These blood-vessel problems cause pain and cold in the extremities; an excessive nerve response causes the blood vessels to constrict. Allergies and tobacco smoke act to trigger the response mechanism.

Niacin, 3000 to 6000 mg a day in divided doses, should

control it. Most patients build up the dose slowly because the niacin flush is rather overwhelming.

VIRUS INFECTIONS □ The key to controlling virus infections is to help the body manufacture interferon, an intracellular antiviral substance. If the body has enough interferon, a virus cannot get started. If a virus gets established and starts spreading to other cells, stopping it is more difficult because it takes more interferon. Vitamin C is known to aid the body in manufacturing this bit of protein, so it makes sense to increase the daily consumption of C to the point where virus infections cannot get established or, if they do, will not last long. (See Respiratory Symptoms.)

VISION □ Primitive people didn't wear glasses (who knows if they needed them or not). But everyone seems to wear glasses nowadays. Vitamin A deficiency usually shows itself as a difficulty seeing objects in dim light; 5000 units a day, a small dose, is recommended as sufficient for everyone. A reasonably good diet would easily provide that, but 25 percent of our population do not get even that amount.

A decrease in visual acuity could be due also to an impaired function of the optic nerve. Vitamins B_1 and B_{12} would help if a neuritis is suspected. B_2 is valuable for indistinct vision or discomfort in strong light. It would help those who regularly must use their eyes in strong light. Iodine (in kelp) and copper help some improve their vision. Most of us get enough copper these days. Zinc is necessary to mobilize the vitamin A from the liver; protein is necessary also. Calcium is necessary for the absorption of A.

Someone did a study on highway patrol officers. The night shift had trouble with lights; their nutrition was poorer also. They were low in A, calcium, zinc, and B vitamins.

Zinc helps eye-hand coordination. Chromium helps the eyes work, but it must be incorporated in the tissues in the last three months of the pregnancy or the baby may be nearsighted. Maybe this is why so many people who were prematurely born need glasses.

(See Eyes.)

VITILIGO □ A condition marked by patchy areas of skin with no pigment. The darker the normal skin pigment, the more obvious are the depigmented areas. Once those pale areas show up, it means the pigment cells are dead. No one as yet has found a satisfactory way to bring back the color.

It is not known what causes vitiligo. Insufficient hydrochloric acid may be partially responsible. Forty percent of vitiligo patients over fifty years of age have low thyroid output. This problem may fall into the category of an autoimmune disease (q.v.).

Paraminobenzoic acid (PABA) has been claimed by some to bring about improvement. Good and adequate nutrition may be helpful to keep it from getting a lot worse.

A recent report used 10 to 20 mg of copper daily plus the PABA. Too much copper can be toxic, however.

W

WARTS □ Dr. Rees B. Rees has stated that the wart virus is a weak antigen that sits and grows on the skin surface, somewhat like a barnacle; the body doesn't really know it is there and cannot make any antibody against it. Treatment must create an inflammation whereby the protection is broken down, allowing the body to produce the immunity.

Twenty percent of warts disappear after one office visit, no matter what the treatment. Treating one wart may make all the rest of them go away because of the development of circulating antibodies. But it is a weak antigen and these antibodies are not strong enough to prevent the future growth of warts. A cellular immunity is suspected, which is why regression of warts is associated with an inflammation.

The missing link may be a need for vitamin A. Along with anything the doctor might want to do (hold the surgery) to create an inflammation—dry ice, acid, liquid nitrogen—a nutritional approach also should be tried. There is no doubt that vitamin A will toughen the skin and allow the warts to drop off. A child might respond in about three to five weeks to an oral dose of 50,000 units a day. Most have no toxic symptoms from that dose, but if double vision, dry scaly skin, and headache appear, stop it. Adults would use 50,000 to 100,000 units.

Vitamin E oil from a capsule directly on the wart, plus a bandage, will speed resolution. (I have the best luck with raw tape, no gauze pad; it causes the surface of the wart to get mungy and deteriorate faster.) Topical vitamin C (with a bandage) acts as an irritant and can help.

Don't forget spunk water. Now tell me why a hypnotist can get rid of warts? Just believe in what you do.

WEAKNESS ☐ Weakness of the muscles is similar to fatigue (q.v.). But I assume the latter to be a generalized feeling, whereas in weakness the muscles only, and not the brain, are affected.

Osteomalacia (adult rickets) makes the muscles weak. Vitamin D and calcium would be required. (See Osteomalacia.)

A neuritis could prevent the nerve impulse from telling the muscle what to do. Vitamin B complex helps this, but B_1, B_6, and B_{12} are more specific. If the hand grip is weak, B_6 would help. (See Carpal-Tunnel Syndrome.) Choline (in lecithin) will help the body make acetylcholine, the chemical responsible for neuromuscular function. (See Myasthenia Gravis.)

Multiple sclerosis would have to be considered. Small strokes can compromise muscle function. Nerves pinched due to a herniated disc or osteoporosis (q.v.) usually give pain also.

Lead and heavy-metal poisoning cause muscle weakness.

See the doctor or neurologist; something is wrong.

Y

YEAST INFECTIONS □ Since the start of the extensive use and overuse of antibiotics from the 1940s, a parallel rise in the occurrence of yeast infection has plagued the doctors' practice. At first it was considered just a mild nuisance, then an irritation, and now a threat to the established practice of curing disease with antibiotics, cortisone, and immunosuppressive drugs, and to the casual use of contraceptive pills. For every medical advance humanity makes, there seems to be a counterproductive force.

Dr. C. Orian Truss was treating a woman ten years ago for a vaginal yeast infection. The nystatin cleared it up in a few days, and at the same time her depression and paranoia disappeared. Treating one problem and clearing up several was something new to his practice. If she quit the medicine, however, she was psychotic again in three days. She is still on this medicine.

He has found that we all carry this yeast, Candida. It grows in our intestinal tract along with fungi, viruses, and bacteria. It will grow and create symptoms if a person's immune system is weakened by antibiotics, cortisone, or hormones. Stress and childbirth may contribute to the imbalance. Carbohydrate ingestion seems to "feed" it, especially yeasty foods—bread, cheese, wine, beer, and even brewer's yeast.

It can cause every symptom listed in this book and more. It triggers autoimmune diseases, schizophrenia, hyperactivity, multiple sclerosis, diarrhea, anorexia, constipation, anything. The most likely situation is that of an older teen or adult female who had antibiotics for infections and acne as a youngster, has used the contraceptive pill alternating with pregnancies, and might have had cortisone occasionally for asthma. She has menstrual irregularities, premenstrual tension, intestinal gas and bowel movement irregularities, and the two most common findings, fatigue and memory loss. Most of the victims simply cannot remember what they did the previous day. There may be headaches, depression, severe allergic symptoms, skin rashes, and decrease in taste and smell sensation. They have little interest in sex.

Dr. Truss feels that the yeast products overwhelm the immune system and that a tolerance or an unresponsiveness develops, in which all of the immune system cells are involved in the antigen-antibody reaction with the yeast's foreign substance. These complexes lodge in cells and cause the illness—in the brain, the intestines, the lungs, wherever.

Apparently particles break off from the yeast in the intestinal tract, are absorbed, and subdue the immune system. When nystatin is used to cut down the yeast population, many allergies simply disappear, perhaps because the drug has freed the immune system for other work in the body.

Since we all have the yeast growing in us, and since most of us have a positive reaction, no test is currently of diagnostic value. It has occurred to me when I have used all my nutritional supports for a woman (usually), including I.V. and I.M. shots, to ask about memory, fatigue, and what happens when the patient drinks wine or beer.

Nystatin, 500,000-unit tablets four to eight times a day, should be continued for four to six weeks if the problem is even suspected. Most victims will cheer up and have a little more energy in just a week or ten days. The nystatin is not absorbed, so suppositories must be used if vaginal candidiasis is present. Liquid or powdered nystatin is preferred if oral or esophageal yeast is suspected.

Some patients note some queasiness, and some will have

an increase in the symptoms for a few days. It is assumed that the drug breaks up the growing yeast in the intestines and the yeast particles cause the temporary increase of symptoms.

All the vitamins and minerals known to improve immunity would be helpful. Vitamin C is increased to bowel tolerance. Zinc (60 mg) and vitamin A (25,000 to 50,000 units) should help the body dump the large load of yeast. Iodine (as in kelp) was all they had in the old days; the dose would be five to ten tablets a day.

PART
3

7

THE NUTRICOPIA OF VITAMINS AND MINERALS

Vitamin A is the vitamin we associate with night blindness. But the whole body appears to need it, especially surface cells. Smokers who have a higher than usual intake of carotene (vitamin A precursor) have a lower incidence of lung cancer. Vitamin A helps to prevent the obstruction of the skin oil follicles that is regarded to be the first step to acne. Vitamin E helps the A work better.

Vitamin A is depleted if a person has been stressed. Stress can lead to respiratory problems (bronchitis and asthma) and gastrointestinal ulcers. Vitamin A can control the diarrhea often associated with Crohn's disease. It stimulates the formation of mucous and may control the symptoms associated with respiratory flu. It has healing and controlling effects on cell membranes; the lipid part of the membrane will undergo oxidation unless protected with A and vitamin E.

Vitamin A seems to be helpful in controlling some cancers. Patients on steroids (as in allergy or autoimmune disease) are protected from some of the disturbing side effects, e.g., loss of immunity.

Vitamin A is needed by the liver to change the protein we eat into protein our bodies can use. It stabilizes the amount of protein in epithelial structures. If not enough is provided, hyperkeratosis, ulcerations of skin, defective taste and smell, and disorders of the inner ear may appear. The cochlea (hearing organ) has 10 times the amount of A that other tissues have. Glaucoma is associated with low levels of vitamin A.

Only 5000 units are needed as a supplement if one is eating some liver powder every week or two, if egg yolk, deep yellow and dark green vegetables, cheese made from whole milk, and butter are being consumed frequently. About 25 percent of our population have low levels of vitamin A in their blood. This dose would be adequate if a person is in good health, resistance to infection is high, and the environment has few pollutants. If the patient is a smoker or cancer is in the family or stress is obvious, the dose should be increased. If the skin is dry and bumpy and night blindness is prominent, the dose should be 20,000 to 30,000 units. Some find 50,000 to 100,000 units is best for them, but this gets into a potentially toxic dose. One must watch for headache, double vision, fatigue, upset stomach, night sweats and loss of body hair.

Vitamin B_1, or thiamine, is essential for a wide variety of functions related to the nervous system. Any of the following conditions could be due to a deficient intake of B_1: muscle cramps, clumsiness, insomnia, anxiety, irritability, depression, increased sensitivity to noise and pain, weight loss, anorexia, learning disability, reduced ambition, memory loss, and increased ingestion of alcohol.

We all need a few milligrams of B_1. It is necessary for the oxidation of carbohydrates in the brain. Some need more than others; 25 to 100 mg is not excessive.

Milling flour removes 85 percent of the B_1; roasting beef reduces B_1 by 35 to 50 percent. Modern processed food is low in B_1. If carbohydrate intake is increased, B_1 must be increased. Without B_1, the body cannot use oxygen or glucose. Whole grains, pork, and peas are loaded with B_1.

Vitamin B_2, or riboflavin, accounts for the yellow color to the urine when a B-complex vitamin capsule is swallowed. It is needed for general health, red blood cell formation, integrity of the skin and eyes, and the function of the nervous system. It is needed for the utilization of carbohydrates, fats, and proteins.

Low B_2 is associated with cataracts, seborrhea, inflammation of mouth tissues, dermatitis, failure to grow, poor vision, fatigue, and depression. The minimum dose would be 25 mg a day if one has cracks at the corners of the mouth; the tongue is smooth and purple; the eyes are sensitive to light, and itch and burn; and one feels worn out or depressed.

Liver, whole grains, eggs, and milk are well endowed with B_2.

Vitamin B_3, or niacinamide, is required by all cells, as it is necessary for the metabolism of carbohydrates, fats, and proteins. A deficiency can cause rough, scaly skin, diarrhea, and a schizophrenic type reaction. Some of those with dysperceptions may be improved with 3000 mg of B_3 daily.

Halitosis, unmanageable hair, canker sores, and hypoglycemic attacks can be corrected with 50 to 500 mg of niacinamide a day. Some people need supplements because their bodies need more than what can be found in liver, peanuts, grains, legumes, and fowl.

Large doses of niacinamide (1000 to 3000 mg) each day help about half the alcoholics who have tried it. Depression, insomnia, headaches, and ringing in the ears may be improved with 100 mg of B_3 three times a day.

Vitamin B₆, or pyridoxine, is one of the busiest vitamins known. It helps the functions of the brain, skin, liver, pancreas, muscles, joints—every ill of the body seems to need B₆ to help the enzymes operate. To find out what B₆ does, volunteers were put on a B₆-deficient diet. In just two to three weeks most of them were irritable, depressed, and mentally confused. Depending on genetic factors or poor absorption or stress or food allergies, a B₆-deficient person might notice the following: acne (especially that seen in women at menstrual-period time), convulsions, asthma and allergies, oxalate kidney stones, infertility, poor stamina, diabetes, edema, halitosis, dandruff, anemia, neuropathy (pain, numbness, tingling), joint pain and stiffness, headaches, hemorrhoids, dental decay, eczema, striae, arteriosclerosis, hyperactivity, autoimmune and degenerative diseases.

B₆ is needed for the digestion and metabolism of carbohydrates, fats, and protein. Extra B₆ is needed if one has diabetes, is allergic, under stress, or eating extra protein for whatever reason.

Dr. Bernard Rimland is our guru when it comes to B₆, as he used 300 to 500 mg per day on autistic children with proven results. B₆ is the coenzyme of the decarboxylase step of both serotonin and catecholamine pathways in the brain. Its use has helped treat hyperactivity, learning disabilities, and depression.

B₆ is the woman's friend, as it helps a liver enzyme metabolize estrogens, whose excess may lead to the irritability, headache, fatigue and puffiness so many women experience at menstrual-period time.

Dr. John Ellis, who discovered that the swollen nerve due to B₆ deficiency caused the carpal tunnel syndrome, tells us that myocardial infarction is seen in those low in B₆, potassium, and magnesium. Deficiencies of these caused muscle spasm and impaired function of the motor nerve impulse.

B₆ has been shown in animal studies to slow blood clotting by interfering with platelet clumping.* It would thus preclude a few heart attacks due to emboli or thrombi.

Some authorities believe that the diseases related to B_6 deficiencies have increased because of the increased use of B_6 antagonists. These include hydrazines found in plant growth regulators, herbicides, medicines (penicillamine, L-dopa, oral contraceptives) and antioxidants in petroleum. INH (isonicotinic hydrazine) is used as a TB inhibitor. Tartrazines are used as a food dye. Tons of it (yellow #5) are in our foods and some is converted in the body to hydrazines.

No wonder that B_6 deficiency is so common in the athlete, the student, those under stress, women, those consuming sugar, and in the elderly.

Vitamin B_{12}, or cyanocobalamine or hydroxocobalamine, comes to mind when one speaks of pernicious anemia. But a wide variety of physical and mental problems are definitely related to a deficiency of B_{12}.

All obstetricians know or should know of its restorative value in postpartum depression. Usually a couple of shots of B_{12} will brighten the outlook of the most tearful new mother.

It makes folate available for some essential metabolic reactions.

A deficiency of B_{12} might lead to fatigue, weakness, unsteadiness (and loss of vibration sense), paresthesia (needles-and-pins sensation) in legs, memory loss, depression, irritability, confusion, visual difficulty, infertility, anemia.

A deficiency should be suspected in a person with any of the above symptoms who also is a vegan vegetarian, or has had his stomach removed, or has had a pancreatic or intestinal disease. One must have enough stomach acid to free B_{12} from the protein ingested. Some of the stomach cells must be capable of secreting enough trypsin and bicarbonate to fur-

* *The Lancet* (1981) 1:1799.

ther digest the protein, and the small bowel must be capable of absorbing the B_{12}.

The metabolic defects of a deficiency of B_{12} are body-wide. Every cell can be affected.

"B_{15}," or pangamic acid, was isolated in 1951 and assigned the name and the number. It has not been proven to be essential; no one has developed a deficiency disease as a result of being deprived of it. It is rightly called dimethylglycine. It has been useful in the treatment of disturbed and autistic children, it cuts the alcoholics craving for ethanol, and it seems to help lift fatigue. It is quite safe. The dose would start at 50 mg two or three times a day. After a month one would try to decide if it were worth continuing or not.

Bioflavonoids or, specifically, Rutin (100 mg) and hesperidin (100 mg) usually taken 2 or 3 times a day along with Vitamin C have proven helpful in controlling capillary permeability and keeping connective tissue healthy. They may cause the red capillaries in the whites of the eyes to disappear, hemorrhoids may shrink, bruises will fade more rapidly. Bursitis and ulcers are felt to heal faster when bioflavonoids and rutin are used. Cataracts are less common in these on high doses of bioflavonoids. Varicose veins disappeared more rapidly if patients are given bioflavonoids with rutin, C, and E. The bleeding following tonsil and adenoid removal is considerably reduced. Spontaneous abortions may be avoided. Some forms of arthritis are helped, because bioflavonoids will slow the manufacture of hyalouronidase. And in those who have had a stroke, this substance will cut the recurrence rate.* Hot flashes are milder with bioflavonoids.

A daily dose of 100 to 300 mg of bioflavonoids is recommended, but with stress or the appearance of any of the above symptoms or signs, the dose should be increased to 500 to 1000 mg daily.

* *Medical World News*, 30, April 1979.

Vitamin C, ascorbic acid, has been shown to be a most valuable aid in controlling bacterial infections, but even more for those caused by viruses. Vitamin C helps the cells produce interferon, a natural antiviral intracellular substance.

Low levels of vitamin C are associated with impaired immunity, gallstones, thrombosis and arterial narrowing in diabetics, bladder cancer, hay fever and allergies in general, anemia, bedsores, anxiety, and drug addiction.

Vitamin C is helpful for fighting cancer and fatigue; shortening the length of labor; reducing the incidence of sudden infant death syndrome; controlling the pain of trauma; alleviating constipation; helping insomnia, glaucoma, urinary infection, almost any virus infection (hepatitis, mononucleosis, common cold, herpes), drug toxicity, snakebite, sunburn; and it also acts as a meat preservative.

It must work through an enzyme system, so when the cancer victim has had chemotherapy and radiation therapy in addition to the surgery, these enzyme systems may not be able to transform the C into an anticancer metabolite. Linus Pauling tells us that vitamin C increases the rate of production of lymphocytes to help fight infection and some cancer. Some malignant tumors release an enzyme, collagenase, which destroys the collagen fibers, weakening the normal tissues and allowing the tumor to spread.

Dr. Robert Cathcart suggests that each person find the proper dose for his or her body by increasing the ingested amount by 1000 mg a day until a dose is found that just barely softens the stools. Then when a stress or infection occurs, the dose is increased to the daily dose given every hour until the situation is under control. This would be used for a bad cold or flu bug. In a more severe illness like hepatitis, mononucleosis, or viral pneumonia, as much as 100 grams (100,000 mg) of vitamin C or more a day may be needed to bring the virus under control. The dose is slowly reduced back to the original maintenance dose as convalescence progresses.

Vitamin C will increase the blood level of high-density lipoprotein, felt to be protective against vascular disease.*

Calcium is needed daily for life. Because it is poorly absorbed, it is recommended that about twice as much be ingested as is excreted in the urine and stool. Since about 400 mg is lost daily, 800 to 1000 mg of calcium should be taken daily, and more during the rapid growth of adolescence and during the times of increased demands of pregnancy and nursing. A quart of milk, translates to about 800 mg of calcium, but there are those who cannot drink milk or if they do, may not absorb it.

A calcium deficiency in the body might make itself known with palpitations, insomnia, muscle cramps, arm and leg numbness, tooth decay, brittle nails, osteoporosis, and rickets. The blood calcium will try to maintain itself at 8.6 to 10.4 mg per 100 ml of serum by removing calcium from the bone when the level is low and replacing it when the intake and absorption are adequate or elevated.

Deficiencies have been found to be common because of decreased ingestion, poor absorption, and possibly inadequate amounts in the food we eat. One explanation is the increased ingestion of phosphorus (in meat and soft drinks) which tends to compete with calcium for absorption.

Exercise will improve calcium absorption. Vitamin C and hydrochloric acid improve absorption. High-fat, high-protein, and high-fiber diets will reduce calcium absorption. Lactobacillus acidophilus helps calcium absorption, as it increases the acidity of the intestinal contents.

Choline is known to help the body make cell membranes and lipoproteins, used in fat transport. It is part of the material surrounding some nerve cells and is in acetylcholine, which is a neurotransmitter. Memory and mental function can be improved with its use.

* *Journal of Human Nutrition*, Feb. 1981.

The average diet has plenty, 500 to 1000 mg. Lecithin is the usual source of supplemental choline, as plain choline is degraded to diethylamine, which has a fishy odor.

It is found in meat, egg yolks, legumes, fish, and cereal.

Chromium has been found to help stabilize the blood sugar in diabetics and hypoglycemics. Chromium increases tissue sensitivity to insulin. The glucose-tolerance factor includes chromium, niacinamide, glycine, cysteine, and glutamic acid. This GTF is found in brewer's yeast and will usually reduce some of the insulin requirements.

Chromium also has a controlling effect on heart attacks; there is less chromium in the main vessel walls of those dying of heart attacks than in those dying of accidents. Chromium is lost from the body with aging.* Chromium is lost when foods are refined. The soil is easily depleted of its chromium, and the plants growing therein will reflect that loss. When glucose in the blood rises, chromium will follow, and then it is easily lost in the urine. Low chromium is associated with elevated cholesterol and myopia.

An average dose is 20 mcg up to 100 mcg. Chromium should be adequate in brewer's yeast, meat, and grains, but because of the deficiency of the soil, it would be wise to take a supplement.

Copper excess seems to be more common than copper deficiency, because of its presence in plumbing systems and pipes bringing water into homes. Water spoiled by acid rainfall increases the leaching of copper out of the pipes.

Copper is essential, however. With iron, it is needed to make hemoglobin. About 75 percent of body copper is in the bones; it contributes to bone and artery stability. It is involved in protein-building enzymes. It helps make fibrin and the elastic connective tissue, collagen. It can be a protection against osteoporosis. A deficiency is associated with stomach

* *Postgraduate Medicine*, 1971.

ulcers and is implicated as a factor in the nonformation of hair pigment, in alopecia, and in some dermatitis cases. High zinc or calcium intake tends to reduce copper assimilation.

Copper levels in women taking contraceptive pills are even higher than the levels usually found in the ninth month of pregnancy. It is needed to convert estradiol and estriol to estrone.

Copper is found in oysters, liver, nuts, and chocolate, but its level may vary in foods from zero to sixty parts per million if the soil is deficient. Many people absorb excess copper from drinks (beer, carbonated, citrus) distributed in metal cans. Copper in intrauterine devices will increase the body's burden of this metal.

Vitamin D is essential for calcium and phosphate levels in bone, blood, and tissues. It is formed when ultraviolet light strikes the skin. Those who live in northern zones or in polluted, cloudy areas, or who spend much time indoors have to compensate with oral ingestion. This would be especially important whenever calcium deficiency is suspected.

Vitamin D stimulates a transport system in the lining cells of the intestines to absorb calcium and phosphorus and maintain an optimum level of these two minerals in the blood. When serum calcium levels fall, an active form of vitamin D is produced that helps mobilize calcium from bone; it is also a factor in the reabsorption of calcium in the kidneys. The vitamin cannot work, however, if the minerals are not present.

Liver, egg yolk, and D-fortified milk are sources of vitamin D; 400 international units (10 mcg) is the standard for all of us, and half of that daily after age twenty is the recommended dose. Rickets, or soft bones, is the childhood result of inadequate vitamin D and is still seen in our country despite vitamin D's addition to most commercially sold cow's milk. The irradiated ergosterol (synthetic D_2) may not be ideal. Many patients report muscle cramps and irritability on homogenized/pasteurized milk and no problems when they drink fresh raw milk. Some believe that this D_2 is responsible for some of the hardening of the arteries seen in milk drinkers. Rickets is called osteomalacia in adults and may be due to a strict vegan diet, no exposure to sunlight (frequent in shut-ins), a low-fat diet, or malabsorption.

Natural Vitamin D_3 (cod-liver oil) appears less likely to calcify the body tissues. A capsule with 10,000 units of A and 400 units of D would be a suggested prophylactic dose. Some have received 2000–6000 units of D (natural) as an aid in controlling chronic anxiety, depression, asthma, arthritis, and the hot flashes, sweats, cramps, and irritability of the menopause. (*A doctor should supervise the patient's intake of these doses.*)

Vitamin D toxicity is rare and usually is due to excessive ingestion of vitamin D supplements. Hypercalcemia and subsequent kidney calcification would be the results. Tens of thousands of units would be needed to cause toxicity. Such large doses are used only in special cases of rickets, and must be supervised by a physician.

Vitamin E has been the subject of much research in the past ten years and has, indeed, been found helpful and even curative in some vascular, muscular, and energy problems. D alpha-tocopheryl acetate is found in wheat germ and soybean oils, in polyunsaturated oils, in grains, liver, beans, and some fruits and vegetables.

Its chief help for us humans is its action as an antioxidant. Vital phospholipids in the cell walls are subject to peroxidation, which creates free radicals and cell death or sickness. Smog, ionizing radiation, and tobacco smoke require extra vitamin E to protect the body from peroxidation. Unsaturated bonds in fatty acids are more susceptible to oxidation, so vitamin E is a necessary accompaniment to the ingestion of polyunsaturated fats (corn, safflower, peanut, and other vegetable oils).

Wherever lack of oxygen or reduced blood supply is a problem, vitamin E will help. It keeps blood from clotting where it is not supposed to clot. It discourages platelet aggregation. It has been valuable in cyanosis, glomerulonephritis, rheumatic fever, thrombophlebitis, ulcers, gangrene, and some autoimmune diseases such as lupus erythematosis. Allergies, arthritis, diabetes, menstrual problems, and migraine have been improved. Dr. Emanuel Cheraskin noted that people taking more than 30 units of E had fewer cardiovascular complaints. The fact that 40 million people have been taking vitamin E supplements may account for the reduction in the heart attack rate in the past five years.

The tendency to cramps—nocturnal, exercise, menstrual—has been reduced with vitamin E. Breast cysts may be reduced with 600 units per day for six weeks. Hemorrhoids have been reduced by oral and local vitamin E. Scar formation is less if vitamin E is rubbed on a wound. E helps warts disappear. It relieves sore nipples and the pain of burns and poison oak.

Taken internally, it will help the atrophic senile vagina sometimes better than estrogens will.

Stress and vigorous physical exercise use up vitamin E rapidly.

Dr. Wilfred E. Shute (Evan's brother) provided the following schedule at a 1977 conference. The dose range is 90 to 4000 units a day. The following amounts of E are suggested along with the standard treatment regimes:

Coronary thrombosis: 450 to 1600 units per day.

Chronic rheumatic heart disease: 90 units daily for one month; 120 units for the second month, and 150 units daily for life.

Angina: 450 to 1600 units a day if the systolic blood pressure is less than 160. A large dose of E sometimes will shoot the blood pressure up to dangerous levels.

Phlebitis: 600 to 1600 units daily.

Hypertensive heart disease: 75 units daily for a month, then 150 units daily for a month. The blood pressure should be monitored frequently and antihypertensive drugs should accompany the E.

Fatty acids are our chief source of energy. The essential ones (EFAs) are linoleic, linolenic, and arachidonic. They must be consumed because they cannot be synthesized by the body. A deficiency may lead to growth failure, reproductive failure, and a scaly rash.

Linoleic acid is a precursor of prostaglandins. Alpha E 2 prostaglandin is a powerful vasodilator and could help lower high blood pressure.

The EFAs are found in fish, corn, whole grains, peanuts, sunflower seeds, and beans.

Folic acid deficiency is fairly common in the United States because of our limited intake of organ meats, yeast, mushrooms, asparagus, spinach, cabbage, broccoli, and kale. It is needed by the enzymes that lead to the synthesis of DNA, and thus is essential for growth and reproduction. Bone marrow, where blood is being formed, and the rapidly growing cells lining the intestinal tract are especially vulnerable to folic acid deficiency. Anemia and malabsorption can result.

Before the laboratory would be able to diagnose a folate deficiency, the victim might notice the restless-leg syndrome, depression, muscular and intellectual fatigue, constipation, and diminished feeling in lower legs. Once megaloblastic anemia appears, folate will have dropped to low, diagnostic levels. B_{12} and folic acid usually are given together because of the fear of undertreating the neuropathy of pernicious anemia.

Folic acid supplementation would be prudent for pregnancy, lactation, early infancy, and adolescence, because the rapidly growing cells are very vulnerable to a deficiency. Extra folate should be taken if cancer, parasites, or infection has been diagnosed. Alcohol interferes with its metabolism; phenytoin (used for seizures) impairs folate function. Women taking contraceptive pills are more likely to develop cervical dysplasia, a precancerous condition; folic acid, 5 mg per day, reverses this cellular growth.

Megaloblastic anemia (large, pale red cells) is the usual laboratory clue that folate deficiency is present. This deficiency is associated with chronic degenerative diseases and may be responsible for their appearance in 40 to 50 percent of cases, especially if forgetfulness, depression, insomnia, and irritability are manifested. Folate can improve the manic-depressive patient. Regional enteritis has been associated with folic acid deficiency; many of these patients have been on a low-residue diet with almost no ingestion of folates and vitamin C. Vitamin C is necessary to turn folic acid to the active folinic acid.

A good dose for a daily supplement is 400 mcg (0.4 mg), but 1 to 4 mg a day might be used for any of the above conditions. Some forms of depression improve with 10 mg a day along with a B_{12} shot (1000 mcg) every two to three days for a week or two; 5 mg of folic acid every day or two has helped some clumsy children become more adroit. Folic acid can upset the histadelic type.

Glutamic acid has been helpful in reducing the alcoholic's craving. It seems to help the hypoglycemic resist sugar. Some claim it helps the retardate and can reduce the frequency of seizures of those with petit mal. It is a fuel for the brain. L-glutamine, 1 to 2 grams a day, is taken daily; this passes into the brain and becomes glutamic acid.

Inositol, one of the B-complex vitamins, is involved in fat metabolism and is able to reduce cholesterol and triglycerides in some patients. It is found in most grains, fruits, and vegetables. Intestinal bacteria can synthesize it.

It has an antianxiety effect, can induce sleep, and has a calming effect on brain waves. The suggested dose to get these benefits is 250 to 500 mg or more.

Iron is needed for the formation of hemoglobin. Iron-deficiency anemia is common in humans. Menstruating women need about 20 mg daily as a supplement if they eat little meat; 30 mg daily is needed if the periods are heavy and the woman is weak and pale. An "average" diet—one that includes some green leafy vegetables, a bite of liver occasionally, at least three eggs a week, and raisins, nuts, and beans—would supply about 12 to 18 mg per day, but only 10 percent of the iron from vegetables is absorbed and about 20 percent from meat gets into the circulation. Iron absorption is enhanced with vitamin C, B_{12}, folic acid, low proteins, high lactose, and a good calcium-to-phosphorus ratio (1:1). B_6 is needed to synthesize hemoglobin.

Less iron is absorbed if the diet is high in phytates, oxalates, phosphates, and antacids. Mineral supplementation with zinc, copper, and manganese will suppress the absorption of iron.

Lecithin is a phospholipid and acts as an emulsifier; it can put fats into solution in the blood for transport. It may reduce cholesterol in some patients. Energy and a sense of well-being have increased in some. Gallstones have been reduced in some.

Lecithin contributes choline to the body and increases the formation of acetylcholine, a neurotransmitter. Those with learning disabilities and Alzheimer's disease have been helped some. *The Lancet* (December 2, 1978) had a report indicating that some of those afflicted seemed to understand better and were more cooperative when on lecithin.

Dr. Lester Morrison used a low-fat diet and 2 tablespoons of lecithin three times a day (36 grams a day) and was able to reduce the patients' cholesterol levels in three months.

Lecithin is found in eggs, which may account for the fact that most of us can eat several eggs a day with no change of the blood cholesterol.

A large amount of lecithin may cause a low serum calcium because it contains so much phosphorus.

Magnesium is now known to be associated with a wide variety of enzyme systems that are involved in some very important functions. A deficiency of magnesium could produce the following: rapid heart rate, hypotension, anorexia, apathy, negativism, irritability, failure to heal, growth failure, retarded dentition, nystagmus, staring, cheilosis, inflamed gums, teeth loss, malabsorption, albuminuria, weakness, sensitivity to noise, paranoia, confusion, auditory hallucinations, paresthesia, tremors, convulsions, and just not feeling well.

Low magnesium in the body has been associated with confusion, disorientation, easy arousal to anger, poor memory, depression, anxiety, sweating, calcium deposits, kidney stones, and sudden death following a myocardial infarction.

Medical World News reported in February 1982 that premenstrual tension may be due to low magnesium. PMT was exaggerated by the calcium from dairy products; if calcium intake went up, more magnesium was needed. A high B_6 intake depletes the body of magnesium.

Magnesium promotes muscle relaxation; hibernating animals have increased amounts of magnesium in the body, especially in the spinal fluid. Stopping milk and increasing magnesium may control tremors and convulsions.

High-altitude endurance is enhanced with magnesium; it relaxes the spastic lung vessels. Bones are more dense if magnesium is increased. Magnesium is lower in osteoporotic bones; Hal Huggins has found that a slight increase in magnesium intake will increase bone density significantly.

Magnesium is found inside the cells, second in concentration to potassium. Magnesium would be lost with the potassium when diuretics are used and when a high-protein diet is followed; the potassium will not return to normal until the magnesium deficiency is corrected.* This could explain the cardiac deaths noted following the use of liquid-protein diet exclusively.†

Magnesium loss is controlled by the kidneys, but if the diet is deficient, or if diarrhea or alcoholism is present, the need for magnesium is increased. Diuretics will allow urinary loss of magnesium. A low magnesium intake plus a high calcium intake will exaggerate the problem, as calcium and magnesium compete for transport into the circulation. Calcium deficiency develops slowly because the bones act as reservoirs of calcium to be drawn upon; in contrast, the magnesium in the tissue cells (muscles, liver, heart) moves to the blood; thus the symptoms of magnesium depletion may be quick and nasty.

When magnesium is deficient in the diet, less appears in the urine but phosphate is increased; this can lead to kidney stones. Oxalate and phosphate kidney stones have been prevented by 420 mg of magnesium oxide daily. Low magnesium ingestion may lead to calcium phosphate deposition in arterial wall plaques; this may be the reason that heart attacks are less common in areas whose inhabitants are ingesting hard water. The magnesium is the protective element.

The daily dose should be 300 to 400 mg. Most take it at bedtime because of its relaxing effects. Dolomite has calcium and magnesium at about the proper ratio, but it is a rock (limestone), and if the stomach acid is diminished the minerals may not be absorbed well. Magnesium oxide should work, but chelated magnesium should work the best.

Magnesium is to chlorophyll as iron is to hemoglobin; any green plant that is edible should supply some. Beans; soy; almonds; sunflower, sesame, and pumpkin seeds; and many tree fruits whose roots were nourished by soil with magnesium are good sources.

* Flink, *Modern Medicine* (Oct.–Nov. 1979).
† Fouty, Letter to the Editor.

Manganese levels in foods vary considerably depending on how much is in the topsoil where the food was grown. It is in seeds, grains, nuts, egg yolk, leafy vegetables, blueberries, and legumes. Calcium and phosphorus impede its absorption. Chelated forms are absorbed better. We all need 2 to 20 mg each day.

Deficiencies are seen in some of those with epilepsy, incoordination, dizziness, ear noises, indifference, diabetes, myasthenia gravis, sterility, growing pains, backaches. Manganese helps the mitochondria of each cell, whose function is to burn fuel and provide energy. It is needed for the synthesis of fatty acids and cholesterol. If a pregnant cat is deprived of manganese, the newborn kittens are unable to right themselves; the otoliths in the inner ear have not formed properly. Manganese is needed to form cartilage, and it is believed to be deficient in disc disease.

Manganese has an effect on memory similar to that of B_6. It stimulates adenylate cyclase activity, which has a regulatory effect on several brain neurotransmitters.

Manganese concentrates in the pancreas, and the concentration is low in diabetics. Manganese supplements improve glucose tolerance.

Molybdenum is found in legumes, grains, and green leafy vegetables. Trace amounts are needed to activate certain enzymes. One of these enzymes is in the plants that produce vitamin C; no molybdenum (to activate the enzyme), no C. The people eating those plants have a higher cancer rate.

A study in New Zealand indicated that the trace amounts of molybdenum in the plants prevented tooth decay.

Pantothenic acid is a cortisol precursor and an important nutrient for allergy sufferers. Coenzyme A, the chief metabolically active form of pantothenic acid, is needed for all energy-requiring processes; it also makes protective antibodies. If there is no pantothenic acid, the adrenals become damaged. Stress depletes coenzyme A. (In a stress test, rats given extra pantothenic acid could swim longer in cold water.) Pantothenic acid helped surgical patients and those who needed x-radiation. It can be used as an antihistamine (100 to 500 mg two to three times a day) with no side effects.

Reproductive failure may be treated with it. It has prolonged some animals' lives.

It is in almost all foods, but freezing, canning, and refining reduce the content by 30 to 50 percent. We all need at least 10 to 15 mg a day; to help exhausted adrenals, one should aim for 500 to 1000 mg a day. Good sources are kidneys, heart, liver, and brewer's yeast.

PABA, or paraminobenzoic acid, is considered one of the B vitamins. It is used mainly in sun lotions to screen out ultraviolet, burning rays. Any sunscreen you use should have PABA in it.

It has helped scleroderma and some painful conditions associated with arthritis. The calcium salt is better form.

PABA plus hydrochloric acid may help vitiligo. Occasionally hair color has been restored with supplements including PABA (100 mg), folic acid (1 mg), pantothenic acid (30 mg), and choline (2000 mg)—all daily.

Phosphorus rarely needs supplementation because it is abundant in most foods. A deficiency would show up as fatigue, rickets, osteoporosis, and decayed teeth. If the vitamin D level is adequate, the calcium-to-phosphorus ratio should be close to 1 : 1; infants need twice as much calcium as phosphorus. High intake of meat and soft drinks, which are full of phosphorus, may provide too much of it in relation to the calcium intake.

Potassium is needed for muscle contraction. The heart muscle needs it to relax between contractions. The nervous system needs it; if intake is inadequate, many will experience apathy, boredom, listlessness, depression, headache, backache, insomnia, nausea, and chronic fatigue. The muscles are weak and flaccid. Constipation is common.

Potassium is depleted by the use of coffee, alcohol, salt, sugar, cortisone drugs, and by the effects of stress. Surgery, diarrhea, ulcerative colitis, and diabetes will lead to potassium loss.

Excessive heat will cause potassium loss, which, if severe, will lead to heatstroke; taking salt (sodium chloride) tablets will make the condition worse. Natives in hot climates eat a larger amount of potassium-bearing foods and have little trouble with heatstroke.

Blacks in the United States have 2 times the high-blood-pressure rate of whites. They have a lower consumption of fresh fruits, vegetables, and salads. Long cooking of foods puts the potassium into the water. In general, the higher the blood pressure, the lower has been the potassium intake.

Insufficient potassium may lead to a slow, weak, irregular pulse. Low levels of potassium and magnesium may lead to inadequate heartbeat or sudden heart stoppage.

If potassium is restricted in relationship to sodium ingestion, and if sugary and salty foods are eaten, the adrenal glands will become exhausted. Allergies, headaches, and edema fluid are common in this situation. Many find weight loss impossible until potassium is increased and sodium is restricted.

Potassium as gluconate or chloride may be necessary for some, but most can get enough (4 to 6 grams per day) from the following: potatoes, endive, nuts, avocadoes, dried apricots, whole grains, bananas, and most fruits and vegetables except commercially canned ones. The commercial refining process leads to a loss of potassium and magnesium.

Vegetarians may need to salt (sodium) their food. But eaters of meat and dairy foods should not salt their food, since they are getting plenty of sodium.

Selenium, like vitamins C and E, acts as an antioxidant. The people of countries where the soil is poor have a high rate of cancer and are 3 times as likely to die of high blood pressure as are those living in selenium-rich areas. Best to eat grain grown in Nebraska or the Dakotas, areas that are high in this trace mineral.

Selenium helps antibody formation and improves vision, skin, and hair. Cataracts are often seen in those low in selenium. Selenium helps the enzyme glutathione peroxidase, a factor in the synthesis of prostaglandins; a deficiency of this enzyme leads to platelet aggregation.

Sulfate fertilizer cuts the uptake of selenium by plants; there is less of it in plants now than there was fifty years ago. Food processing destroys 50 percent of the selenium that is taken up.

Dr. Gerhard Schrauzer recommends 250 to 350 mcg of selenium a day. Japanese women, whose diet provides about this amount of selenium, have one-fifth the rate of breast cancer of women in the United States.

Silicon is part of bone tissue and artery walls and of connective tissues in general. Fiber is high in silicon, and this may provide some degree of protection against arthritis and arteriosclerosis.

Sodium excess may be responsible for migraine, insomnia, hives, epilepsy, high blood pressure, and nervous tension.

The average U.S. citizen puts about 10 to 15 grams of sodium chloride into his body daily. Sugar ingestion along with excessive salt makes the blood pressure rise faster and sooner than just salt alone.

A low-salt diet means eliminating the obvious salty foods (potato chips, pickles, the saltcellar from the table), and limiting intake to about 4 to 6 grams per day.

Only very cooperative patients will follow a *very* low-salt diet: no bread, pastry, meat, eggs, and dairy products. This amounts to less than 1 to 2 grams of salt and is very flat and dull.

Primitive people have few or no blood pressure problems; their daily intake is less than 1 to 2 grams a day. The amount of sodium in cow's milk is about 4 times that of human milk. A frozen Swanson's three-course turkey dinner contains more than 4 grams of salt. Two ounces of Kraft processed American cheese contain more than 2 grams of salt.

A high sodium intake may account for a poor response to diuretics. The drinking water in Chicago has about 120 mg sodium per liter. In hard-water areas it would be best to soften only the water connected to the hot-water line, for washing bodies, clothes, and dishes. Use hard water (calcium and magnesium) for cooking and drinking. Bisodol, sodium bicarbonate, Alka-Seltzer, and many other drugs are high is sodium.

Sulfur is in every cell of animals and plants. It is a component of skin, hair, and nails, and is involved in collagen synthesis. It works closely with B-complex vitamins.

If the level is low in the body, anemia and hair loss may occur, but a deficiency of sulfur is rare, because it is found in protein foods, cereals, eggs, peanuts, onions, and other common foods.

These sulfur-containing foods may work along with zinc to control psoriasis.

Zinc is a part of many enzyme systems with a wide variety of actions. Zinc deficiency is common in our country because it is depleted in the soil and is largely destroyed by commercial food processing.

A deficiency might show as any of the following: slow growth, delayed sexual development, cancer, delayed wound healing, acne, acrodermatitis enteropathica, distorted taste, enlarged prostate, below-average sperm count, boils, hair loss, learning disabilities, hyperkeratosis, toxemia of pregnancy, pica, stretch marks, brittle hair, sore joints, dysmenorrhea, and eczema.

We need 15 mg of zinc almost every day, but it is hard to get that minimum. There are only 6 mg in 3 ounces of liver; a similar amount of peanut butter has about 3 mg; and these are two of the better sources. A supplement, therefore, seems prudent.

Zinc will stop some scalp and body odors. Low intake is also associated with Crohn's disease, cystic fibrosis, decreased sex drive, rheumatoid arthritis, canker sores, and genital herpes.

Older people are often zinc deficient because they usually eat less meat, a good source. Commercial milk formulas are low in zinc. Vegetarians have trouble getting the right dose because the phytates in their diet bind with zinc, preventing absorption. Eating unleavened bread reduces the available zinc due to the same phenomenon. Galvanized pipes and tubs are made of zinc, but are used little now in the preparation of food, hence less zinc in the diet. Oral contraceptive pills reduce the zinc in the serum. Calcium will compete with zinc for admission into the body, therefore calcium supplements should be taken at a different time than zinc. Zinc is usually taken with meals, and calcium and magnesium at bedtime with vitamin C.

Skin ulcers heal faster with zinc. Burn patients get out of the hospital in half the usual time if given a zinc supplement. In doses of 50 mg twice a day, zinc increases T lymphocytes, increases the skin reaction to invading bacteria, and increases the production of antibodies.

Zinc and vitamin A work together. The zinc mobilizes A from storage in the liver. They are usually taken together for the treatment of acne, eczema, and psoriasis.

EPILOGUE: BE WELL

MY HOPE as I wrote this book was to encourage you, the reader, to change your eating and exercise habits just enough to show yourself and your doctor that there is truth in the old saw, "You are what you eat." If you can reduce your high blood pressure by cutting out salt and sugar, by exercising and taking garlic capsules, the doctor may have to agree that there is something to this food and supplement "treatment."

But more important than impressing and educating your doctor is what you will do for yourself. Your doctor cannot live inside your body and perceive your stomach, your back, your brain, your world. You are the expert, because you are the one your body serves. You are getting the messages. The doctor reads your body only when he can diagnose a pathological condition. You should have figured out your nutritional needs when you got the first gas pain, muscle twinge, rapid pulse episode, or sense of fatigue on awakening.

My wish is that you will become skilled in recognizing little tilts or slips from the norm (not the average) and compensate before they grow to be diseases requiring medical or surgical treatment. You are in charge of the area of your health between normal well-being and palpable pathology. You will embarrass the doctor if you only have a symptom which he cannot connect with a classifiable disease. Most of your symptoms will interest only you, and you must take care of them. When or if they become signs of disease, then you will need the doctor's diagnosis, judgment, prognosis, recommendations, and maybe medicine and surgery. You still have some choices at this late moment.

Almost all I have written here is based on medical literature. Anecdotal case histories are from my (and other like-minded doctors') files. If orthodox doctors cannot believe at least some of this, they are not keeping up with their own medical literature. What we learned in school is not always the last word.

Medicine is an art. Holding the patient together with sympathy and understanding is called a placebo by some and psychotherapy by others. It is also the essence of medical practice. But it works a lot better if each cell of the body and the brain has the correct amount of energy, amino acids, vitamins, and minerals.

REFERENCES

Preface and Chapters 1, 2, and 3

Airola, Paavo, N. D., Ph.D.: *How to Get Well*, Health Plus Pub., Phoenix, 1974.
Bland, Jeffrey, Ph.D.: *Your Health Under Siege*, Stephen Greene Press, Brattleboro, Vt., 1981.
Cheraskin, E., M.D., D.M.D., W. M. Ringsdorf, D.M.D., and Arline Brecher: *Psychodietetics*, Bantam Books, New York, 1974.
Cheraskin, E., M.D., D.M.D., W.M. Ringsdorf, D.M.D., and J.W. Clark, D.D.S.: *Diet and Disease*, Keats Pub. Co., New Canaan, Conn., 1968.
Gerras, Charles, Exec. Ed.: *The Encyclopedia of Common Diseases*. Rodale Press, Emmaus, Pa., 1976.
Hodges, Robert, M.D.: *Nutrition in Medical Practice*, W. B. Saunders, Philadelphia, 1980.
Hoffer, Abram, Ph.D., and Morton Walker, D.P.M.: *Orthomolecular Nutrition*, Keats Pub. Co., New Canaan, Conn., 1978.
Hunter, Beatrice Trum: *Consumer Beware!* Simon & Schuster, New York, 1971.
Kamen, Betty: *Kids Are What They Eat; What Every Parent Needs to Know About Nutrition*, Arco, New York, 1983.
Lesser, Michael, M.D.: *Nutrition and Vitamin Therapy*, Grove Press, New York, 1980.
Nutrition Search, Inc.: *Nutrition Almanac*, McGraw-Hill, New York, 1979.
Pfeiffer, Carl C., Ph.D., M.D.: *Mental and Elemental Nutrients*, Keats Pub. Co., New Canaan, Conn. 1975.
Selye, Hans, M.D.: *The Stress of Life*, McGraw-Hill, New York, 1956.
Stitt, Paul A.: *Fighting the Food Giants*, Natural Press, Manitowoc, Wis., 1980.

Chapter 4

Bio-science Laboratories: *The Bioscience Handbook*, 13th ed., Bio-science Laboratories, Van Nuys, Calif., 1982.

Cheraskin, E., M.D., W.M., Ringsdorf, et al.: The "Ideal Total White Cell Count," Nutr. Perspect. 1: #1, pp. 41–44, Jan. 1978.

Chapter 5

Bland, Jeffrey, Ph.D.: "Aging and the Reduction of Illness," Northwest Academy of Preventive Medicine Newsletter, September 1980, pp. 3–5.

Hoffer, Abram, M.D., and Morton Walker, D.P.M.: *Nutrients to Age Without Senility,* Keats Pub. Co., New Canaan, Ct., 1980.

Kugler, Hans, Ph.D.: "Combination Theory of Aging," Lecture, 1978.

"Nutrition of the Elderly," *Dairy Council Digest,* 48:1 (1977).

"Old Age," *Outlook Magazine,* Washington University School of Medicine, 1980.

Scott, M.L.: "Understanding Vitamin E," *Federation Proceedings* 39 (1980), pp. 2736-2739.

Sheldon, Williams: *Somatotyping the Adult Male,* Harper and Row, New York, 1980.

Winick, Myron, M.D.: "Aging and Diet," *Modern Medicine,* February 1978, pp. 69–72.

Chapter 6

Abdominal Discomfort

American Journal of Gastroenterology 75 (1981), pp. 192–196.

Burkitt, Denis, M.D.: "Effect of Dietary Fiber on Stools and Transit Times and Its Role in the Causation of Disease," *Lancet,* December 1972, p. 1229.

Ingelfinger, F. J., M.D.: "For Want of an Enzyme," *Nutrition Today,* September 1968, pp. 2–10.

"Role of Lactose," *Dairy Council Digest* 45:5 (1974).

Roth, L. J. A., M.D.: "Problems of Gas," *Medical World News,* April 1975, pp. 92–107.

Aches

Journal of Orthomolecular Psychiatry 9:4 (1980), pp. 237–249.

Pfeiffer, Carl C.: *Mental and Elemental Nutrients,* Keats Pub. Co., New Canaan, Conn., 1975.

Acne

Leyden, James J.: "Acne," *Dermatologica,* October 1981, pp. 51–52.

Michaelson, Gerd, M.D., et al.: "Oral Zinc in Acne," *Archives of Dermatology* 113 (1977), pp. 31–36.

Shefrin, David, N.D.: *Naturopathic Physician's Handbook/Cookbook,* Sun Chief Enterprises, Missoula, Mo., 1980.

Addiction

Libby, A. E., and Irwin Stone, Ph.D.: "The Hypoascorbemia-Kwashiorkor Approach to Drug Addiction Therapy: A Pilot Study," *Journal of Orthomolecular Psychiatry* 6:4 (1977).

Aggressive Behavior

Bagley, Robert, Ph.D.: "Diet and Behavioral Problems," *Journal of Orthomolecular Psychiatry* 10:4 (1981), pp. 284–298.

Brazelton, T. Berry: *On Becoming a Family*, Delacorte Press, New York, 1981.

————: Speech in Portland, Ore., December 1981.

Reed, Barbara: *Food, Teens and Behavior*, Natural Press, Manitowoc, Wis., 1983.

Robins, Lee, Ph.D.: *Deviant Children Grow Up*, Williams & Wilkins Pub. Co., Baltimore, 1966.

Roy, Maria, ed.: *Domestic Violence: A Critical Analysis*, Van Nostrand Reinhold, New York, 1982, pp. 76–90.

Schauss, Alexander: *Diet, Crime and Delinquency*, Parker House, Berkeley, Calif., 1980.

Yaryura-Tobias, José A., A. Chang, and F. Nezroglu: "A Study of the Relationship of Serum Glucose, Insulin, Free Fatty Acids, and Free and Total Tryptophan to Mental Illness," *Biological Psychiatry* 13:2 (1978), pp. 234–254.

Alcoholism

Hague, William, M.D., and Robert Howard, M.D.: "Alcoholics May Perceive Life in a Different Fashion," *Journal of the American Medical Association* 229 (1974), pp. 630–631.

Krasner, M., et al.: "Ascorbic Acid Saturation and Ethanol Metabolism," *Lancet* 2 (1974), pp. 693–695.

Lemere, Frank, M.D.: "What Causes Alcoholism?" *Journal of Clinical and Experimental Psychopathology* XVII:2 (1956), pp. 202–205.

Lieber, Charles S., M.D.: "Alcohol and Malnutrition in the Pathogenesis of Liver Disease," *Journal of the American Medical Association* 233:10 (1975), pp. 1077–1082.

————, "Metabolic Basis of Alcoholic Toxicity," *Hospital Practice*, February 1977, pp. 73–80.

Williams, Roger J.: *The Prevention of Alcoholism Through Nutrition*, Bantam, 1981, Appendix I.

Allergies, Sensitivities, and Intolerances

Alvarez, Walter, M.D.: *The Neuroses*, Saunders, Philadelphia, 1952.

Alvarez, Walter, M.D.: "Puzzling Nervous Storms Due to food Allergy," *Gastroenterology* 7 (1946), p. 241.

American Dietetic Association: *Allergy Recipes*, A.D.A., 620 N. Michigan Ave., Chicago, IL 60611.

Anah, C., L. Jarike, and H. Baig: "High Dose Ascorbic Acid in Nigerian Asthmatics," *Tropical and Geographical Medicine* 32:132 (1980).

"Asthma," *Medical World News*, 12 March 1978, pp. 50–60.

Badr-el-Din, M. D., et al.: "Beta-adrenergic Receptors in Asthmatic Bronchitis," *Annuals of Allergy* 46 (1981), pp. 336–337.

Coca, Arthur F., M.D.: *The Pulse Test*, Arco Publishing, New York, 1972.

Conrad, Marion: *Allergy Cooking*, Thomas Y. Crowell, New York,

Crook, William G., M.D.: *Your Allergic Child*, Medcom Press, New York, 1973.

Deamer, William, M.D.: "Pediatric Allergy: Some Impressions Gained over a 37-Year Period," *Pediatrics* 48:6 (1971), pp. 930–935.

————: "Recurrent Abdominal Pain," *C.M.D.* 40 (1973), pp. 130–154.

Frazier, C. A., M.D.: *Coping with Food Allergies,* New York Times Book, Co., Quadrangle, New York, 1975.

Fries, Joseph H., M.D.: "Food Allergy," *Annals of Allergy* 46 (1981), pp. 260–263.

Gierrard, John W., M.D.: *Food Allergy,* Charles C Thomas, Springfield, Ill., 1980.

Golos, Natalie, Frances Golos Golbitz, and Frances Spatz Leighton: *Coping With Your Allergies,* Simon & Schuster, New York, 1979.

Johnstone, Douglas E., M.D.: "Some Aspects of the Natural History of Asthma," Annals of Allergy 49 (1982), pp. 257-264.

Mandell, Fran Gare, M.D., and Jill Bomser: *Dr. Mandell's Allergy-Free Cookbook,* Simon & Schuster, New York, 1981.

Mandell, Marshall, M.D. and L. W. Scanlon: *Dr. Mandell's 5-Day Allergy Relief System,* Thomas Y. Crowell, New York, 1979.

Miller, Joseph B., M.D.: *Food Allergy,* Charles C Thomas, Springfield, Ill., 1972.

Norman, Philip S., M.D.: "Allergies," *Drug Therapy,* January 1980, pp. 127–130.

Philpott, William, M.D., and Dwight Kalita: *Brain Allergies,* Keats Pub. Co., New Canaan, Conn., 1980.

Randolph, T. G., and R. W. Moss: *An Alternative Approach to Allergies,* Lippincott & Crowell, New York, 1980.

Rapp, Doris J., M.D.: *Allergies and the Hyperactive Child,* Simon & Schuster, New York, 1979.

————: *Allergies and Your Family,* Sterling Pub. Co., New York, 1980.

Rinkel, H. J., T. G. Randolph, and M. Zeller: *Food Allergy,* Charles C Thomas, Springfield, Ill., 1950.

Rowe, A. H., M.D., and A. H. Rowe, Jr.: *Food Allergy, Its Manifestations and Control and the Elimination Diet,* Charles C Thomas, Springfield, Ill., 1972.

Sokol, W. M., M.D.: *Allergies, Hospital Medicine,* May 1977, pp. 10–34.

Speer, Frederic, M.D.: *Allergy of the Nervous System,* Charles C Thomas, Springfield, Ill., 1970.

————: "Tracking Down Food Allergies," *Medical Opinion,* August 1975, pp. 48–51.

————, and Robert Dockhorn: *Allergy and Immunology in Children,* Charles C Thomas, Springfield, Ill.

Steinfield, H. R., M.D., ed.: *Hypersensitivity Problems,* Ross Laboratories, 1975.

Wilson, C. W. M., M.D.: "Food Sensitivities," *Annals of Allergy* 44 (1980), pp. 302–307.

Zuskin, E.: "Allergies," *Allergy and Clinical Immunology* 51:18 (1973).

Alopecia

Baden, Howard P., M.D.: "Hair Loss," *Consultant,* August 1977, pp. 29–34.

Seidman, Michael, M.D.: "Reversal of Baldness," *Cutis* 28 (1981), pp. 551–553.

Anemia

Laboratory Aids, 13th ed., Bio-Science Laboratories Pub., Van Nuys, Calif. 1982.

Pritchard, N.: "Iron Stores of Normal Adults Replenished with Oral Iron," *Journal of the American Medical Association* 190 (1964), pp. 897–901.

REFERENCES

Anorexia

Bruch, Hilda, J.D.: *Anorexia Nervosa, Pediatric Herald* 13:8 (1979).
Crisp, A. M., M.D.: "Anorexia Nervosa," *Procedures of the Royal Society of Medicine* 70 (1977), pp. 686–690.
Hoffer, A., M.D.: editorial, *Huxley Institute Newsletter,* Spring 1981.

Anxiety

Cadie, M: "Anxiety and Mononucleosis," *British Journal of Psychiatry* 128 (1976), pp. 559–561.

Arthritis

Brown et al.: "Anti-inflammatory Effects of Some Copper Complexes," *Journal of Medicinal Chemistry* 23 (1980), p. 729.
Chao, I. T., M.D.: "Food Incompatibility," *Journal of Allergy and Clinical Immunology,* 1981.
Childers, Norman, Ph.D.: "A Relationship of Arthritis to the Solanaceae (Nightshades)," *Journal of the International Academy of Preventive Medicine,* November 1982, pp. 31–37.
"Differential Diagnosis of Arthritis," *Pediatrics Digest,* December 1970, p. 13.
Ellis, John, M.D.: *Vitamin B₆, The Doctor's Report,* Harper & Row, New York, 1973.
Fries, J. F., M.D.: "Rheumatic Diseases," *Modern Medicine* 15:28 (1981), pp. 153–154.
"Gold and Rheumatoid Arthritis," *Journal of Rheumatology* 5 (1978), pp. 68–74.
"Histidine Deficiency in Rheumatoid Arthritis," *Hospital Practice,* August 1981, p. 47.
"Juvenile Rheumatoid Arthritis Called Hereditary," *Pediatric News,* September 1977, p. 16.
Kaufman, William, M.D.: *The Common Form of Joint Dysfunction,* Hildreth & Co., Brattleboro, Vt., 1949.

Autoimmune Diseases

Grouse, L., M.D., Ph.D.: "Histocompatibility Complex," *Journal of the American Medical Association* 246:8 (1981), pp. 873–876.

Breast Cysts

Miller, Joseph B., M.D.: "Relief of Premenstrual Symptoms," *Journal of the Medical Association of the State of Alabama* 44 (1974), pp. 57–60.
Ross, M.D., et al.: *Lancet,* April 1981, p. 858.

Cancer

Brown, B.: *Cancer Victory Bulletin,* 1981.
Burack, W. Richard, M.D.: "Lies and Statistics," *Medical World News,* August 1979, p. 59.
Burkitt, Denis, M.D.: "Effect of Dietary Fiber on Stools and Transit Times and Its Role in the Causation of Disease," *Lancet,* December 1972, p. 1229.

Cameron, E., M.D., and Linus Pauling, Ph.D.: *Vitamin C and Cancer,* Pauling Institute, Menlo Park, Calif., 1979.

"Cancer and Food Fat," *Medical World News,* October 1977, p. 82.

Cancer Control Society, Newsletter, 2042 No. Berendo St., Los Angeles, Calif. 90027.

Cathcart, R. F., M.D.: "The Method of Determining Proper Doses of Vitamin C for the Treatment of Disease by Titrating to Bowel Tolerance," *Journal of Orthomolecular Psychiatry* 10:2 (1981), pp. 125–132.

Chowka, Peter B.: "Cancer and Diet," *Nutritional Journal,* 1979.

Hagstead, Mark: quoted in the Portland *Oregonian,* 1981.

Huemer, Richard, M.D.: "Vitamin A and Cancer," *Journal of the International Academy of Preventive Medicine* 5:1 (1979), pp. 59–64.

Jensen, O. M.: "Colonorectal Cancer," *Israel Journal of Medical Sciences* 15 (1979), pp. 329–334.

Klenner, F. R., M.D.: "Significance of High Intake of Ascorbic Acid in Preventive Medicine," *Journal of the International Academy of Preventive Medicine* 1:1 (1974), pp. 45–69.

LeShan, L.: "Psychological States as Factors in the Development of Malignant Disease: a Critical Review," *Journal of the National Cancer Institute* 22 (1959), p. 1.

Monthly Memo, *International Academy of Preventive Medicine,* June 1981, pp. 3–4.

"Norwegian Cancer," *Lancet,* 18 October 1980.

Passwater, Richard, Ph.D.: *Cancer and Its Nutritional Therapies,* Keats Pub. Co., New Canaan, Conn., 1978.

————, *Selenium, As Food and Medicine,* Keats Pub. Co., New Canaan, Conn., 1980.

"Stress and Cancer," *Journal of the American Medical Association* 238:4 (1977), p. 301.

Claudication

Dotter, Charles, M.D.: "Transluminal Angioplasty," in Abrams, ed., *Angiography,* Little, Brown, Boston, 1983.

Colitis

Siegel, J., M.D.: "Inflammatory Bowel Disease," *Annals of Allergy* 47 (1981), pp. 92–94.

Convulsions

Philpott, William, M.D. and Dwight Kalita, Ph.D.: *Brain Allergies,* Keats Pub. Co., New Canaan, Conn., 1980.

Coronary Artery Disease

Antial, M., et al.: "Fat Globule Membrane," *Lancet* 1:602 (1980).

Chehak, Anastasia: *Fat in Foods* chart.

Cheraskin, E., M.D., D.M.D., William Ringsdorf, D.M.D., and Arline Brecher: *Psychodietetics,* Bantam Books, New York, 1974.

Cheraskin, E., M.D., D.M.D., and W. M. Ringsdorf, D.M.D.: The ECG and Supplements," *Journal of the International Academy of Preventive Medicine* VI:2 (1981), pp. 11–19.

"Cholesterol," *Dairy Council Digest* 50:6 (1979).

"Diet Modification," *Circulation* 58:381A (1978).

"Experts Link Disease and Diet," *Journal of the American Medical Association* 237:24 (1977), p. 2593.

Flynn, M. A., Ph.D., and G. B. Nolph, M.D.: "Effect of Eggs on Cholesterol," *American Journal of Clinical Nutrition* 32 (1979), pp. 1051–1057.

Ginter, Emil: "Pretreatment of Serum-Cholesterol and Response to Vitamin C," *Lancet,* November 1979, pp. 958–959.

Goodnight, Scott, Jr., M.D., et at.: "Polyunsaturated Fatty Acids, Hyperlipidemia and Thrombosis," *Arteriosclerosis* 2 (1982).

"Greece's Coronary Rate," *Medical World News,* March 1982, pp. 78–79.

Gruberg, E., and S. Raymond: "Beyond Cholesterol," *Atlantic Monthly,* May 1979, pp. 59–65.

MacDonald, I.: "Dietary Carbohydrates Effect in Lipoprotein," *Nutrition Reports International* 17 (1978), pp. 663–668.

Majeski, Edward, Ph.D.: "Cholesterol, " Bio-Science Forum, *The Condenser,* Bio-Science Lab 9:1 (1978).

Mannerberg, Dom, M.D., and June Roth: *Aerobic Nutrition,* Elsevier Dutton, New York, 1981.

Nichols, A. B., M.D., et al.: "Lipids and Dietary Habits," *Journal of the American Medical Association* 236 (1976) pp. 1948–1953.

Oster, Kurt A., M.D.: lecture at the New York Academy of Sciences, 1980.

Phillips, R. L., M.D., et al.: "Heart Disease in Vegetarians," *American Journal of Clinical Nutrition* 31 (1978), pp. S191–S198.

"Recent Decline in Heart Disease Mortality," *Annals of Internal Medicine,* October 1979.

"Type A Debate," *Medical World News,* February 1975, pp. 103–104.

Williams, C. L., M.D., and E. Wynder: "A Blind Spot," *Journal of the American Medical Association* 236 (1976), pp. 2196–2197.

Cystic Fibrosis

Wallach, Joel, D.V.M.: "Cystic Fibrosis," *Journal of Nutritional Consultants,* 1980, pp. 40, 57, 58, 59.

Degenerative Diseases

Bland, Jeffrey, Ph.D.: *Your Health Under Siege,* Stephen Greene Press, Brattleboro, Vt., 1981.

Philpott, William, M.D., and Dwight Kalita, Ph.D.: *Brain Allergies,* Keats Pub. Co., New Canaan, Conn., 1980.

Diabetes

Anderson, James, M.D., and Kay Ward: "High Carbohydrate, High Fiber Diets for Insulin-Treated Men with Diabetes," *American Journal of Clinical Nutrition* (1979), pp. 2312–2321.

Chehak, Anastasia, R.D.: personal communication.

Flood, Thomas, M., M.D.: "Diet and Diabetes," *Hospital Practice*, February 1979, pp. 61–69.

Garritsen, George C.: "Diabetic Hamsters and Diet," pamphet, Upjohn Co. Research Laboratory.

Philpott, William, M.D., and Dwight Kalita, Ph.D.: *Brain Allergies*, Keats Pub. Co., New Canaan, Conn., 1980.

Dizziness

Proctor, Bruce, M.D.: *Medical World News*, June 1981, pp. 27–28.

Dreams

Pfeiffer, Carl C., Ph.D., M.D.: *Mental and Elemental Nutrients*, Keats Pub. Co., New Canaan, Conn., 1975.

Eyes

Lane, B. C., O.D.: "Elevation of Intraocular Pressure with Daily, Sustained Closework Stimulus to Accommodation, Lowered Tissue Chromium and Dietary Deficiency of Ascorbic Acid." *Documenta Ophthalmologica* 28, 3rd International Conference on Myopia, Copenhagen & The Hague, 1981, pp. 149–155.

Female Hormones

Adams, P. W., M.D.: editorial, *British Medical Journal*, October 1976.

Fertility

Cressman, Paul: "Reproduction Under Siege," *CHIMO*, December 1981, pp. 22–31.

Fiber

Bronribb, A. J. M., M.D.: "Diverticular Disease and High Fiber Diet," *Lancet* 1 (1977), pp. 664–666.

Burkitt, D. P., M.D.: "Economic Development—Not All Bonus," *Nutrition Today*, October 1976, pp. 6–13.

Burkitt, D. P., M.D., et al.: "Dietary Fiber and Disease," *Journal of the American Medical Association* 229:8 (1974).

Cleave, T. L., M.D., G. L. Campbell, and N. S. Painter: *Diabetes, Coronary Thrombosis, and the Saccharine Disease.* John Wright & Sons, New York, 1969.

"Fiber," *Journal of the American Medical Association* 238:16 (1977), pp. 1715–1716.

Jenkins, D. V.: "Dietary Fibers and Glucose Tolerance," *British Medical Journal* 1 (1978), pp. 1393–1394.

Kritchevsky, D.: "Effects of Fiber on Cholesterol," *Nutrition Reports International* 9 (1974), pp. 301–308.

REFERENCES

Glaucoma

See "Eyes"

Gout

Baum, John, M.D.: "Modern Concepts in the Treatment of Gout," *Drug Therapy,* September 1978, pp. 23–24.

Hair

Fredericks, Carleton: speech in New Orleans, 1981.

Headaches

Miller, Joseph, M.D.: "Migraine, an Allergic Syndrome," *Annals of Allergy* 47 (1981), p. 122.
Munro, Jean, and Jonathan Brostoff: "Food Allergy in Migraine" *Lancet,* July 1980, pp. 1–4.
Rapp, Doris, M.D.: *Allergies and Your Family,* Sterling Pub. Co., New York, 1980.
Speer, F., M.D.: "Allergic Factors in Migraine," *Modern Medicine* 39 (1971), pp. 100–106.
Thonnard-Neumann, Ernst, M.D., and Leonard Neckers, Ph.D.: "Immunity in Migraine," *Annals of Allergy* 47 (1981), pp. 328–332.

Heart Rate

Cheraskin, E., M.D., and W. M. Ringsdorf, D.M.D.: "The ECG and Supplements," *Journal of the International Academy of Preventive Medicine* VI:2 (1981), pp. 11–19.

Herpes I

Cathcart, Robert: "Vitamin C and Herpes," *Proceedings of the Orthomolecular Medical Society,* Annual Meeting, 1977.

Herpes II

Felman, Yehudi, M.D., and James A. Nikitan, M.A.: "Herpes Genitalis," *Cutis* 30 (1982), pp. 442–454.

Hives

Gordon, Hyman, M.D.: "Hives," *Consultant,* November 1975, pp. 92–94.
"Hives," *Skin & Allergy News* 6:4 (1975).
"Hives," *Skin & Allergy News* 7:1 (1976).

Hyperactivity

Feingold, Benjamin, M.D., *Why Your Child Is Hyperactive,* Random House, New York, 1974.

Hypertension

"Angiotensin Blockers," *Current Prescribing,* Special Report, October 1977, pp. 19–39.
"Blood Pressure of Vegetarians," *Preventive Medicine,* March 1978.
Chehak, Anastasia, R.D.: Sodium and Potassium Charts.
"Diet and Blood Pressure," *Dairy Council Digest* 52:5 (1981).
Hiner, L. B., M.D., and Gruskin, A. B., M.D.: "Physiology of Blood Pressure," *Pediatric Annals* 6 (1977), pp. 19–32.
Laragh, John H., M.D.: "Hypertension," *Drug Therapy,* January 1980, pp. 71–88.

Hypoglycemia

Fredericks, Carlton, Ph.D.: *Low Blood Sugar and You,* Grosset & Dunlap, New York, 1970.
Hudspeth, William J.: "Low Sugar, a Fad Disease?" *Psychology Today,* October 1980.
Philpott, William, M.D., and Dwight Kalita, Ph.D.: *Brain Allergies,* Keats Pub. Co., New Canaan, Conn., 1980.
Schneider, Stephen, M.D.: "Hypoglycemia," *Modern Medicine,* April 1980, pp. 54–68.

Infections

Biesel, William R., M.D.: "Nutrient Effects on Immunologic Functions," *Journal of the American Medical Association,* January 1981, pp. 53–58.
Infant Nutrition, newsletter, Health Learning Systems, Inc., Bloomfield, N.J., 1980–1981.
Katz, Michael, M.D., and E. R. Stehm, M.D.: "Host Defense," *Pediatrics* 59 (1977), pp. 490–494.
Quie, Paul G., M.D.: "Overwhelming Infections," *Consultant,* September 1979, pp. 35–44.
Scott, M. L.: "Vitamin E," *Federation Proceedings* 39 (1980) pp. 1736–1739.
South, M. A., M.D.: "Lacunar Defects in Immunity," *Cutis,* September 1981, pp. 239–247.
Thoine, Jess, M.D.: "Biotin," *New England Journal of Medicine,* April 1981.
"Vitamin E Relieves Cystic Breast Disease," *Journal of the American Medical Association* 244, September 1980, pp. 1077–1078.
Weissman, Gerald, M.D.: "PHagocytosis," *Infectious Diseases,* November 1978, pp. 4, 18, 19.
Young, Lowell, M.D.: "Infection in the Compromised Host," *Hospital Practice,* September 1981, pp. 73–84.

Kidney Stones

Thom, J. A., et al.: "Influence of Carbohydrate on Calcium Excretion," *British Journal of Urology* 50 (1978), pp. 459–464.

Labyrinthitis

Deweese, David, M.D.: "Labyrinthitis," *Newsletter of the Speech and Hearing Society,* University of Oregon Health Sciences Center.

REFERENCES

Lead Poisoning

Journal of Orthomolecular Psychiatry 7:2 (1978).
Moore, M. R., M.D., et al.: *Lancet 1* (1977), 717–719.
Pediatrics Digest, July 1977, pp. 17–20.

Memory Impairment

Gibbs, Marie, M.D.: "Memory," *Medical Tribune & Medical News,* March 1979.
Pfeiffer, Carl C., Ph.D., M.D.: *Mental and Elemental Nutrients,* Keats Pub. Co.,
    New Canaan, Conn., 1975.
Truss, C. Orian, M.D.: "Restoration of Immunologic Competence to Candida Albi-
    cans," *Orthomolecular Psychiatry* 9:4 (1980), pp. 287–301.

Ménière's

"Ménière's," *Journal of the American Medical Association* 240:16 (1978), pp. 1699–
    1705.

Multiple Sclerosis

Brody, J. A. M.: Epidmiology of Multiple Sclerosis and a Possible Virus Etiology,"
    Lancet 2 (1972), pp. 173–176.
Huggins, Hal. A., D.D.S.: "Mercury: A Factor in Mental Disease?" *Journal of Ortho-
    molecular Psychiatry* II:1 (1982), pp. 3–16.
Johnson, K. P. and B. J. Nelson: "Multiple Sclerosis: Diagnostic Usefulness of Cere-
    brospinal Fluid," *Annals of Neurology* 2 (1977), pp. 425–431.
Klenner, Frederick, M.D.: *Nerve Pathology,* privately printed, Reidsville, N.C.
———, "Multiple Sclerosis," *Journal of Applied Nutrition* 25 (1973), p. 384.
Mandell, Marshall, M.D., and L. W. Scanlon: *Dr. Mandell's 5-Day Allergy Relief
    System,* Thomas Y. Crowell, New York, 1979.
Stone, I., Ph.D.: "Inexpensive Interferon Therapy of Cancer and Viral Diseases,"
    Journal of the International Academy of Preventive Medicine 6:2 (1981), pp.
    57–66.
Swank, Roy, M.D.: *The Multiple Sclerosis Diet Book,* Doubleday, Garden City, New
    York, 1977.
Trese, T., D.O.: "Multiple Sclerosis," *Journal of the American Osteopathic Associa-
    tion* 79 (1979), pp. 259–266.

Muscle Symptoms

Cheraskin, E., M.D., D.M.D., W. M. Ringsdorf, D.M.D., and F. H. Medfor, D.M.D.:
    "The musculoskeletal Disease-Proneness Profile," *American Chiropractic As-
    sociation Journal of Chiropracty* 14:5 (1977), pp. 41–51.

Myasthenia Gravis

"Myasthenia Gravis," *Journal of the American Medical Association* 238:13 (1977),
    pp. 1338, 1343.

Obesity

Barnes, Broda, M.D.: *Hypothyroidism, The Unsuspected Illness*, Thomas Y. Crowell, New York, 1976.

Bruch, Hilda, M.D.: "Misuse of Eating," *Pediatric News*, August 1979, p. 38.

Danowski, Thaddeus S., M.D.: "The Management of Obesity," *Hospital Practice*, April 1976, pp. 39–46.

Dunphy, Donal, M.D.: "Obesity in Pediatric Practice," Ross Laboratory Roundtable, 1971.

Research from National Institutes of Health, *Journal of the American Medical Association* 243:6 (1980), pp. 519–520.

Schlauf, George Edward, M.D.: "Cutting Calories is Not the Answer," *Consultant*, January 1973, pp. 164–165.

Sheldon, William: *Somatotyping the Adult Male*, Harper and Row, New York, 1980.

"Treating Obesity," *Medical World News*, August 1971, pp. 20–36.

Osteoporosis

Albenese, Anthony A., Ph.D.: "Osteoporosis," *Medical Tribune & Medical News*, May 1975, p. 5

Bogdonoff, M. D., M.D.: "Osteoporosis," *Drug Therapy*, September 1981, pp. 71–73.

Frame, Boy, M.D.: "Osteoporosis, Questions & Answers," *Journal of the American Medical Association* 237:20 (1977), p. 2234.

Linkswiler, Hellm, M., Ph.D., and Michael B. Zemel, M.S.: "Calcium to Phosphorus Ratio," *New York State Journal of Medicine*, February 1980.

Marsh, A. G., Sc.D.: "Vegetarianism and Osteoporosis," *Journal of the American Dietetic Association* 76 (1980), pp. 148–151.

Wallach, Stanley, M.D.: "Management of Osteoporosis," *Hospital Practice*, December 1978, pp. 91–98.

Pregnancy

Brewer, Gail S.: *What Every Pregnant Woman Should Know*, Penguin Books, New York, 1979.

Brewer, Thomas, M.D.: *Metabolic Toxemia*, rev. ed., Keats Pub. Co., New Canaan, Conn., 1982.

Cathcart, F. R., M.D.: "The Method of Determining Proper Doses of Vitamin C for the Treatment of Disease by Titrating to Bowel Tolerance," *Journal of Orthomolecular Psychiatry* 10:2 (1981), pp. 125–132.

Klenner, F. R., M.D.: "Significance of High Intake of Vitamin C in Preventive Medicine," *Journal of the International Academy of Preventive Medicine* 1:1m (1974), pp. 45–69.

Pauling, Linus, M.D.: *Vitamin C and the Common Cold*, W. H. Freeman & Co., San Francisco, 1970.

Stone, I, Ph.D.: *The Healing Factor: Vitamin C Against Disease*, Grosset & Dunlap, New York, 1972.

Psoriasis

"Psoriasis, an Autoimmune Disease," *Skin & Allergy News*, September 1977.

Roenigk, Henry H., M.D.: "Psoriasis," *Modern Medicine*, October 1977, pp. 59–76.

REFERENCES

Respiratory Symptoms

Truss, C. Orian, M.D.: "Tissue Injury Induced by Candida Albicans," *Journal of Orthomolecular Psychiatry* 7 (1978), pp. 17–37.

Schizophrenia

Hall, Kay, M.A.: "Orthomolecular Therapy," *Journal of Orthomolecular Psychiatry* 4:4 (1975).

Hawkins, David and Linus Pauling (eds.): *Orthomolecular Psychiatry: Treatment of Schizophrenia*, W. H. Freeman and Company, San Francisco, California, 1973.

Hoffer, Abram, M.D., and H. Osmund: *How to Live With Schizophrenia*, University Books, New York, 1974.

Pfeiffer, Carl. C., M.D.: *Mental and Elemental Nutrients*, Keats Pub. Co., New Canaan, Conn. 1975.

Philpott, W. M., M.D., and Dwight Kalit *Brain Allergies*, Keats Pub. Co., New Canaan, Conn., 1980.

Watson, George, M.D.: *Nutrition and Your Mind*, Harper and Row, New York, 1972.

Skin Problems

Jillson, Otis, F., M.D.: "Pruritus," *Cutis* 28 (1981), pp. 335–339.

Kligman, A. M., M.D.: "Early Destructive Effects of Sunlight on Human Skin, *Journal of the American Medical Association* 210 (1969), pp. 2377-2380.

Lynch, Peter J., M.D.: *Skin & Allergy News*, August 1977.

Ringsdorf, W. M., D.M.D., and E. Cheraskin, M.D.: "Diet and Dermatosis," *Southern Medical Journal* 69 (1976), p. 732.

Stress

Cousins, Norman: "Stress," *Journal of the American Medical Association* 242:5 (1979), p. 459.

"Nutrition and Stress," *Dairy Council Digest* 42:3 (1971).

"Nutritional Demands Imposed by Stress," *Dairy Council Digest* 51:6 (1980).

Rosch, P. J., M.D.: "Stress and Illness," *Journal of the American Medical Association* 242:5 (1979), pp. 427–428.

"Stress in the Gravida," *Pediatric News* 15:3 (1981), p. 21.

Wolf, S., M.D., and H. Goodell: *Stress and Disease*, Charles C. Thomas, Springfield, Ill., 1968.

Surgery

Henzel, John, M.D., Marion De Weese, M.D., and Edgar L. Licati, Ph.D.: "Zinc Concentrations Within Healing Wounds," *Archives of Surgery* 100 (1970), pp. 349–357.

Moss, Gerald, M.D.: *Surgery, Gynecology and Obstetrics* 148:81 (1979).

Thurlow, Peter, M.S.: *Surgical Forum,* 1980.

Temporomandibular Joint Dysfunction

Barrett, Patrick, D.D.S.: Personal communication, 1978.
Goodheart, George, D.C.: "T.M.J.," September 1977, pp. 18–19.
Greene, Charles, D.D.S.: "T.M.J.," *Journal of the American Medical Association* 224:5 (1973), p. 622.

Thyroid Problems

Barnes, Broda, M.D.: *Hypothyroidism, The Unsuspected Illness*, Thomas Y. Crowell, New York, 1976.
Gaskin, Joe H., M.D.: "Hypothyroidism in Adults," *Drug Therapy*, September 1981, pp. 41–48.
"Hypothyroidism," *Geriatrics* 36:5 (1981), p. 79.
Liener, Irvin: *Toxic Constituents of Plant Foodstuffs*, Academic Press, New York, 1969.
Yao, Yulin, M.D.: "Thyroid Function Tests," *Hospital Practice*, September 1981, pp. 149–164.

Ulcers

Clayman, Charles B., M.D.: "Carbonate," *Journal of the American Medical Association* 244:22 (1980), p. 2554.
Cleave, T. L., M.D., G. L. Campbell, and N. S. Painter: *Diabetes, Coronary Thrombosis, and the Saccharine Disease*, John Wright & Sons, New York, 1969.
Editorial, *Medical Tribune & Medical News*, May 1972.
Rebhun, J.: "Duodenal Ulceration in Allergic Children," *Annals of Allergy* 34 (1975), pp. 145–149.

Warts

Rees, Rees B., M.D.: "Warts—a Clinician's View," *Cutis* 28 (1981), pp. 175–180.

Yeast Infections

Truss, C. Orian, M.D.: "The Role of Candida Albicans in Human Illness," *Journal of Orthomolecular Psychiatry* 10 (1981), pp. 228–238.
———: *The Missing Diagnosis*, published privately by Dr. Truss, P.O. Box 26508, Birmingham, Alabama, 35226

Chapter 7: The Nutricopia

Vitamin B₆

Bartos, F.: University of Oregon Health Sciences Center *International Journal of Nutrition Research*, December 1981. *Journal of Sports Medicine and Physical Fitness*, June 1981.
"B₆ and Platelet Adhesiveness," editorial comment, *Lancet* 1 (1981), pp. 1299–1300.
Ellis, John, M.D., *Vitamin B₆: The Doctor's Report* (Harper & Row)

McConnell, Ben H., M.D.: "Little Strokes and Bioflavonoids," *Medical World News*, April 1979.

Vitamin C

Anah, C., L. Jarike, and H. Baig: High Dose Ascorbic Acid in Nigerian Asthmatics," *Tropical and Geographical Medicine* 32:132 (1980).

Cathcart, R. F., M.D.: "The Method of Determining Proper Doses of Vitamin C for the Treatment of Disease by Titrating to Bowel Tolerance," *Journal of Orthomolecular Psychiatry* 10:2 (1981), pp. 125–132.

Klenner, F. R., M.D.: "Significance of High Intake of Ascorbic Acid in Preventive Medicine," *Journal of the International Academy of Preventive Medicine* 1:1 (1974), pp. 45–69.

Journal of Human Nutrition, February 1981.

Journal of Orthomolecular Psychiatry 8 (1979).

Pauling, Linus, and Evan Cameron, Ph.D.: *Proceedings of the National Academy of Sciences of the U.S.A.* 73 (1976), pp. 3685–3689.

Siegel, B. V.: "Interferon Production," *Nature* 254 (1975), pp. 531–537.

Stone, I., Ph.D.: *The Healing Factor, Vitamin C Against Disease*, Grosset & Dunlap, New York, 1972.

"Vitamin C in Exercise Asthma," *Journal of the American Medical Association* 243 (1981), p. 548.

Chromium

Mayer, Jean, Ph.D.: "Chromium in Medicine," *Postgraduate Medicine* 49 (1971), pp. 235–236.

Vitamin D

Reich, C., M.D., "Allergies and Diseases of the Central Nervous System," *Journal of Orthomolecular Psych.* 4(1975), pp. 269–273.

Vitamin E

Cheraskin, E., and W. M. Ringsdorf: "Daily Vitamin E Consumption and Reported Cardiovascular Findings," *Geriatrics Digest* 8:3 (1971).

Shute, Wilfrid E., M.D.: "The Vitamin E Story," in *The Complete Book of Vitamins*, ed. C. Gerras, Rodale Press, Emmaus, Pa., 1977.

———: Health Preserver, Rodale Press, Emmaus, Pa., 1977.

Williams, H. T. G.: "Alpha Tocopherol in the Treatment of Intermittent Claudication," *Surgery, Gynecology, and Obstetrics* 132 (1971), p. 662.

Fatty Acids

Progress in Food and Nutrition 4:5 (1980).

Folic Acid

Bolez, M. E., M.D.: "Folate and Neurological Disorders," *Canadian Medical Association Journal* 115 (1976), pp. 217–233.

Butterworth, Charles:"Cervical Dysplasia," Journal of the American Medical Association 244:7 (1980).

Lecithin

"Lecithin in Alzheimer's," letter to the editor from P. Etienne et al., Douglas Hospital, Montreal, Canada, Lancet 2 (1978), p. 1206.
Morrison, Lester: "Lecithin," Geriatrics, 1958.

Magnesium

Flink, Edmund, M.D.: "Can You Spot Magnesium Deficiency and Toxicity?" Modern Medicine, October–November 1979, pp. 48–55.
Fouty, Robert, M.D.: Letter to the editor, Journal of the American Medical Association 240:24 (1978).
Huggins, Hal, D.D.S.: Minerals for the Teeth and Body, privately printed, Colorado Springs, Co.

Molybdenum

"Teeth and Molybdenum," Soil Science Society of American Journal, 1975.

Selenium

Passwater, Richard, Ph.D.: Selenium, As Food and Medicine, Keats Pub. Co., New Canaan, Conn., 1980.
Schrauzer, Gerhard, N., M.D.: "Selenium and Cancer, a Review," Bioinorganic Chemistry 5 (1976), pp. 275–281.

Index

Dyspnea, 227

Ear disorders, 222–225, 253, 299–300, 307, 384
Ectomorphs, 320
Eczema, 16, 134–136, 362, 365
Edema, 186, 225–226, 235
Eggs, 124, 190, 201, 205
Elavil, 18, 211
Elderly, 63–76
    checkups for, 20–21
    diet for, 75–76
    emotional problems of, 65–67, 72
    nutrition of, 63–76
    physical problems of, 63–64, 72–74, 91, 185–186
Electroencephalograph (EEG), 188, 255, 278, 360
Ellis, John, 154, 400
Embolism, 226–227
Emphysema, 227–228
Endometrial cancer, 171
Endometriosis, 228
Endomorphs, 320
Endorphins, 98, 99, 132, 230, 341
Enzymes, 84, 129–130, 150, 163, 208, 306, 358
Eosinophils, 23, 277
Epilepsy, 188–189, 274
Epinephrine, 130, 131, 134
Esophagus, 90, 254
Essential fatty acids (EFAs), 199, 350
Estradiol, 162
Estrogens, 27, 162, 171, 235, 308, 337, 340
Estrone, 162
Ethyl alcohol, 114
Exercise, 65, 69, 173, 228–230, 299, 321, 326, 341
Eye disorders, 222, 230–231, 318, 389–390

Fainting, 374–375
Fasting, 143, 232, 261, 326, 327
    allergies detected by, 124–125, 153, 182, 183, 232, 280, 361
Fatigue, 50–51, 76, 99, 233–235, 275
Fats, 24, 191–194, 196, 199, 372
    in diet, 71, 74, 200, 254, 279
Fatty acids, 198–199, 200, 205, 324, 325, 326–327, 328, 408
Feingold, Ben, 260
Female hormones, 26, 235–236, 305–306
Fertility, 236–237
Fiber, 168, 173, 203, 213–214, 222, 237–242, 256, 280, 388
Finberg, Laurence, 40

Fingernails, 314–315
Fleege, Herbert, 385
Flu, 106, 216
Folic acid, 18, 40, 52, 62, 76, 89, 133, 142, 149, 210, 217, 236, 247, 329, 360, 409–410
Food allergies, 120–124, 153, 166, 181, 182, 209, 214, 216–217, 220, 232, 251, 252, 253, 260, 261, 280, 299, 302, 317, 324, 343, 351, 355, 364, 368, 377, 384
Foods for Healthy Kids (Smith), 165
Foot problems, 166–167, 181, 363
Formaldehyde, 124
Fractures, 242
Fredericks, Carlton, 248
Free radicals, 155
Fungus, 242–243

Gallstones, 200, 243–244
Gangrene, 244
Garlic, 267, 292
Gastric cancer, 171–172
Genetic factors, 7–9
    in disorders, 101, 111, 138, 151, 192, 193, 196, 197, 212, 244, 250, 319–320, 321, 334–335, 350, 358, 360, 363, 370
    in health, 7–13
    questions about, 9–13
    in young adults, 46–47
Genital herpes, 257–258
Gibbs, Marie, 306–307
Ginter, Emil, 201
Glaucoma, 244–245
Globulin, 28
Glucocorticoids, 27
Glucose, 275, 276, 281, 287, 320, 324, 325, 326, 372
Glucose tolerance test, 214, 272, 274, 277–278, 281
Glutamic acid, 303, 410
Goiter, 245–246
Gold therapy, 156
Gout, 246
Granulocytopenia, 287
Greenwald, Peter, 168
Growth, human, 246–247

Habits, unhealthy, 54–55
Hair, 247–248
    loss of, 137–139, 248
    tests on, 29–30, 33, 142, 155, 266, 312, 340
Halitosis, 249
Hands, cold, 181
Hay fever (allergic rhinitis), 118
Headaches, 249–253, 275
    diet and, 5, 6, 253

444

Thrombi, 196
Thrombosis, 377–378
Thymosin, 73
Thymus gland, 73, 286, 291–292, 314
Thyroid gland, 27, 97, 128, 226, 233–234, 245, 247, 248, 277, 322, 328, 330, 374, 375, 378–384, 390
Tics, 384
Tinnitus, 384
T lymphocytes, 286, 287, 288
Tongue, 384–385
Tonsils, 286, 343
Tooth decay, 385–386
Trabecular bone, 336
Transferrin, 288
Tremors, 384
Triglycerides, 24–25, 96, 191, 192, 193, 196
Truss, C. Orian, 307, 354, 392, 393
Tryptophan, 293
Tumors, 175
Twitches, 384
Tyrosine, 162

Ulcerative colitis, 183, 184, 304
Ulcers, 386–388
Uric acid, 25, 246, 299
Urinalysis, 29
Urinary tract infection, 296–297
Urine, 53
Uterine bleeding, 309
Uterine (endometrial) cancer, 171

Vaccines, 97, 157
Valium, 19, 21, 52, 56, 110, 272
Varicoceles, 388
Varicose veins, 388
Varicosities, 388
Vascular problems, 263–264, 388–389
Vegetarian diet, 33, 173–174, 204, 219, 247, 266, 335
Venereal disease (see Herpes II)
Vertebrae, 91–92
Vertigo, 222, 299, 307
Very-low-density lipoprotein (VLDL), 191, 192, 193, 194
Virus, 310–311, 355, 389, 390
Vision, 222, 230–231, 318, 389–390
Vitamin A, 73, 95–96, 139, 171, 175–176, 230–231, 261, 289, 291, 309–310, 315, 318, 349, 352, 354, 371, 389, 391, 397–398
Vitamin B complex, 4, 16, 40, 41–42, 46, 51, 52, 57, 112, 132, 150–151, 159, 205, 215, 236, 248, 252, 281, 293, 328–329, 354, 374
Vitamin B$_1$, 209, 231, 341, 373, 398–399
Vitamin B$_2$, 399

Vitamin B$_3$, 113, 154, 209, 342, 360, 399–401
Vitamin B$_6$, 16, 76, 132, 154–155, 166, 167, 176, 203, 205, 209, 223–224, 226, 234, 235, 302, 306, 317, 358, 359, 362, 400
Vitamin B$_{12}$, 18, 52, 76, 94, 136, 142, 149, 166, 210, 219, 234, 288, 360, 401–402
Vitamin B$_{15}$, 112–113, 402
Vitamin C, 16, 41–42, 51–52, 92, 99, 151, 166, 174, 175, 201–202, 231, 234, 244, 245, 256, 287, 303, 341, 344, 346, 359, 367–368, 388, 403–404
   infection treated with, 131–132, 290–291, 343, 352–356, 373, 389
Vitamin D, 33, 52, 58, 133, 332, 335–336, 406–407
Vitamin E, 52, 74, 176–177, 199–200, 202, 215, 227, 228, 229, 243–244, 248, 256, 281, 308, 367, 371, 374, 377, 388, 391, 407–408
Vitamins, 69, 114, 136, 287, 289, 306, 397–419
Vitiligo, 390

Wallach, Joel, 206
Warts, 354, 390–391
Watson, George, 361
What Every Pregnant Woman Should Know (Brewer), 346
Wheat germ oil, 314
Wheat products, 124
Wolfe, S., 372
Women:
   contraception used by, 203, 235–236, 253, 305, 347
   disorders in, 144–146, 148, 162–163, 219–220, 223, 226, 228, 235–237, 243, 256, 257–258, 308–310, 315, 333

Xanthomas, 192
X-rays, 173, 175

Yaryura-Tobias, José, 102
Yeast infections, 6, 128, 185, 354, 392–394
Young adults, 42–52
   genetic factors in, 46–47
   life expectancy and, 47–49
   nutrition of, 42–52
   physical problems of, 42–45

Zinc, 30, 31, 96–97, 113, 139, 167, 215, 234, 281, 289, 301, 305–306, 346, 354–355, 360, 366, 367, 371, 373, 375, 389, 418–419